FILLER

ILLUSTRATIVE MANUAL OF INJECTION TECHNIQUES

80 Illustrations
128 Photographs
29 Videos

For Lorenzo and Alessandra
For those I love, and who love me in return
For my students

FILLER
Illustrative manual of injection techniques

Editing: Rachele Villa
English translation: Studio Melchior, Turin
Design and layout: Massimo D'Onofrio - www.grafic-house.com
Illustrations: Davide Gamberini
Video: Macro, Naples

Printing: Starprint srl
1st edition - English version: June 2021

PUBLISHER
Griffin srl unipersonale
Via Ginevrina da Fossano 67/A - 22063 Cantù (Como)
Tel. + 39 031.789085 - Fax + 39 031.6853110
customerservice@griffineditore.it
www.griffineditore.it

ISBN 978-88-97438-62-5

QR Code VIDEO System

To watch the videos, scan the QR codes using the camera on your device or download a QR Reader app.

PRESENTATION

My friend Giuseppe Sito and I have been working with facial filler injections for over 15 years.
The range of these products has never stopped evolving and today we have high-tech fillers that allow us to offer our patients a multitude of subtly personalised treatments. The new formulas based on hyaluronic acids open up countless possibilities to fulfil the varying expectations of patients.
The introduction of the cannula has represented another important step forward. Our patients are constantly developing new requirements, favouring a natural result which is almost invisible to the eyes of those around them, while performing a tangible action on the signs of ageing. Younger patients participate in our meetings in order to address the signs of ageing before they actually occur. These patients tend to gather a lot of information online: they are open to the enhancement of their beauty, willing to undergo an engaging experience and take advice from the community.
The concept that never changes from patient to patient is the personalisation of the treatment and experience.
The generally accepted concept: beauty is part of a natural gesture of well-being. The new concept: preserving beauty, caring for it, enhancing it thanks to fillers, has become more accessible.
My friend Giuseppe's book will give aesthetic doctors the opportunity to comprehend the new injection techniques and understand which filler to choose, without losing sight of the natural result and the patient's expectations. Of course, as is already the case during our courses, Giuseppe and I always stress the need for a thorough knowledge of 3D anatomy, of the foundations that welcome these filler injections. While anatomy is always the same, the 3D approach has revolutionised the injection therapy protocol. This has been made possible thanks to the acknowledgement of the dynamic aspect of the face.
Lastly, the artistic dimension of treatment is essential, and Italy has been the

birthplace of great aesthetes for centuries. The tradition is continued in this work written by Professor Sito, whose experience and expertise are recognised at national and international level.

Every time we meet, we learn something from each other, and it is an honour for me today to write the presentation to this outstanding broker of knowledge.

Professor Patrick Trevidic
Plastic Surgeon and Anatomist in Paris

PREFACE

I started practicing "the art of fillers", because it really is an art when performed by the right hands, at the beginning of the Nineties, after attending a famous edition of a congress by the American Academy of Facial Plastic Surgery in San Francisco. I was lucky enough to meet Arnold Klein, an American dermatologist who already had a studio with nine different chairs and injected more syringes than the whole of Austria put together, in person; and with him, Mark Rubin, then a young Californian dermatologist with an enormous amount of experience, who later published his famous classification of facial peelings.
The subject piqued my interest immediately and, with some initial fears, I began injecting the only substance that was allowed in Italy, good old collagen, of which there were, however, only three formulations, which we had to make do with for everything. I was not the first in Italy, but I was definitely among the first, and, with a bit of technique developed with a touch of imagination and daring, I quickly became consultant to the Collagen Company, the only American company that produced collagen, which competed in Italy with the infamous silicone, a competition easily won by virtue of the extensive damage caused by silicone.
A few years later I progressed to hyaluronic acid, which continues to be the market leader today and, above all, leader of our treatments, which are effective, satisfying and harmless. I became consultant to Qmed, good old Restylane and then to many other manufacturers, and I believe there is no syringe of hyaluronic acid or other substances (none of which ever permanent, heaven forbid), that I have not used, always with the philosophy of *primum non nocere*.
I must have injected thousands and thousands of vials, fortunately with little or no side effects, and never any that have been permanent. A question of talent? To a certain extent perhaps, yes, but above all, because I have always chosen the right product for the right area, using exclusively products listed in proven bibliography, never improvising. And, of course, training courses, monothematic courses, congres-

ses all over the world and lectures, lessons at all the schools of Aesthetic Medicine in Italy and beyond, but never a book.
Despite the fact that, on several occasions, the thousands of students who followed me asked me for a book to accompany my explanations. Maybe I just wasn't ready and didn't have a clear idea of exactly what it was that I wanted to write.
But now the time is right. I know now that what we aesthetic doctors lack is a book of practical notions that describe exactly "where, how and what", a book that takes us by the hand and, with the right illustrations, explains how far we have to go and what we have to create. Because the use of fillers is an art which drives us and helps us to create, to reveal the beauty that is already in our patients, bringing it back to the surface, in the same way that a sculptor uses a chisel to shape marble, which is only apparently lifeless.
Writing however, didn't seem to be enough, so I have added some high definition videos to each chapter, to really show you how and where to place your hands and syringe, so that every movement is safe, giving us all, myself included, the satisfaction of seeing a work of art come to life.
And it is with this desire to reveal beauty that I hope you will be able to tell me: "You have written about and shown us exactly the same things that you have always told us".

Professor Giuseppe Sito
Aesthetic Doctor and Surgeon

THE AUTHOR

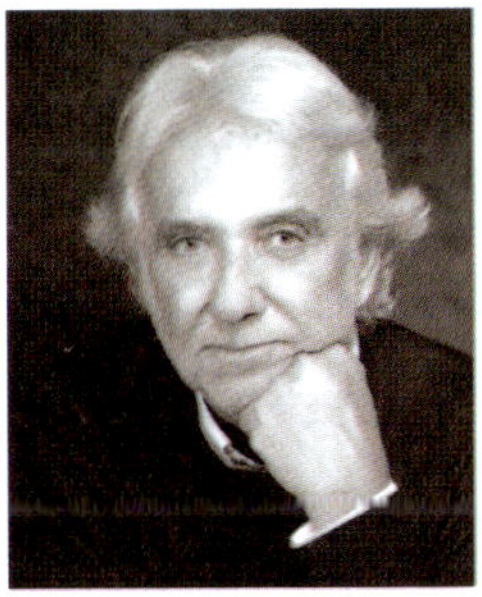

Giuseppe Sito

Born in Naples, he graduated with honours from the University of Naples. He then obtained diplomas as a specialist in General and Endocrine Surgery at the same university, and in Urology at Rome's Università Cattolica del Sacro Cuore. He attended courses in Aesthetic Surgery at the Société de Chirurgie Esthétique in Paris, obtaining the relevant diploma.

He is an adjunct professor at the Second University of Naples.

He is scientific director of Università Pegaso for the 1st and 2nd level master's degrees in Aesthetic Medicine and the Advanced Training Course in Aesthetic Medicine.

He is a member of the Società Italiana di Chirurgia Plastica Estetica.

He is a full member of the Société Française de Chirurgie Esthétique in Paris, the Società Italiana di Chirurgia Estetica and the Società di Chirurgia Italiana, as well as an emeritus member of the American Academy of Facial Plastic Surgery.

He teaches at Agorà - Postgraduate School of Medicine specialising in aesthetic medicine in Milan.

He is a member of the scientific committee of the International Face2Face Congress held regularly in Cannes.

He teaches at the Scuola di Perfezionamento Universitario in Chirurgia Plastica ed Estetica of the University of Pavia.

He is the author of a technique, called the "Protocollo Sito", published in the leading Italian and international journals of aesthetic surgery, and has spoken about the technique at international congresses in the United States.

He is the author of over 100 publications and consultant to numerous publications in the field of Aesthetic Medicine.

He is legal medical consultant, specialised in Aesthetic Medicine, for the Court of Naples.

CONTRIBUTING AUTHORS

Lucia Calvisi

Surgeon specialised in Dermatology at the University of Cagliari. She has perfected her professional training working mainly in the field of aesthetic medicine, participating actively in the most prestigious national and international congresses and maintaining an active collaboration with the University of Brooklyn, New York.
She currently teaches at the Università telematica Pegaso and is the author of numerous national and international publications.

Luana Consolini

Doctor of Biological Sciences, she graduated from the University of Bologna, Department of Biological, Geological and Environmental Sciences - BiGeA.
She is the author of several publications in the field of aesthetic medicine and has worked with various medical journals. She has worked for many years as technical-scientific contact for companies operating in the field of aesthetic medicine.

Alberto Diaspro

Surgeon specialised in maxillo-facial surgery at the University of Turin. He obtained a Diploma in Aesthetic Medicine at the Agorà Postgraduate School of Milan, a master's degree in Aesthetic Medicine and Therapy at the University of Camerino and a master's degree in Facial Plastic Surgery at Rome's "Tor Vergata" University.
He is a member of the European Academy of Facial Plastic Surgery (EAFPS).
He is a member of the Associazione Italiana Chirurgia Estetica e Funzionale della Faccia (AICEF).
He is a member of the Società Italiana di Chirurgia Maxillo-facciale (SICMF).
He is currently Medical Director at Rigeneralab, Centro di Medicina Rigenerativa, in Turin.

CONTENTS

1

INSTRUMENTS AND PREPARING THE PATIENT

Welcoming the patient

So here we are. We have taken a filler course and bought the book. We have chosen all the necessary fillers, never just one for all seasons, and now we are ready to get started.

Needless to say, our clothes and hair will have to be tidy and our hands and nails clean; the studio, because we should always talk in terms of studios or clinics, never beauty salons or similar, must be comfortable, well lit, better if equipped with a direct beam lamp that lights up the patient's face and all its faults, be they real or imaginary. Cool in summer and well-heated in winter.

The consultation should start with the collection of the anamnesis, paying particular attention to previous local or general anaesthetics, allergies or previous aesthetic medical treatments. Be wary of patients who are too well-informed and have already been to more than one aesthetic doctor. Those are the ones who are never happy and who could cause problems later on. Learn to observe the patient carefully as soon as they enter the studio. Notice whether a woman is overly made up, if she bears the scars of previous treatments on her face, if she is wearing a short skirt or low neckline, and try to gain a rough idea of what she is going to ask for and, above all, how great her expectations are.

Let the patient ask for what they want without ever offering anything. Avoid falling into the trap of: "Doctor, what do you think I should have done?". A long time ago, I suggested a badly needed face-lift to a 75-year-old patient. All she said was: "A facelift for me? But there's absolutely nothing wrong with me!". I never saw her again.

And then, when all the talking is over, we can move onto the couch, which must be comfortable, so that the patient can relax and enjoy stretching out, on a brand-new white paper sheet. The table holding all our "weapons" should be placed just slightly above the patient's head so that they won't be frightened by the sight of needles or anything else.

After thoroughly cleansing the area to be treated (one of the worst enemies of asepsis is make-up), examine the face, dividing it into quadrants. Use a white light with a direct beam, followed by Wood's light, to identify any lentigo or hyperpigmentation; check for the presence of capillaries that might cause bothersome bruises, informing the patient of their presence, and examine the facial defects that the patient wants you to treat. Bear in mind that it must always be the patient alone who decides they want the treatment.

After disinfecting the face, pull on a pair of gloves, which need not be sterile unless you are going to perform invasive manoeuvres. Hold a piece of gauze in your free hand, avoiding the use of cotton wool, which always leaves annoying fluff behind, to clean up any blood and apply pressure to the bleeding vessels.

Choosing the anaesthetic

I prefer not to use local anaesthetic, unless I am working on the lips, but I do keep some on my table. No area of the face is so sensitive as to feel unbearable pain, except, as I've already said, the lips, where I usually block the infraorbital nerve or apply a cream with a high

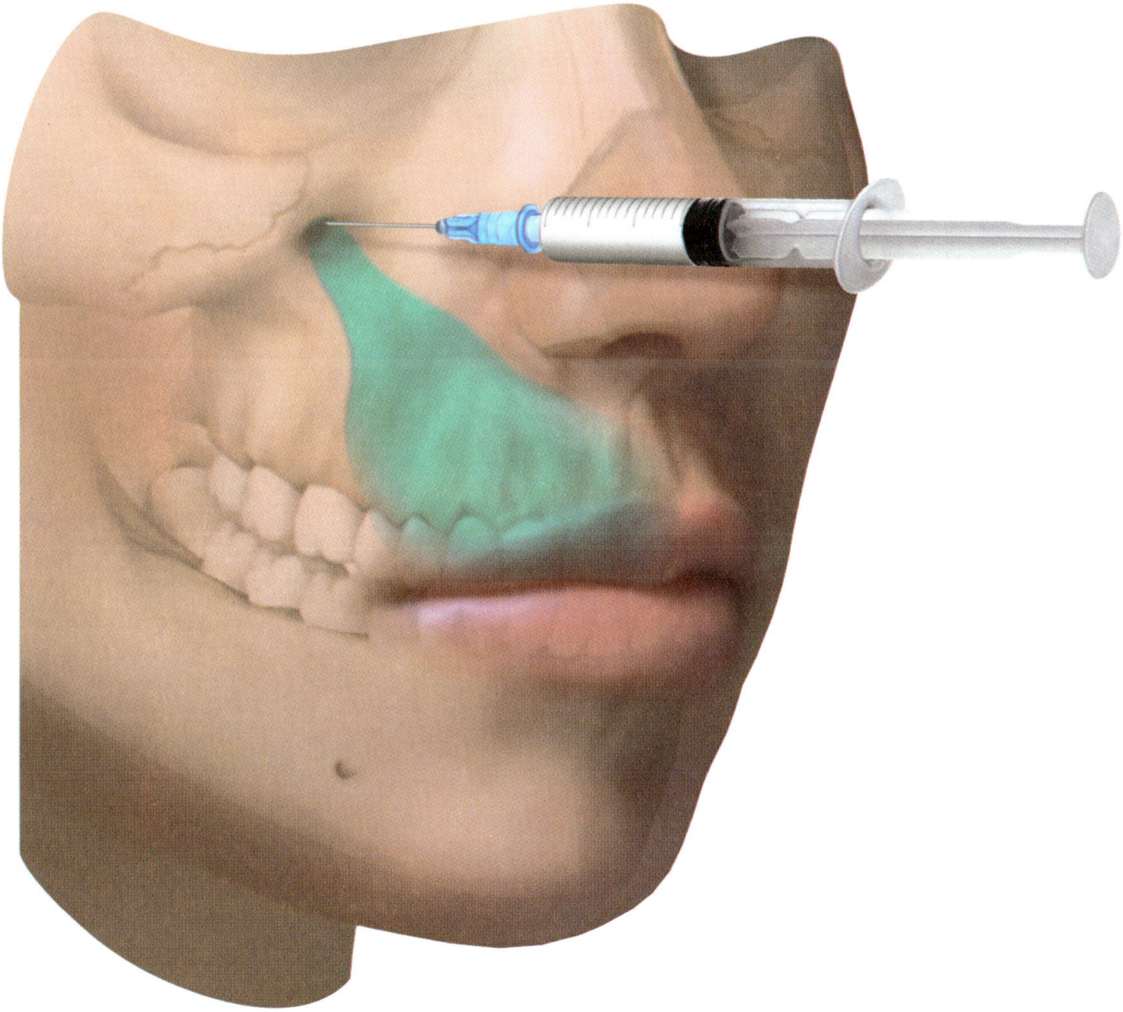

Figure 1 Blockage of the infraorbital nerve in the point where it emerges

concentration of lidocaine (33%), which takes effect within about ten minutes.
The infraorbital nerve stems from the maxillary branch of the trigeminal nerve. It runs through the infraorbital canal of the maxillary bone and exits at the infraorbital foramen, level with the third upper tooth. The landmark is the palpable infraorbital foramen level with the third upper tooth, in the so-called canine fossa (figs. 1 and 2). The tip of the needle must be inserted parallel with the palate into the infraorbital canal and the local anaesthetic, usually lidocaine with adrenaline 1 or 2%, pushed as distally as possible. After the injection, vigorously massage the deposit in a circular motion for 30 seconds, to help it circulate more effectively in the canal. This type of blockage usually covers the whole upper lip area and sometimes the nasal alae, lasting an hour or so.
Infiltration of the lower lip is usually less painful than that of the upper lip.

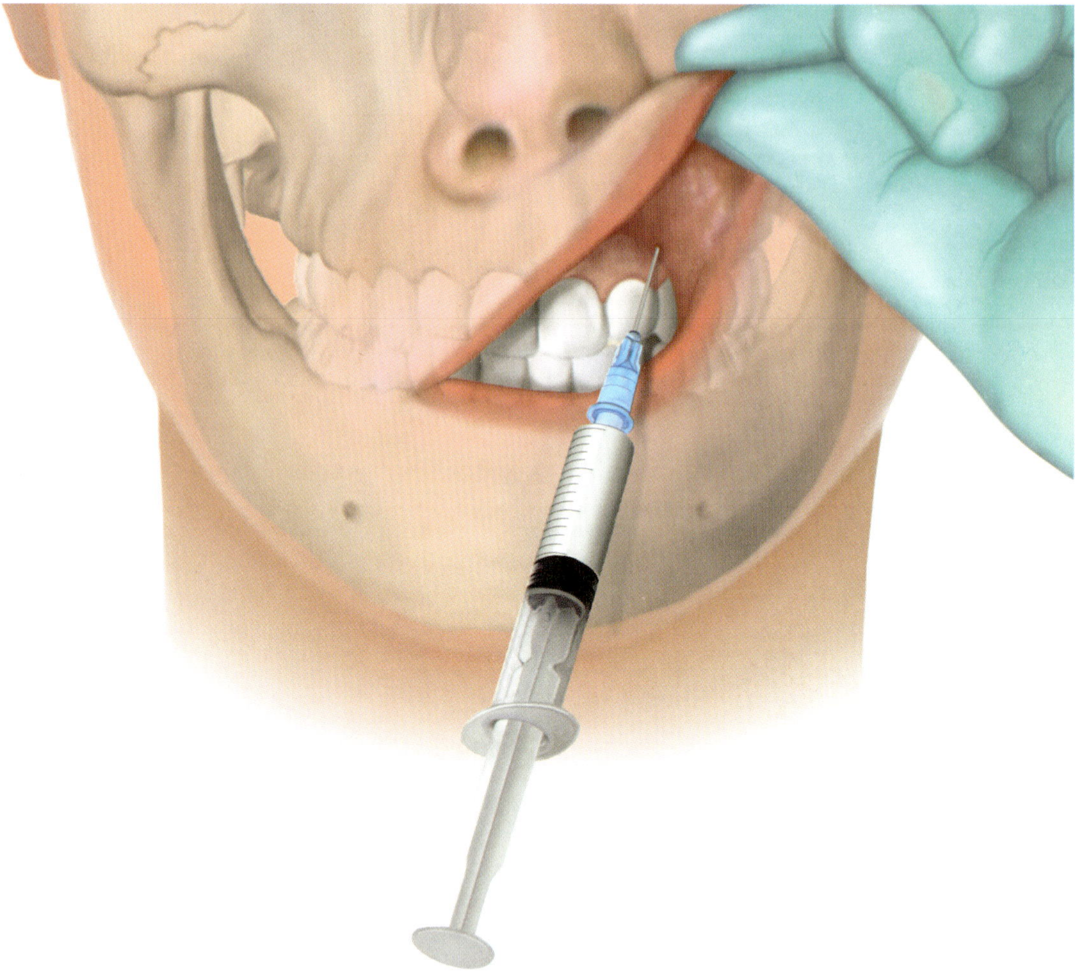

Figure 2 Infraorbital nerve blockage technique

The mental nerve, which is the terminal branch of the alveolar nerve, is blocked at the level of the mental foramen, located below the second lower premolar (figs. 3 and 4). The injection must be performed by introducing the needle into the main mental foramen, which is slightly rostral in relation to the mental foramen, approximately halfway up the mandibular branch.

For those who prefer to use anaesthetic gel only, I suggest the officinal formula of lidocaine 33% in ointment, which can be prepared by a good pharmaceutical laboratory. Its application will provide sufficient analgesia, without causing the tissue disruption that sometimes occurs with infiltrative anaesthesia and will last just over half an hour. It starts taking effect on the lips and mucous membranes in general after about ten minutes, sometimes less.

It goes without saying that patients prefer anaesthetic in gel form to injections.

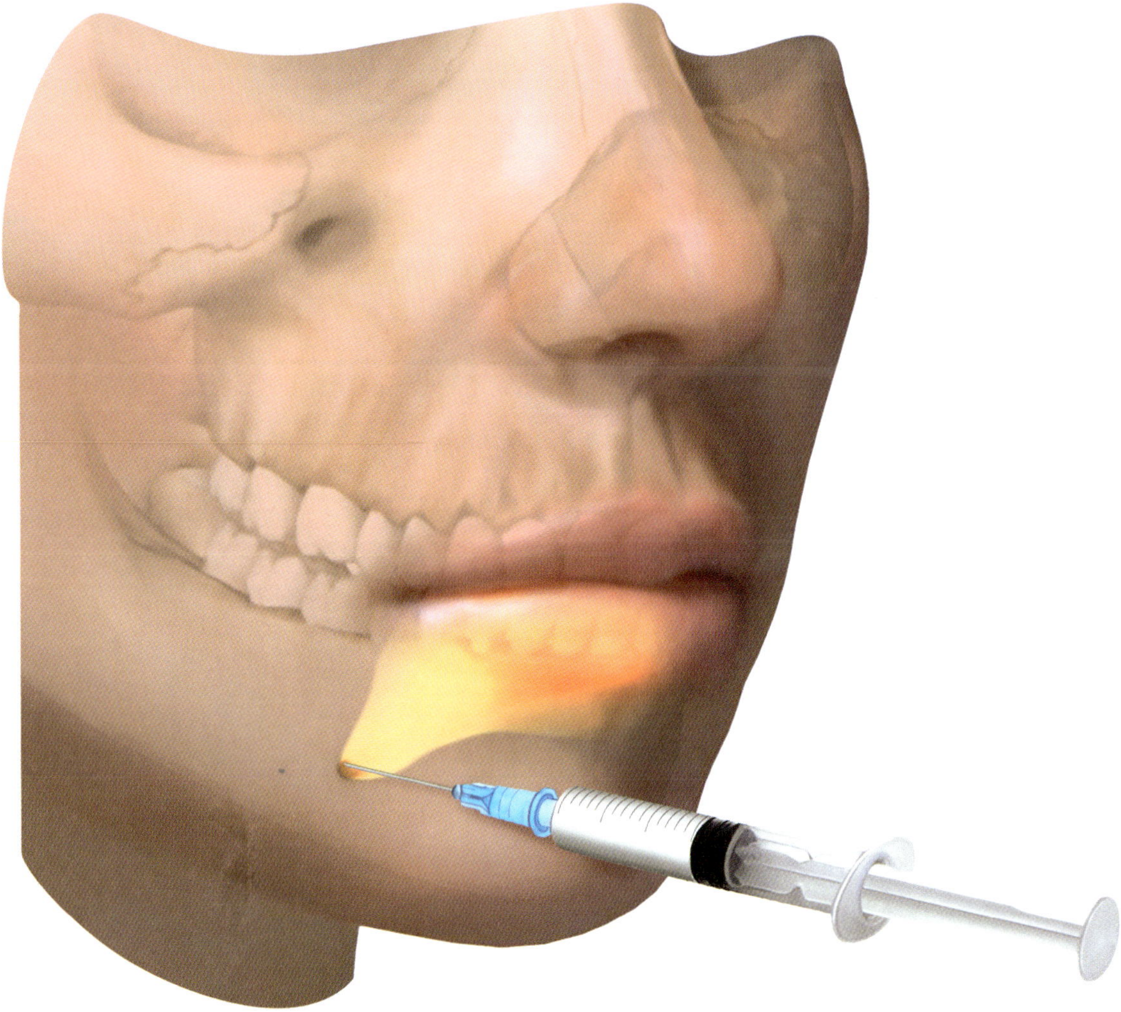

Figure 3 Blockage of the mental nerve in the point where it emerges

Accessory instruments

There are also some non-essential but useful accessory tools. These include a mirror. There are all kinds of mirrors, but I personally would not recommend a magnifying mirror, which enlarges good results but defects too, so a 1:1 ratio mirror is better. Give it to the patient before beginning treatment so that they can tell you exactly what they want and can see the results afterwards. The dermographic pencil is always an essential aid and some patients like to be able to use it themselves to indicate the areas on which to intervene. Let them do it, as this will be helpful for you.

You can also supply a small fan for the patient to use during the application of a peeling treatment. The patient will be distracted by directing the air flow towards the area where they feel most discomfort and this is an easy way for you to ensure perfect neutralization.

A pair of clippers or a decapsulator will

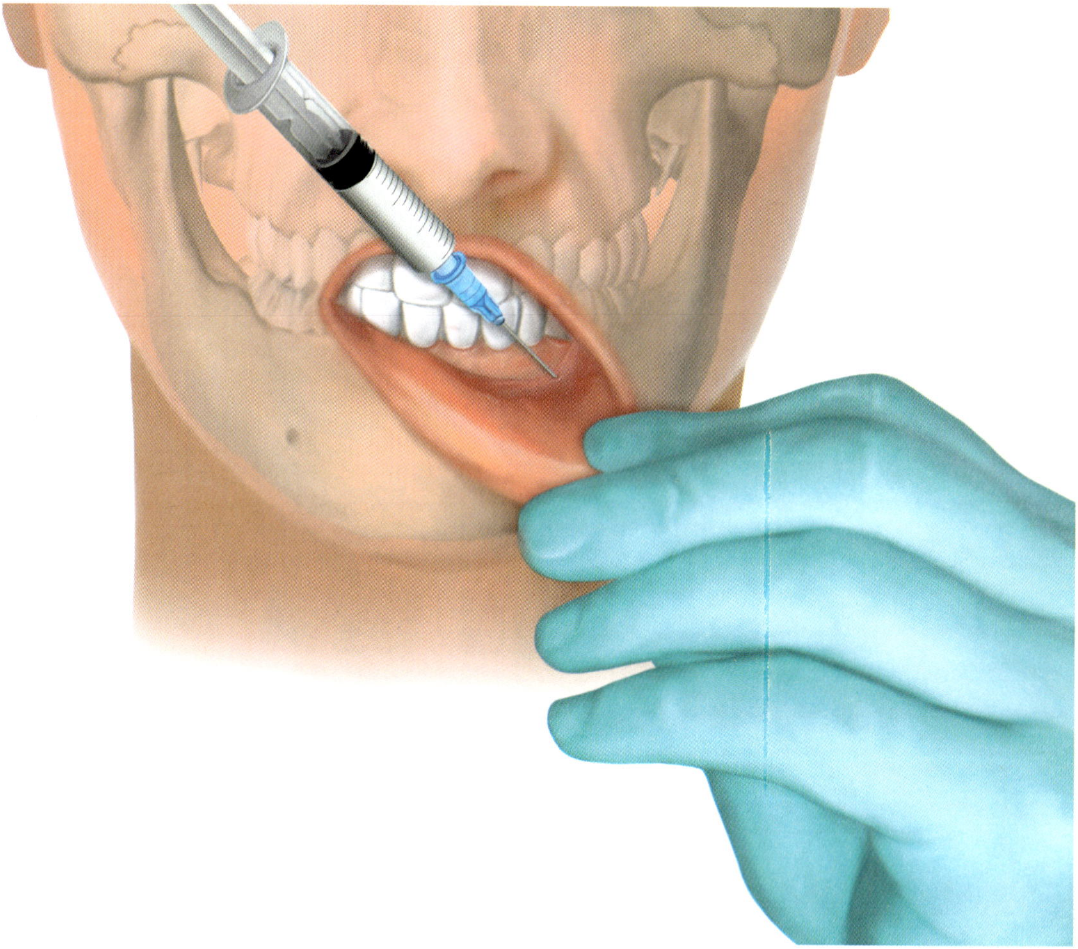

Figure 4 Blockage of the mental nerve below the 5th tooth in the lower dental arch

help you open bottles of toxin and use every last drop.

A mini freezer for making ice cubes is also very useful: it is inexpensive, takes up little space and ice cubes are much colder than the refrigerated plastic blocks usually given to us as gifts by manufacturers.

Bibliography

1. Kapi E. Surgeon-Manipulated Live Surgery Video Recording Apparatuses: Personal Experience and Review of Literature. Aesthetic Plast Surg. 2017 Jun;41(3):738-746.
2. Food and Drug Administration, HHS. Medical Devices; General and Plastic Surgery Devices; Classification of the Microneedling Device for Aesthetic Use. Final order. Fed Regist. 2018 Jun 8;83(111):26575-7.
3. Wang JV, Zachary CB, Saedi N.

Counterfeit aesthetic devices and patient safety in dermatology. J Cosmet Dermatol. 2018 Jun;17(3):396-397.
4. van Loghem JAJ, Humzah D, Kerscher M. Cannula Versus Sharp Needle for Placement of Soft Tissue Fillers: An Observational Cadaver Study. Aesthet Surg J. 2017 Dec 13;38(1):73-88.
5. Lee GS. Use of AccuVein™ for preventing complications from accidental venipuncture when administering dermal filler injections. J Cosmet Laser Ther. 2015 Feb;17(1):55-6.
6. Ballin AC, Brandt FS, Cazzaniga A. Dermal fillers: an update. Am J Clin Dermatol. 2015 Aug;16(4):271-283.

2

CHEEKBONES

The game of beauty

Deciding what is beautiful or establishing the specific rules of beauty is far from easy. Yet there seems to be a unanimous agreement that facial beauty should consist of an alternation of hollows and curves, almost as though part of a game, the "game of beauty".

When it comes to the curves, cheekbones are undoubtedly those most evident in the Caucasian race, and when they disappear due to trauma, age, bone resorption, etc., we tend to rebuild them as quickly as possible.

In the recent past, and even today in particularly severe facial traumas or congenital agenesis, all kinds of malar implants, particularly those made of silicone or Gore-Tex, have been used in thousands and thousands of patients.

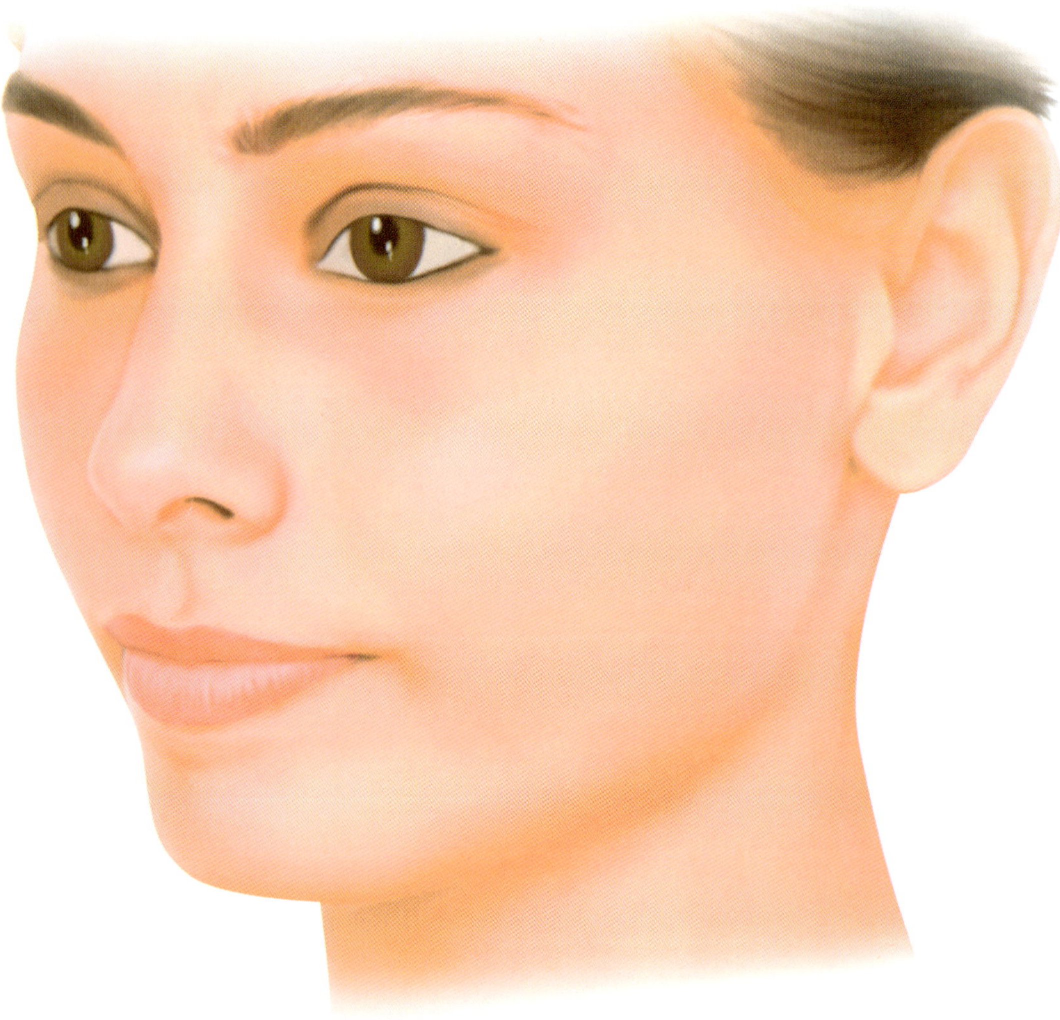

Figure 1 Graphic reconstruction of the ideal face

VIDEO 1

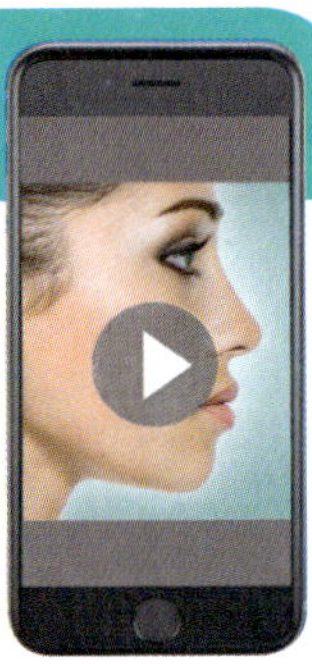

Anatomy of the zygomatic region seen from the side

VIDEO 2

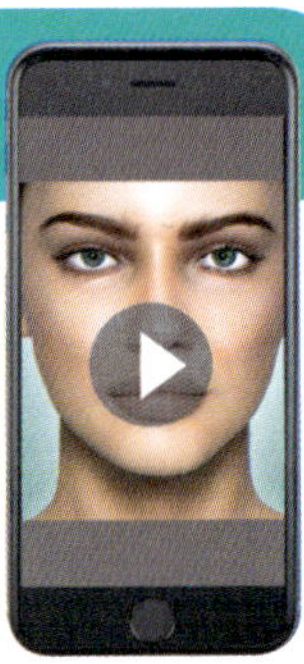

Frontal anatomy of the zygomatic region

Up until the end of the Nineties, when the use of fillers, especially hyaluronic acid, in aesthetic medicine became fully established, reconstruction or even just augmentation of the zygomatic region was achieved exclusively with implants. They were relatively easy to insert but caused post-op swelling which often took as long as thirty days to disappear, leaving patients forcibly incapacitated. Sometimes the results failed to live up to patients' expectations and, due to the particular delicacy of the neighbouring structures, removal was not always simple, occasionally being accompanied by significant complications.

But in 1999, the author of this book presented his original technique for the aesthetic correction of the malar region at the International Congress of Aesthetic Medicine in Monte Carlo. Following some modifications, the work was subsequently presented at congresses and courses all over the world. But let us go back to the anatomical description of the area.

Anatomy of the malar region

The malar region, which is symmetrical, belongs to the middle third of the face and consists mainly of the zygomatic bone, a paired bone articulated with the maxilla, the palatine bones, the zygomatic process of the temporal bone, the lacrimal bones, the ethmoid and the nasal conchae (fig. 2).

The zygomatic region is described as deep and is surrounded by and made up of bone structures as described above, soft tissue, the parotid gland, muscles and Bichet's (or buccal) fat pad (fig. 3).

The skin is mobile, richly vascularized and filled with sebaceous and sweat glands; the subcutaneous layer is variable and forms the Buccal fat pad over the zygomatic bone.

This is a fatty structure in the shape of a biconvex sphere, usually measuring between 6.7 and 12.3 cm^2, but averaging at 10.4 cm^2, and with an average weight of 6.3 g. Everyone has this structure and it tends to become atrophic or sag inside the cheek as we grow older, shrinking significantly. The fat pad usually sits between the masseter and buccinator muscles. The muscle structures are, moving from the surface inwards, the platysma, the masseter and the buccinator.

Referring to the opening remarks, it should be stressed that the zygomatic region, which lends so much beauty to the face, can be affected by illnesses that determine its agenesis. The most important of these is undoubtedly

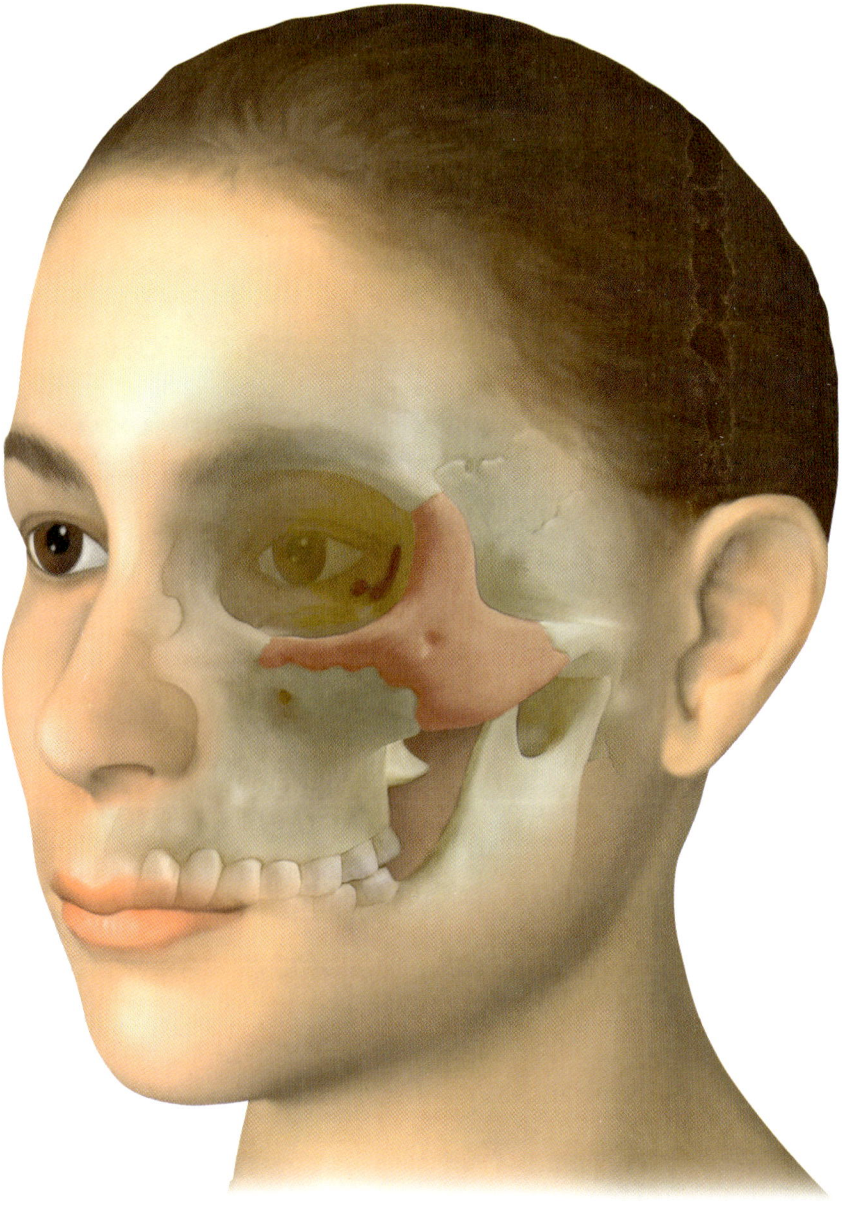

Figure 2 The various planes of the zygomatic region

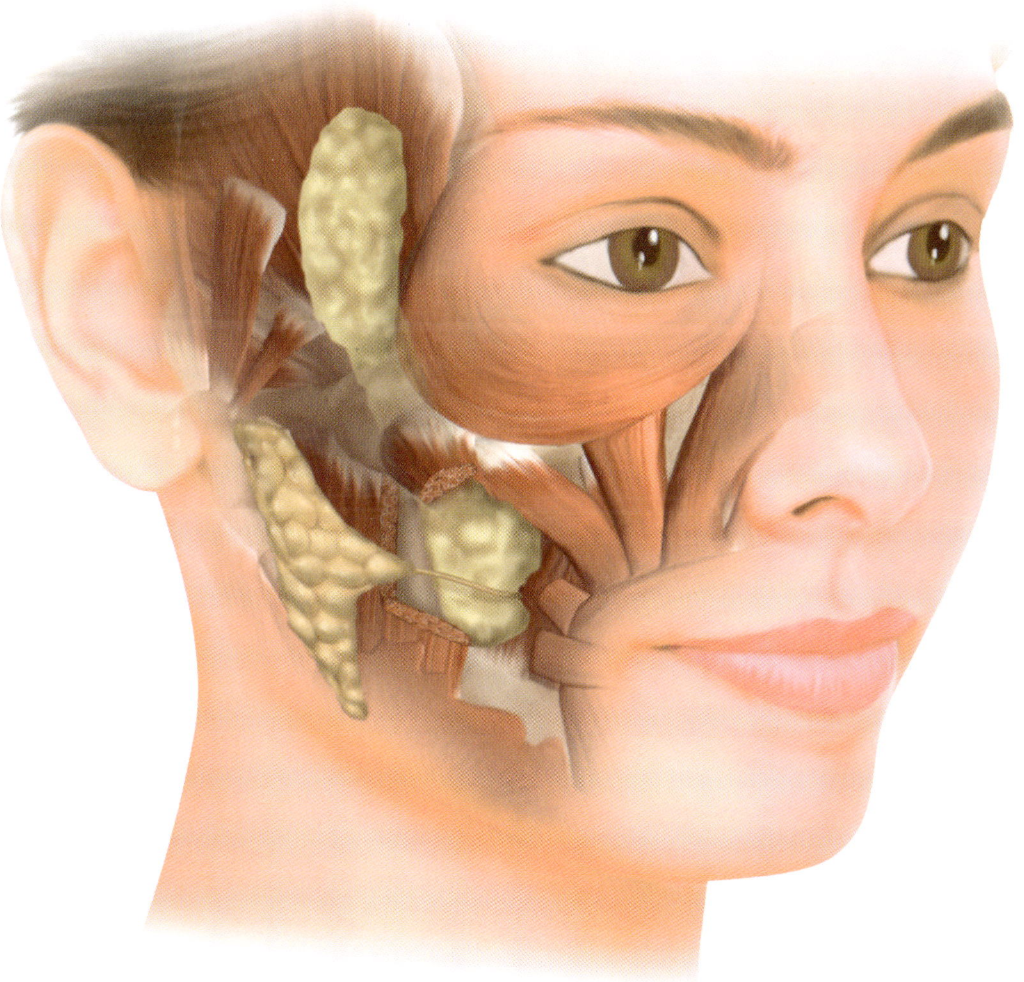

Figure 3 The ratios of the zygomatic region with the Buccal pad and the parotid gland

Treacher Collins syndrome (Franceschetti syndrome), caused by trauma or even just aesthetic deficits.
Of course, in the case of trauma or illness, one does not want and should not presume to treat them only with filler injections, which, however well-performed, are always of a transitory nature. In aesthetic situations, on the other hand, it is necessary to abandon the idea of surgery with additive malarplasty and use fillers without any hesitation.
Until not so long ago, and particularly when synthetic collagen was in use, fillers were suitable for and adaptable to more or less everything. Only in recent years has there been a significant differentiation, which has now become so marked that a different filler is available for almost every facial region.
In the case of non-surgical malarplasty, or if you want to have surgery subse-

quently, and in this case the use of the filler can be very useful to offer a surgical preview for the benefit of both patient and surgeon, there are at least two possible options.
Since the zygomatic protrusion consists largely of bone, injections of calcium hydroxyapatite, a synthetic material already well-known to maxillofacial practitioners, who have been using it in bone reconstruction for decades, are used. In aesthetic medicine it comes in syringes, along with a small amount of lidocaine (0.75%), like most fillers, and is injected deeply, onto the surface of the bone. Bear in mind that hydroxyapatite is also used today as a coating for certain dental implants to promote osseointegration, confirming its deep use in direct contact with the bone.
Numerous hyaluronic acids are used successfully in malarplasty, and all of them fall within the category of the so-called volumizing hyaluronic acids.
They must definitely be included among those with a high G', i.e. a good level of "hardness" and volumizing capacity, a high G", i.e. viscosity, and obviously a low tan delta. Remember that these parameters describe the biochemistry of the filter.

Zygomatic correction

Before approaching a zygomatic correction, it is usually a good idea to draw or outline the area of augmentation, which will correspond mainly to the frontal zygomatic protuberance.
The drawing is carried out using a dermographic pencil, a "weapon" which is always found on the desk of a doctor who performs this procedure. The patient should be seated on the couch looking straight ahead and the drawing must be absolutely symmetrical.
There are at least two techniques. The first one, which is simpler and more widely used, is called Hinderer's technique, modified by the Author, and consists in drawing two lines, one from the labial commissure to the ipsilateral canthus and the other from the tragus to the ipsilateral nasal ala. There is an ellipse at the intersection between the two lines, with the major axis on the tragal line, which is almost always around 4 cm (fig. 4).
One or two boluses will then be injected deeply in the area circumscribed by the ellipse, probably on the periosteum, and then be massaged vigorously to shape the implant. The purpose of the drawing is also to check for any asymmetries and point them out to the patient, who is unlikely to have noticed them before, in order to avoid any complaints afterwards, when the increase in volume will have made them more noticeable.
The second drawing, which is much more complex and consequently hardly ever used, is that of Powell. In this case, a line is drawn from the lateral canthus to the commissure, with another from the tragus to the nasal ala, along with a vertical line from the bridge of the nose to the nasal tip and a line from one tragus to the other (fig. 5). As you can see, this is not a simple drawing and its value is yet to be proven.
The infiltration can be carried out with a needle, directly into the region identified, or with a cannula, the utility of which is unknown, recommending a

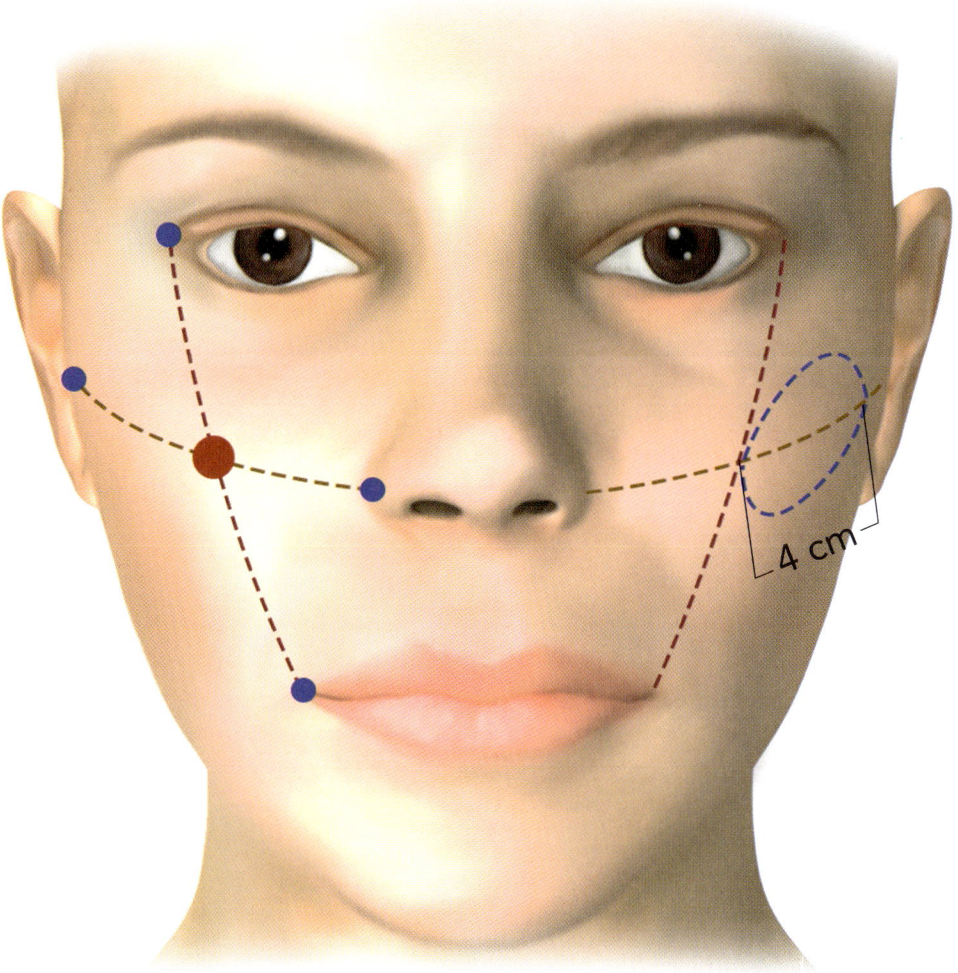

Figure 4 Drawing identifying the zygomatic region to be infiltrated

VIDEO 3

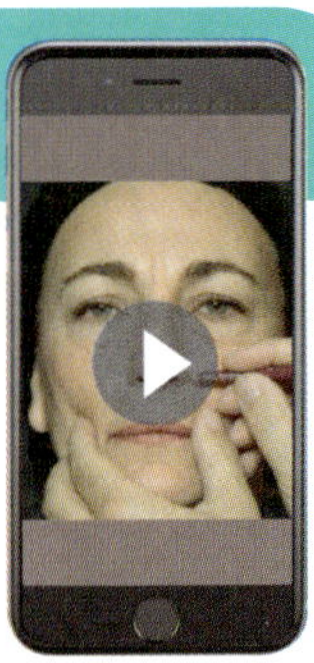

Drawing in preparation for the zygomatic correction

VIDEO 4

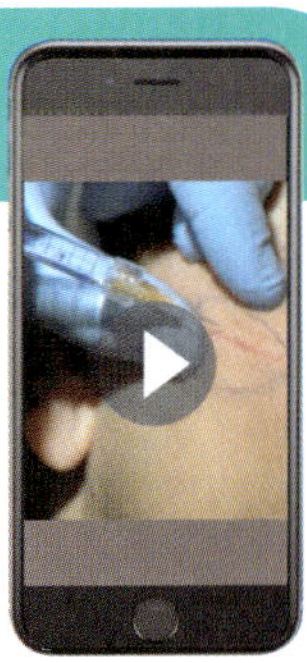

Zygomatic correction technique

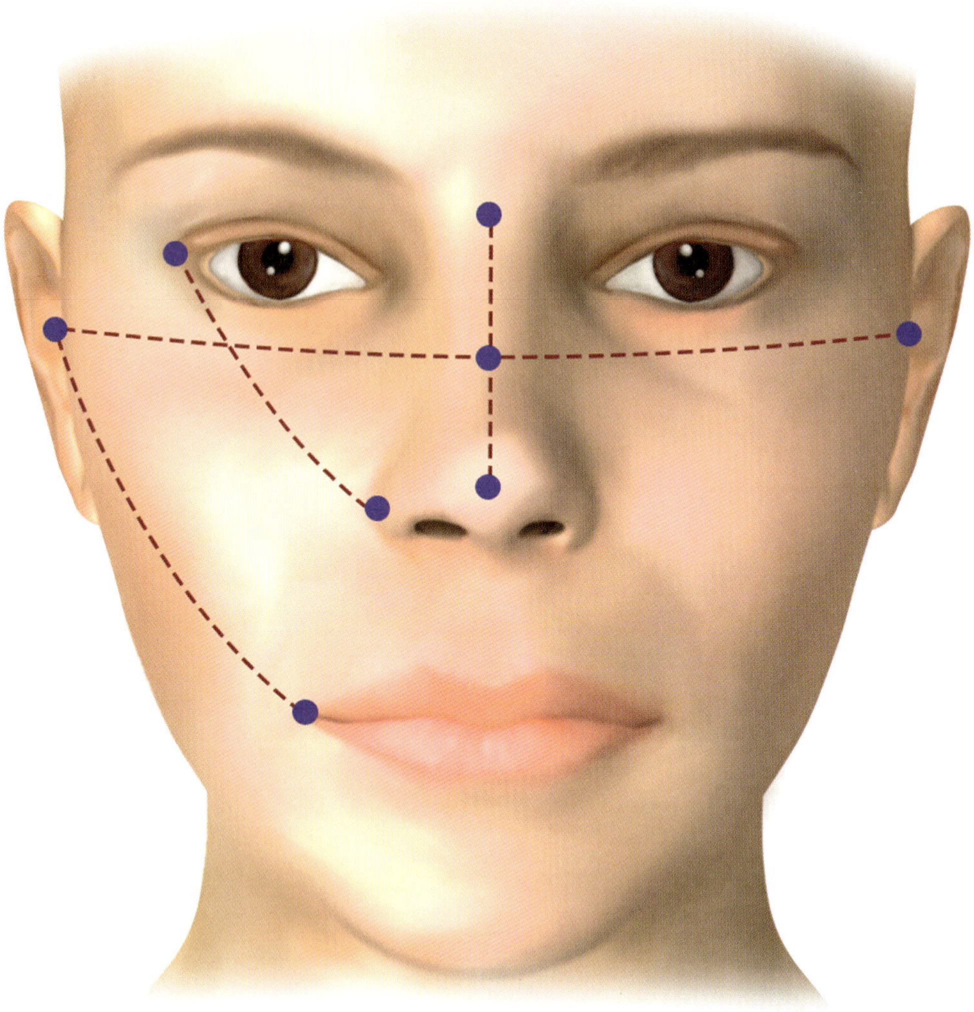

Figure 5 Drawing of Powell

diameter of 25 or 27 G. It will be introduced from a pre-tragal entry point, where there are no fine structures that need to be preserved (fig. 6).
Bruising and other side effects are very rare, while patient satisfaction is always extremely high.
I would just like to say a few words about the dose to be used. Syringes all contain 1 cc of filler nowadays, this being considered the correct dose for malarplasty, using one for each cheekbone.
In actual fact, however, 2 cc for both cheekbones can constitute an overcorrection which is not always appreciated, so we can consider the correct "dose" to be about 1.6-1.8 cc for both cheekbones in a single treatment.
The Author's advice is to start with 1 cc, split between the two cheekbones, and then see the patient after 20-30 days to carry out any necessary retouching.

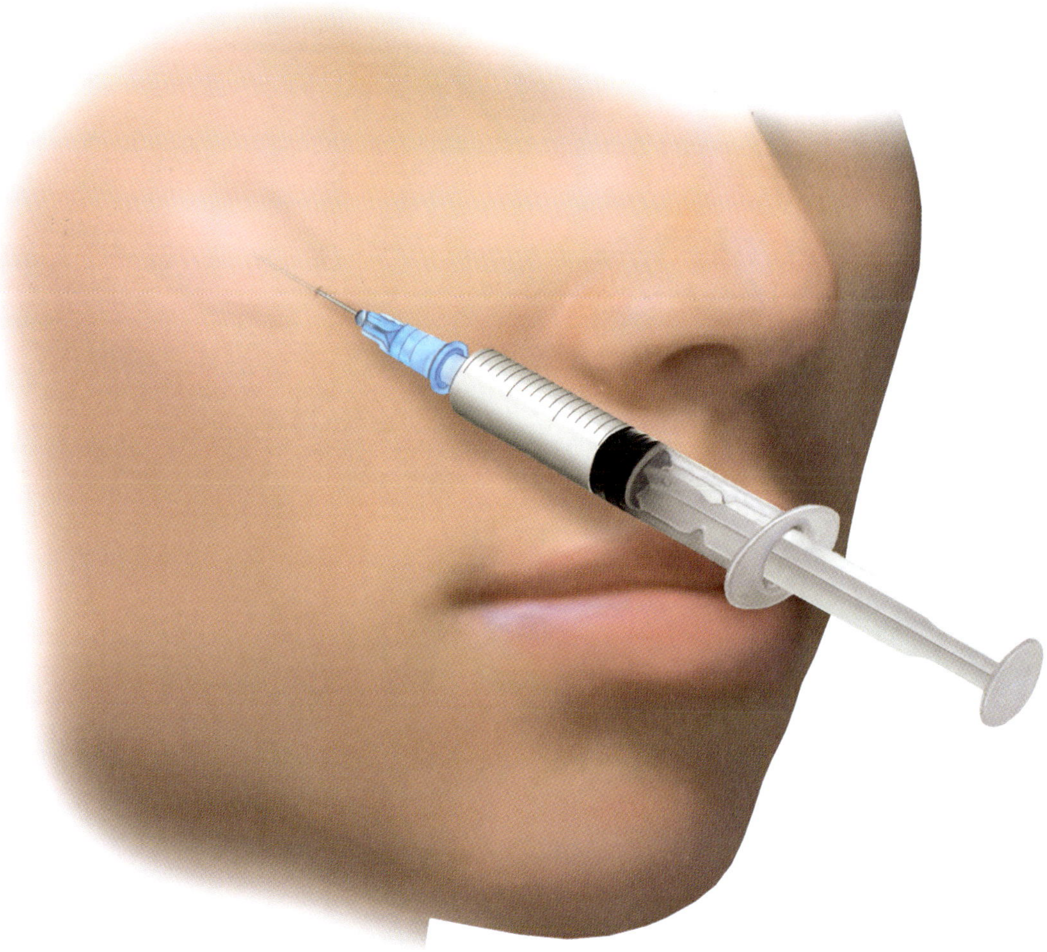

Figure 6 Implant technique

A half-dose (0.5 cc) will allow the patient to see the effect and save some money, which is never a bad thing. Not all patients are willing to spend thousands of euros for full face corrections which, while being widely publicised, leave the face badly swollen and have a limited duration.

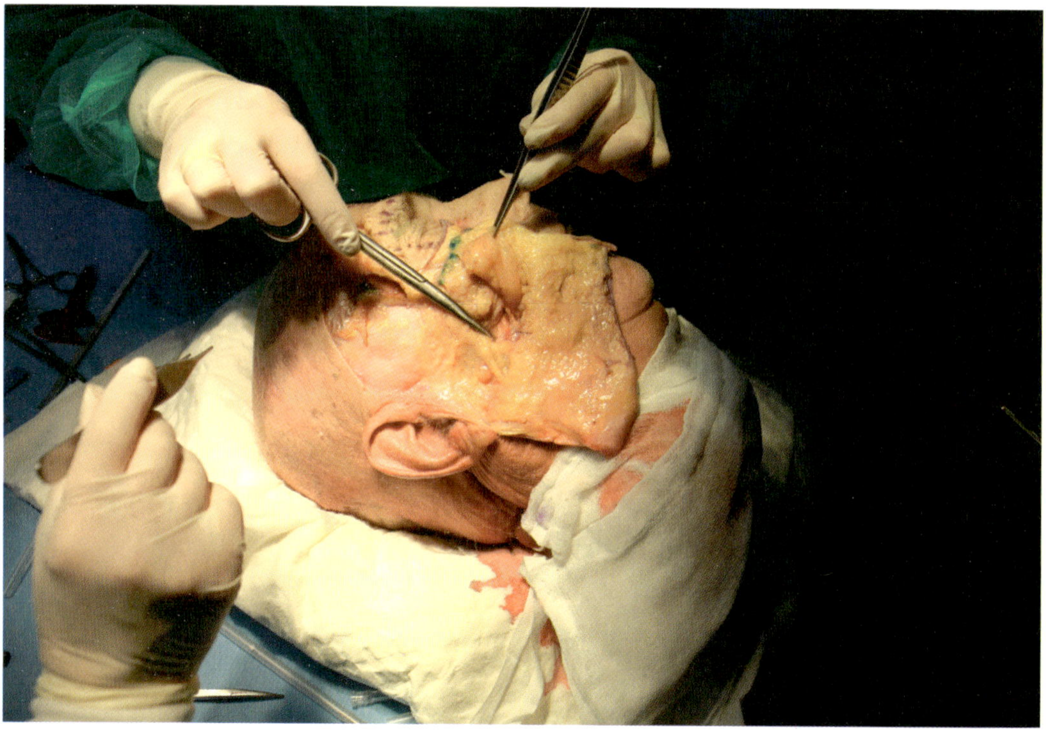

Buccal pad in an anatomic preparation

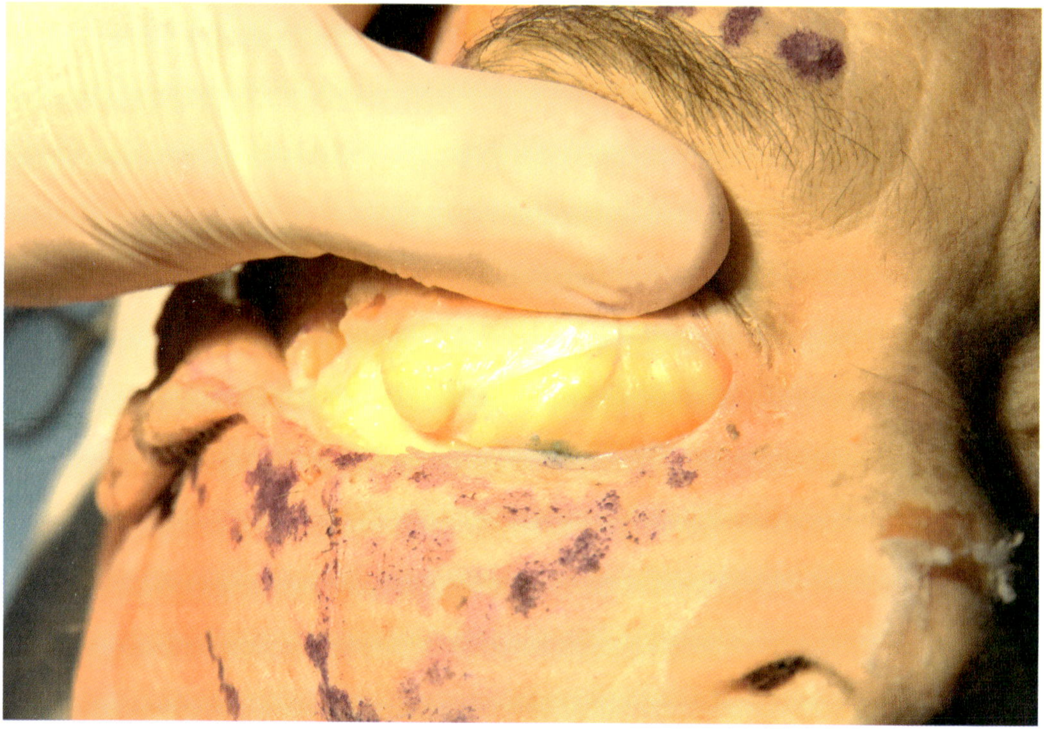

Anatomic preparation with the Buccal pad

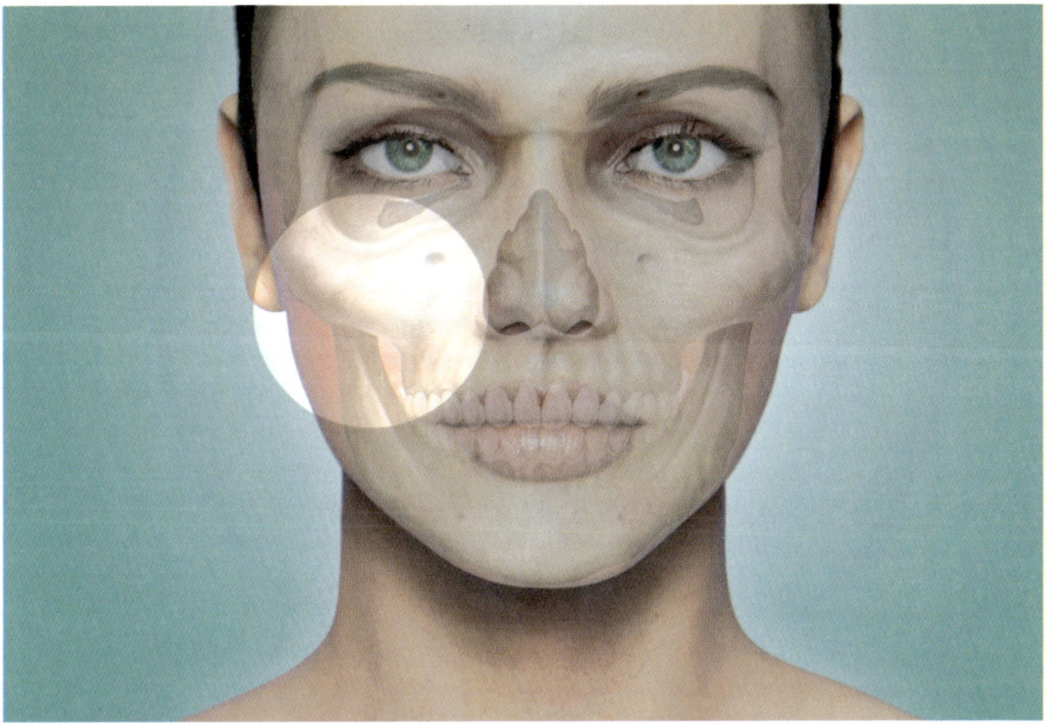

Graphic anatomy of the zygomatic region, frontal view

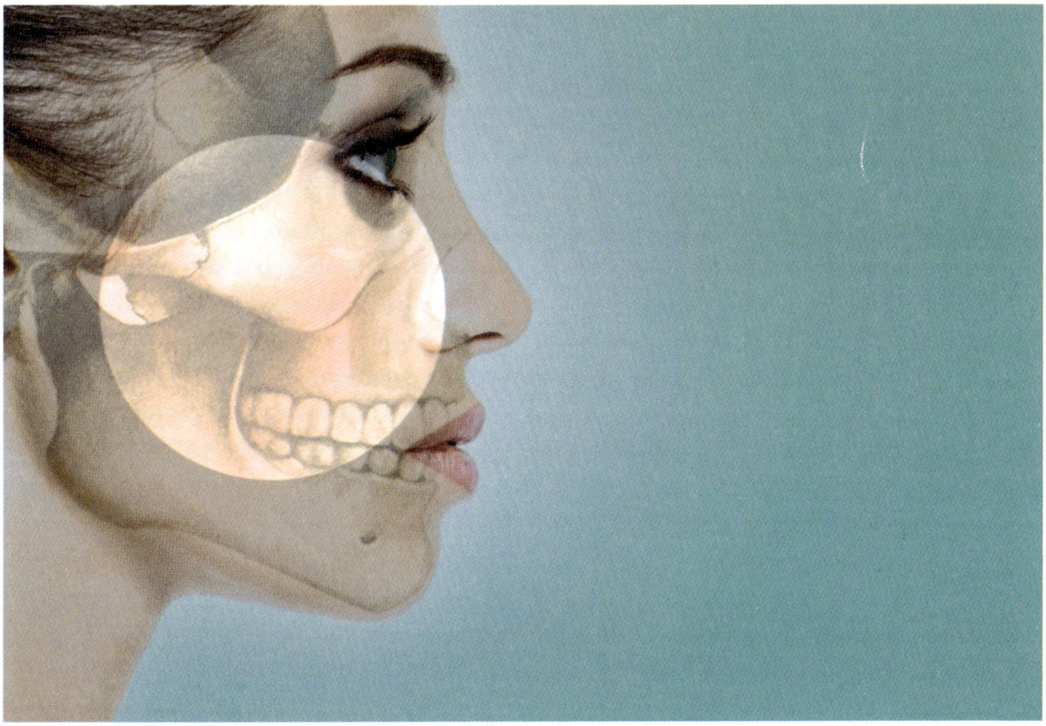

Graphic anatomy of the zygomatic region, lateral view

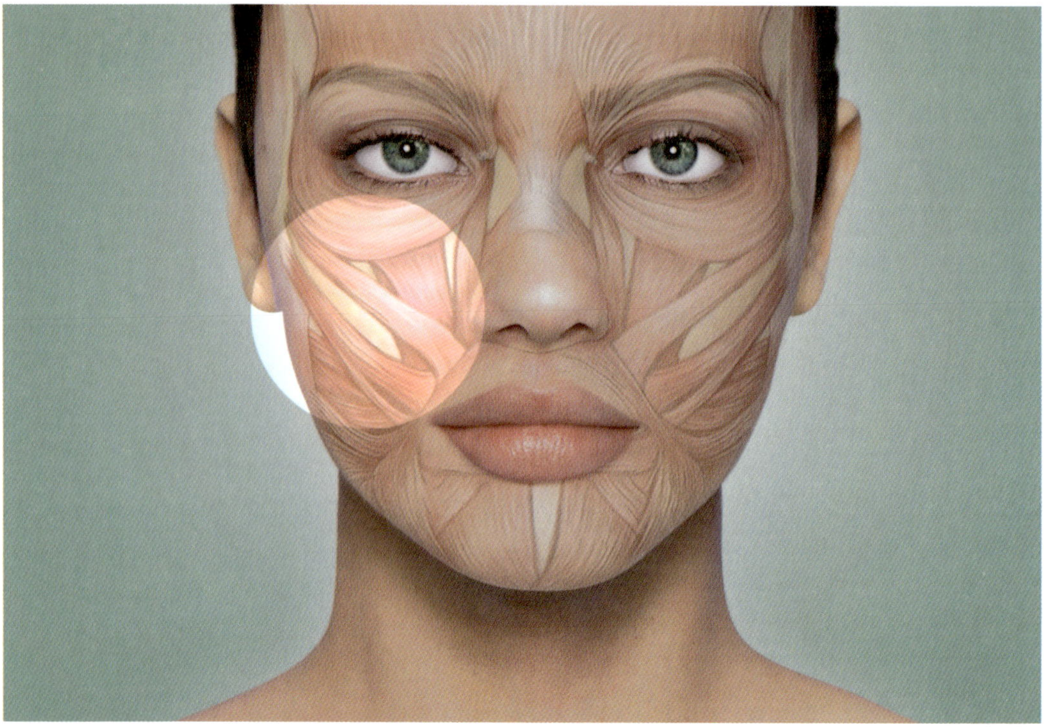

Graphic anatomy of the zygomatic region, frontal view

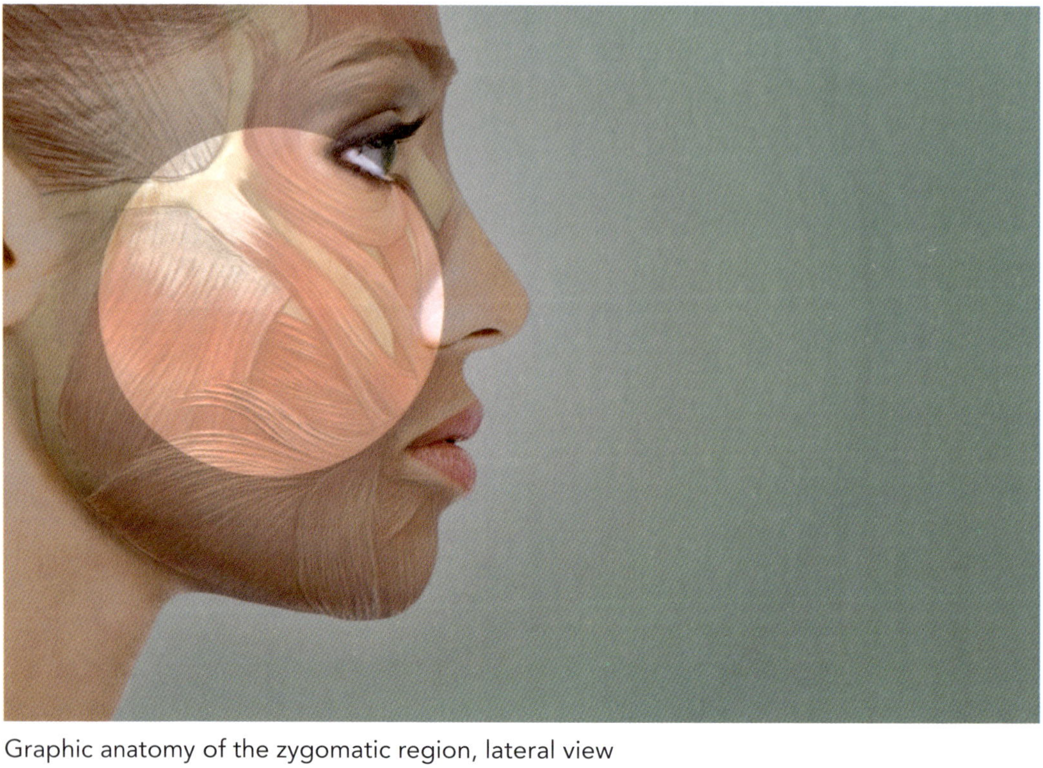

Graphic anatomy of the zygomatic region, lateral view

CLINICAL CASES

CLINICAL CASE 1

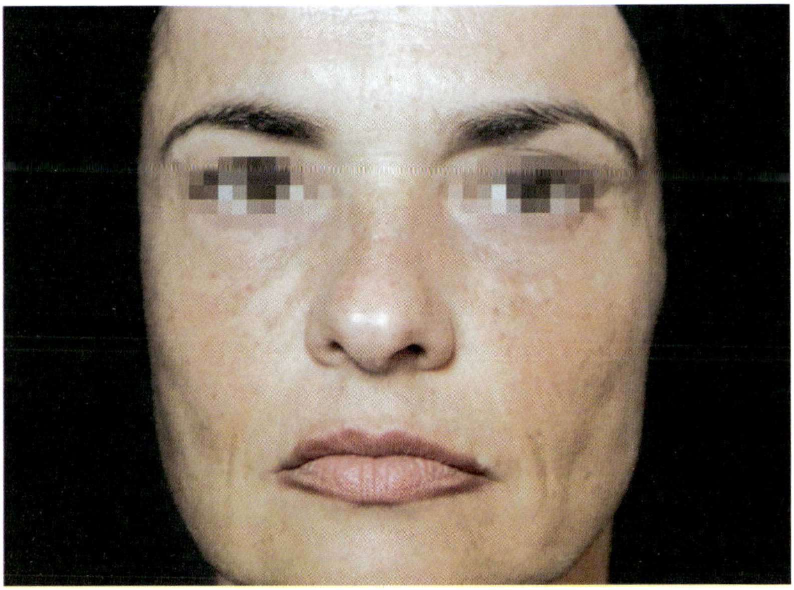

BEFORE

<

VIDEO 5

Zygomatic region: morphing before and after

AFTER

>

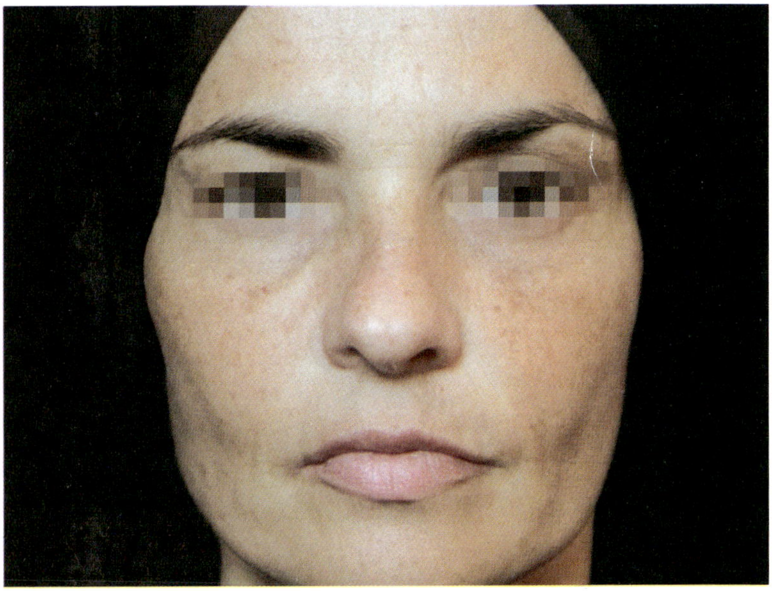

48-year-old patient. Four pregnancies, rather wasted face and with evident hypoplasia of the zygomatic region. Treated with 1 cc of high G′ HA on the periosteal plane, and 1 cc of softer filler (lower G′) on top of the other (multilayer technique), in two separate boluses subsequently merged into a single bolus thanks to vigorous massage.

CLINICAL CASES

CLINICAL CASE 2

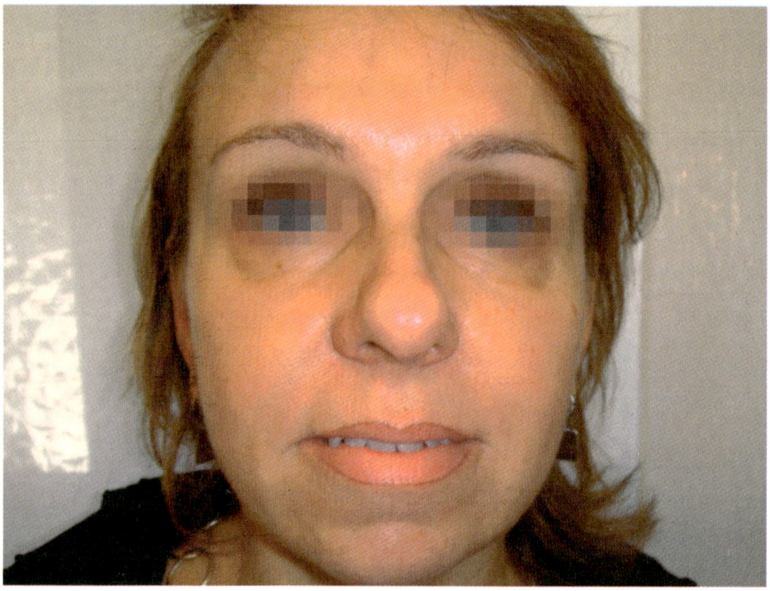

BEFORE

<

AFTER

>

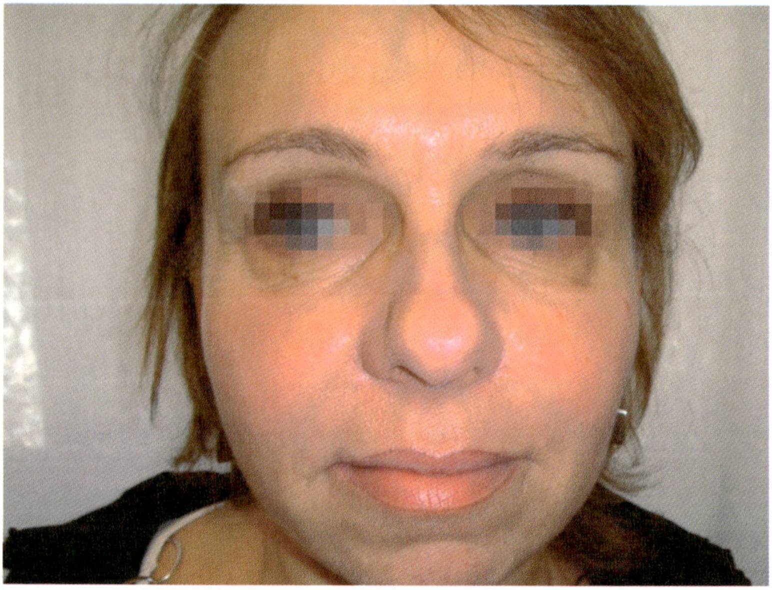

52-year-old patient with modest hypoplasia of the zygomatic region. Treated with HA in the past but never in the cheekbone area. Treated with 1.7 cc of high G′ HA. The patient was extremely satisfied, has returned several times and continues to have treatment.

CLINICAL CASES

CLINICAL CASE 2

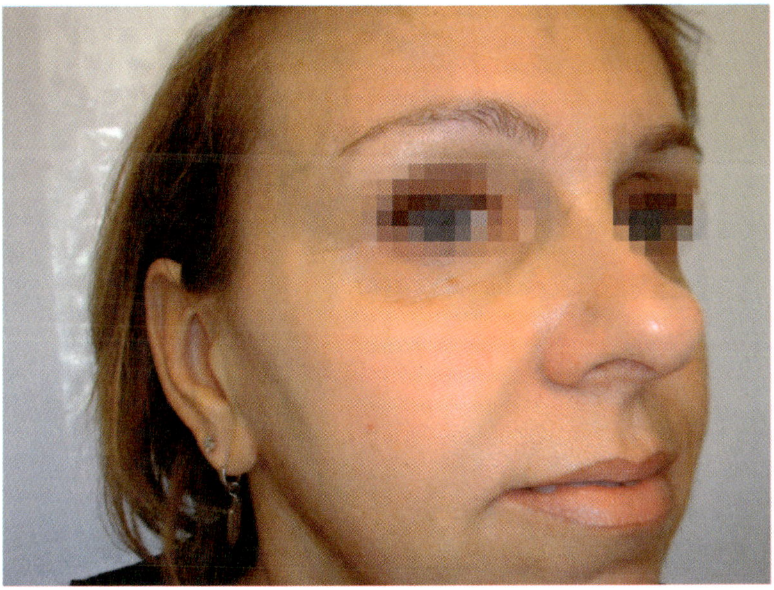

BEFORE

<

AFTER

>

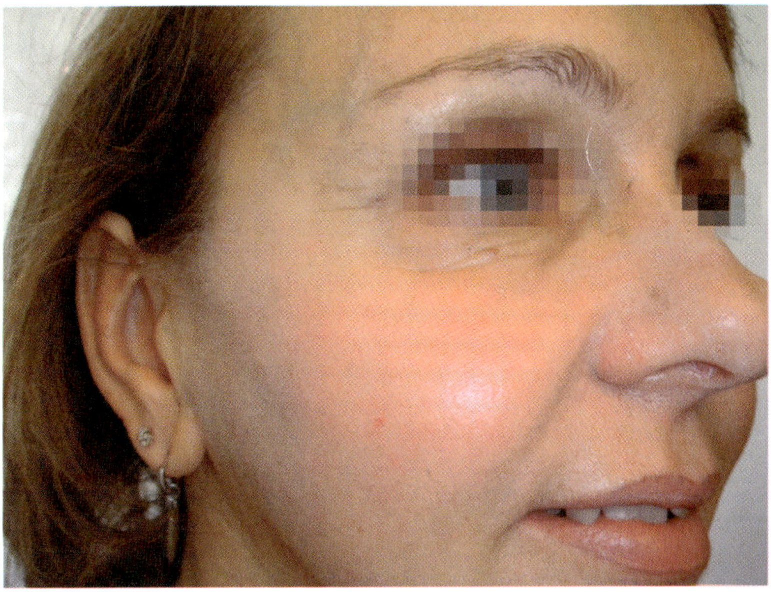

The same patient seen from an angle

CLINICAL CASES

CLINICAL CASE 3

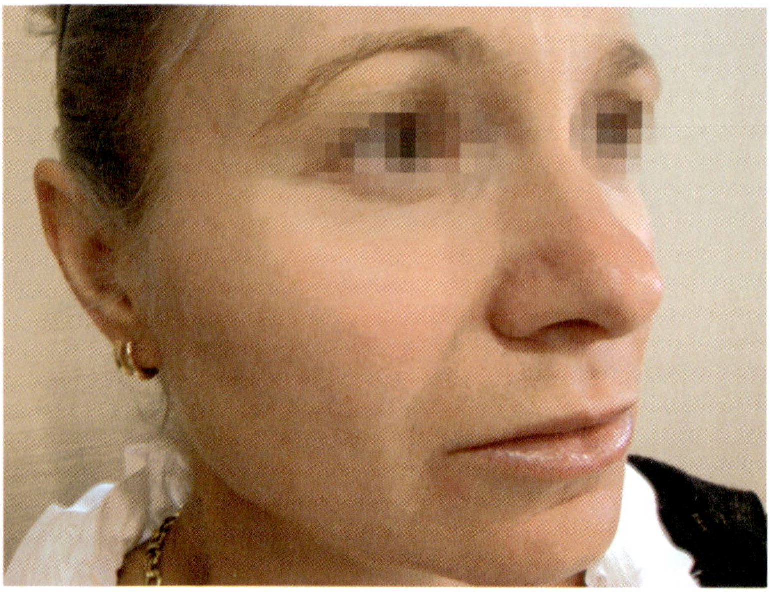

BEFORE

<

AFTER

>

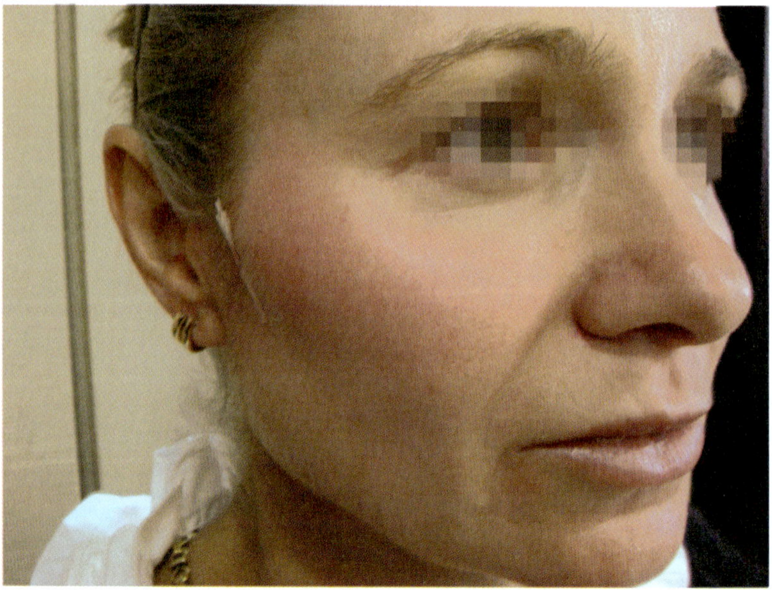

50-year-old patient who had very high and protruding cheekbones when young and wanted to regain the effect. 1 cc of high G′ HA filler was injected on the periosteal plane, with the injection of 1 cc of medium density filler with a medium G′ on top of the other (multilayer technique), during the same session, to add softness.

CLINICAL CASES

CLINICAL CASE 4

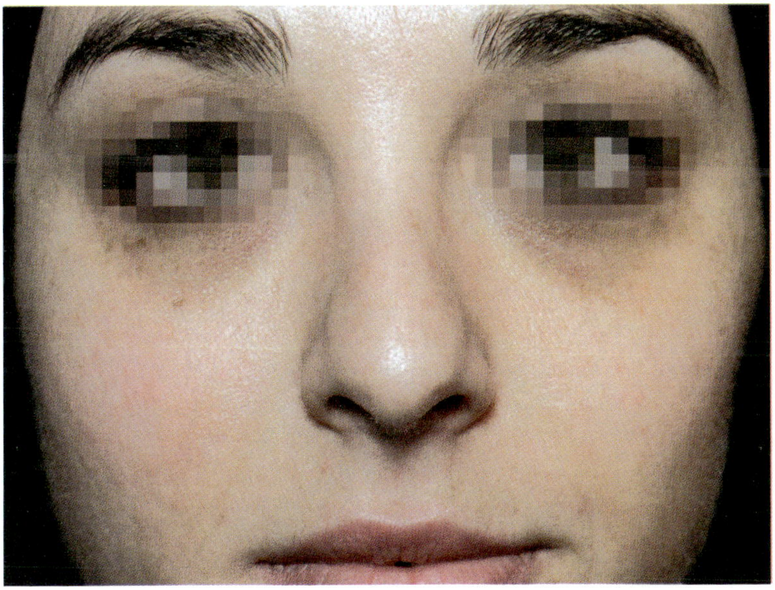

BEFORE

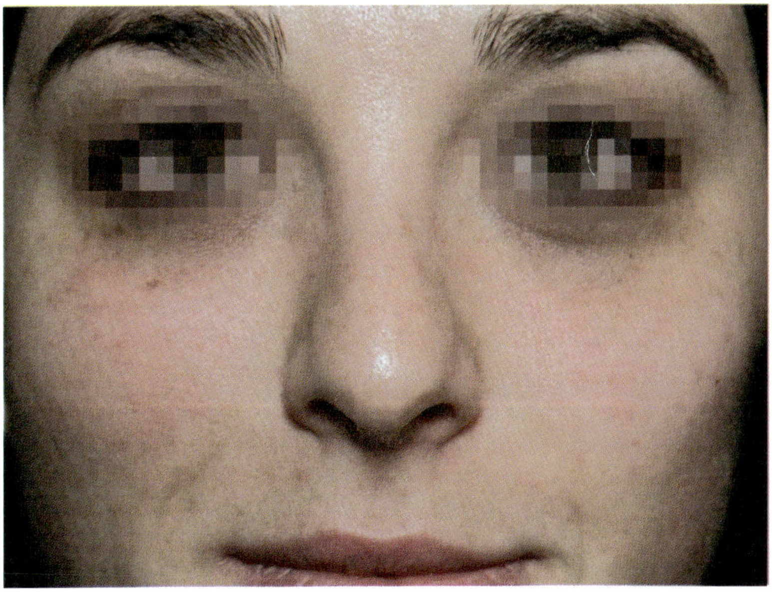

AFTER

28-year-old patient with congenital hypoplasia. Treated with HA in the past but never in the cheekbone area. 1 cc of calcium hydroxyapatite was injected into each side. The patient was very satisfied.

3

TEAR TROUGH

Lucia Calvisi, Alberto Diaspro and Giuseppe Sito

Anatomy of the tear trough

Understanding and knowing the anatomy of the tear trough is essential to achieve optimal correction of this area, which is characterised by some of the thinnest skin on the whole body, just 0.2 mm thick (1), with a layer of smooth muscle cells and practically non-existent subcutaneous tissue.

The lower eyelid region is one of the areas that shows greatest signs of ageing and plays a significant role in the ageing of the entire face.

Consequently, the correction of imperfections in the infraorbital region has become a particularly significant component of surgical and non-surgical facial treatments, given the vast improvements that can be achieved with minimal intervention. Several methods have been proposed for its treatment: lower blepharoplasty, autologous fat implantation, laser or plasma resurfacing and chemical peeling.

Loeb (2) gave a first description of this region in 1961, using the term "nasojugal groove", indicating the furrow extending from the medial edge of the eyelid to the cheek. However, it was Flowers (3) who called it the "tear trough" in 1969.

Haddock et al. described it as the region that extends from the medial canthus of the eye to the midpupillary line. Alongside this we speak more properly of the palpebromalar groove or palpebromalar junction (fig. 1).

Deformity of the tear trough can be due to congenital causes, i.e. it can be present from birth, or it can be acquired and manifest itself slowly as time goes by.

In dissections on corpses, Muzaffar et al. have described the retentive ligament of the orbicularis muscle of the lower eyelid, which originates from the orbital septum and joins the membrane that envelops the supraperiosteal fat of the cheekbone (4-8).

The medial fascia of the retentive ligament of the orbicularis is variable and is indirectly connected to the medial canthus. DMCF (Deep Medial Cheek Fat) corresponds to the medial margin of the SOOF (Suborbicularis Oculi Fat). Its progressive atrophy as we age causes the appearance of an area of visible transition between the fatty parts of the eyelid and the cheek, defining a deeper and more marked tear trough.

The malar septum is a very important anatomical structure in tear trough treatments with fillers. It is a thin septum which originates from the periosteum of the orbital rim and is inserted into the cutaneous plane, dividing the SOOF into an upper and lower portion: before reaching the skin, it crosses the orbicularis muscle of the eye and connects with the surface fat of the cheek, fitting into the dermis about 3 cm below the external canthus.

It is an impermeable membrane that prevents the spread of liquids from the orbital region to the cheek. There are two main arteries in this anatomical region: the infraorbital artery and the angular artery.

The infraorbital foramen, the splanchnocranium exit site of the homonymous artery and vein, is easily located medially along the midpupillary line, about 1 cm below the orbital rim.

A bruise due to blood vessel dama-

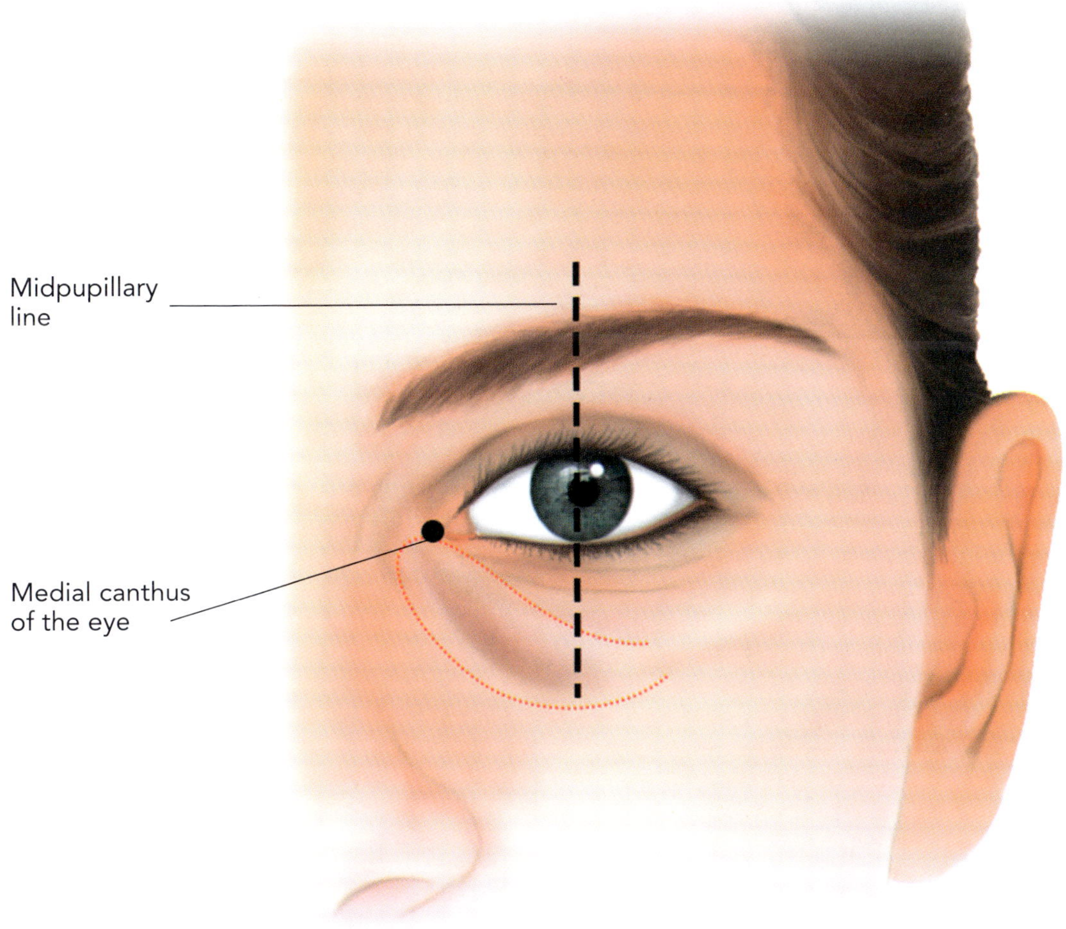

Figure 1 Identifying the tear trough

ge here can lead to increased pressure on the soft tissue, with lymphatic insufficiency and stasis of fluid in the malar region.
The angular artery, a branch of the facial artery, runs from the mandibular ridge obliquely and medially towards the medial canthus, anastomosing with the supratrochlear and supraorbital arteries and the glabellar region.
Accidental intravascular injection of hyaluronic acid into this blood vessel can have catastrophic consequences in the event of occlusion of the ophthalmic artery or the central artery of the retina, the terminal branches, which can lead to amaurosis.

Tear trough classifications

As we age, the weakening of the orbicularis muscle and the ligament, bone thinning and fat herniation lead to the formation of tear trough deformity.
This determines the formation of a trou-

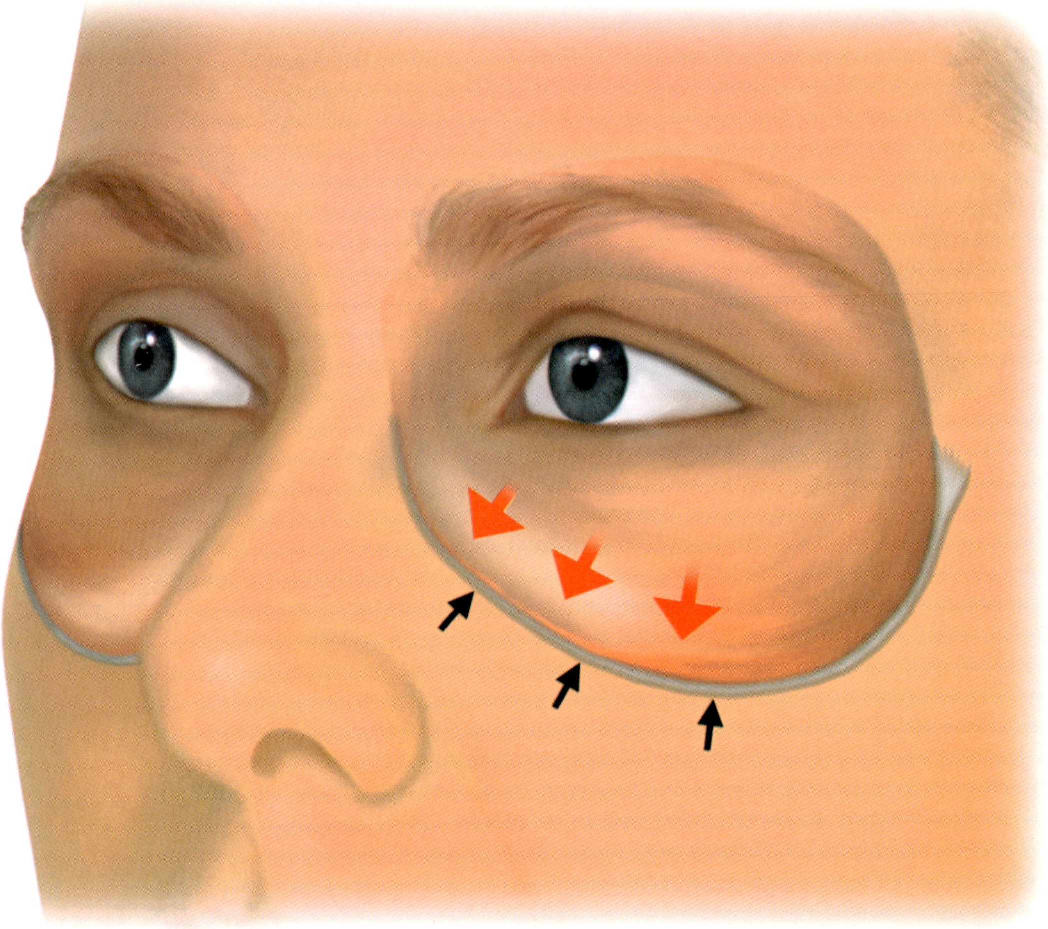

Figure 2 Drooping of the third fascia of the orbicularis muscle

gh, usually of a purplish colour (the dark circles that represent the pathological aspect of the tear trough, but which, unlike the tear trough itself, are not always present), for which various classifications have been proposed (fig. 2).
In particular, in 2010, Hirmand (9) proposed a classification based on clinical assessment, distinguishing between three different levels of tear trough deformity (tab. 1; fig. 3).
A new type of classification is currently being considered however (10). This is particularly useful for discriminating between cases that can be treated with injections and those that cannot (tab. 2).
This new classification is essential, as not all types of tear trough can be injected with dermal fillers, which are only suitable in types II and III. Types I and IV are not good candidates for dermal fillers.
In actual fact, type I does not represent a tear trough deformity at all, and type IV is the consequence of alterations in

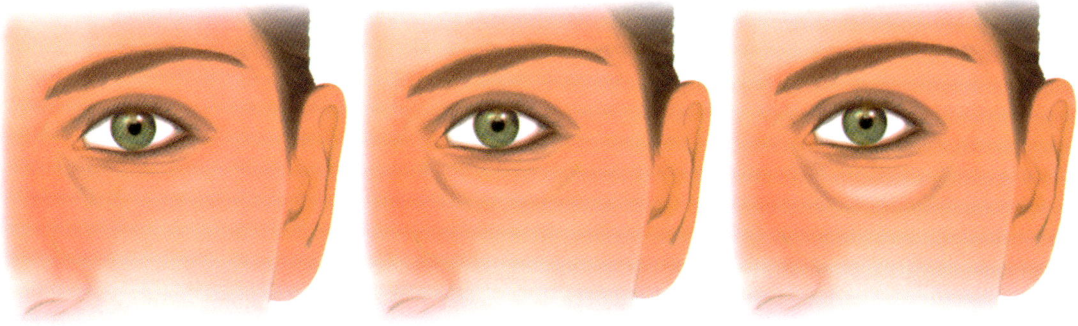

Figure 3 Different types of tear trough identified in Hirmand's classification in 2010

TABLE 1 – TEAR TROUGH: CLASSIFICATION BASED ON CLINICAL ASSESSMENT

Class 1	Patients who suffer a loss of volume limited to the medial portion of the tear trough. These patients may also experience modest flattening that extends to the central part of the cheek
Class 2	Patients in whom the loss of volume also occurs in the lateral part of the orbital zone as well as the medial part; they may experience a moderate loss of volume in the central part of the cheeks with flattening of the upper part
Class 3	Patients who have a complete depression along the palpebral line, both medially and laterally

the periorbital anatomical structures. Consequently, the injection of fillers would only make up for the reduction in malar fat without restoring the loss of orbicularis muscle tone (fig. 4).

Pre-treatment assessment

The deterioration of the tear trough is secondary to herniation of the orbital fat, atrophy of the skin and subcutaneous tissue, weakening of the orbicularis muscle and laxity of the orbital-palpebral ligament ORL (Orbital Retaining Ligament), together with the loss in volume of the pre-zygomatic fatty tissue.

If we tilt the patient's head forward (tilt test), gravity causes the tissues to droop and highlights the trough to be treated. When we pinch the lower eyelid (snap test), it should reposition itself on the conjunctival plane in no more than two seconds; if it takes longer, this indicates the presence of eyelid laxity which could prevent treatment with hyaluro-

TABLE 2 – TEAR TROUGH: NEW CLASSIFICATION

Type I	Prominence	This is due to the herniation of superficial infraorbital fat. Clinically, this is manifested by the formation of a bag on the lower eyelid
Type II	Depression	This is due mainly to a reduction of the malar fat and alterations in the skin Quality (actinic damages and cutaneous laxity)
Type III	Prominence-depression	Prominence-depression The bag is caused by the weakening of the orbicularis muscle of the eye and retentive ligament of the muscle. The depression, on the other hand, is the result of the loss of malar fat and skin alterations
Type IV	Prominence-depression-prominence-depression	The upper bag is caused by loss of tone of the palpebral portion of the prominence-depression orbicularis muscle of the eye; the upper depression is a consequence of the traction effect of the retentive ligament of the orbicularis muscle; the lower bag is due to the loss of elasticity of the muscle, while more caudal depression is caused by fat atrophy and skin alterations
Type V	Mixed	This is the combination of different types

nic acid. The presence of an orbicularis muscle with a hypertrophic tarsal portion can cause dislocation of the injected implant: this becomes particularly visible if we ask the patient to smile (smile test).

Types of treatment

Hyaluronic acid injections have been used to rejuvenate the periorbital region since 2004. Despite the increased use of hyaluronic acid fillers throughout the face, due to its anatomical complexity this region remains a difficult area and must be treated by experienced practitioners.

The treatment of the periorbital region has been in enormous demand in recent years, which is why various methods have been developed to rejuvenate it.

Patients today want methods that are less and less invasive, allowing them to

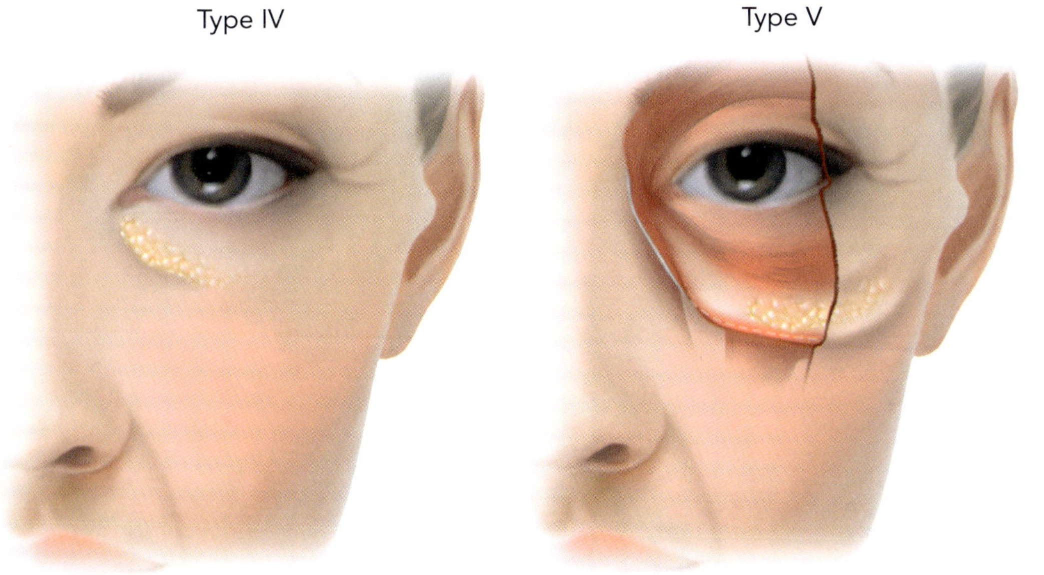

Figure 4 Tear trough and palpebral bags

resume their social life and relationships as soon as possible. So aesthetic medicine is preferred over traditional blepharoplasty when appropriate.

Methods currently used to rejuvenate the area, regardless of the material used, restore the convexity of the cheekbone region and consequently treat the tear trough area. Don't forget that the beauty of the face is represented by the alternation of convexities and concavities: the tear trough represents a slight concavity, or hollow, followed by the evident convexity, or curve, of the cheekbone.

Numerous materials have been described in literature to fill the tear trough area: lipofilling (11-14), calcium hydroxyapatite (15,16), different types of hyaluronic acid (17-20), but very often the materials used and mentioned in literature have proved to be too permanent or not permanent at all in consideration of a region with such distinctive characteristics as the periorbital area. If the patient is a good candidate for medical treatment, based on the new classification described above, i.e. type II or III, the material currently preferred is hyaluronic acid. Different types of hyaluronic acid have been mentioned in literature for the treatment of this area [Belotero® Balance, Merz Pharmaceuticals GmbH, Frankfurt, Germany; Juvederm® Volbella (HA, 15 mg/mL; Lidocaine, 0.3%), Allergan, Inc.; CLEVIEL Fine (HA, 15 mg/ mL; Lidocaine, 0.3%); Teosyal® PureSense Redensity [II] manufactured by Teoxane Laboratories; Restylane].

Regardless of the personal choice of one material rather than another, when dealing with an area as delicate as this, the hyaluronic acid chosen must have a low viscosity and a very low G', otherwise the risk of swelling is high.

Tear trough treatment methods

The injection must always be performed at supraperiosteal level, under the orbicularis muscle, using either the needle or cannula injection technique, depending on individual preference (21).

If you prefer to use the needle, greater attention must be paid to the infraorbital artery and nerve. The needle is used to infiltrate the midpupillary line at a point that can be identified by exerting pressure on the eyeball in order to highlight the last fibres of the orbicularis muscle; at this point the needle is directed medially, protecting the vascular bundle with a finger (fig. 5).

The cannula technique, preferably using a 25 G, which is less traumatic than finer cannulas, envisages a localised entry point where the line passing through the external canthus and the lateral extension of the tear trough meet. The cannula is introduced perpendicularly to the cutaneous plane and, when contact with the bone plane is felt, inclined medially and pushed underneath the orbicularis muscle and in a medial direction until it reaches the orbital rim, where small amounts of hyaluronic acid are injected using a retrograde linear technique.

The choice between needle or cannula depends on the doctor's preference, but the latter usually prevents bruising, which can also lead to compression of the lymphatic vessels and consequent swelling.

In both cases, the technique should be performed in the least traumatic way possible. The cannula also minimises the risk of intravascular injection: to prevent injury to the vessels, it is best to perform the injection more medially in relation to the internal canthus. The hyaluronic acid should be gently massaged during the procedure to ensure better distribution.

It is essential not to overcorrect, preferring to inject small amounts of product, between 0.3 and 0.5 cc per side, retouching after 15 days if it is necessary. In addition to the above, it is important to stress the importance of a suitable product which is only minimally hydrophilic and is anti-edemigenous, as the area is susceptible to severe swelling which, while being quick to recede, would defeat the aesthetic purpose.

Another recommendation concerns the amount of product to be injected: never more than 0.3-0.4 cc per side, precisely to avoid both an accumulative effect, which would simulate ugly bags under the eyes, and to prevent swelling. And let's not forget that this is a very delicate area: the more you touch it, the more it is likely to bruise.

VIDEO 1

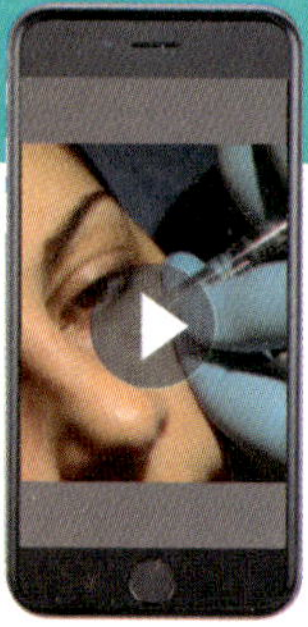

Tear trough: technique

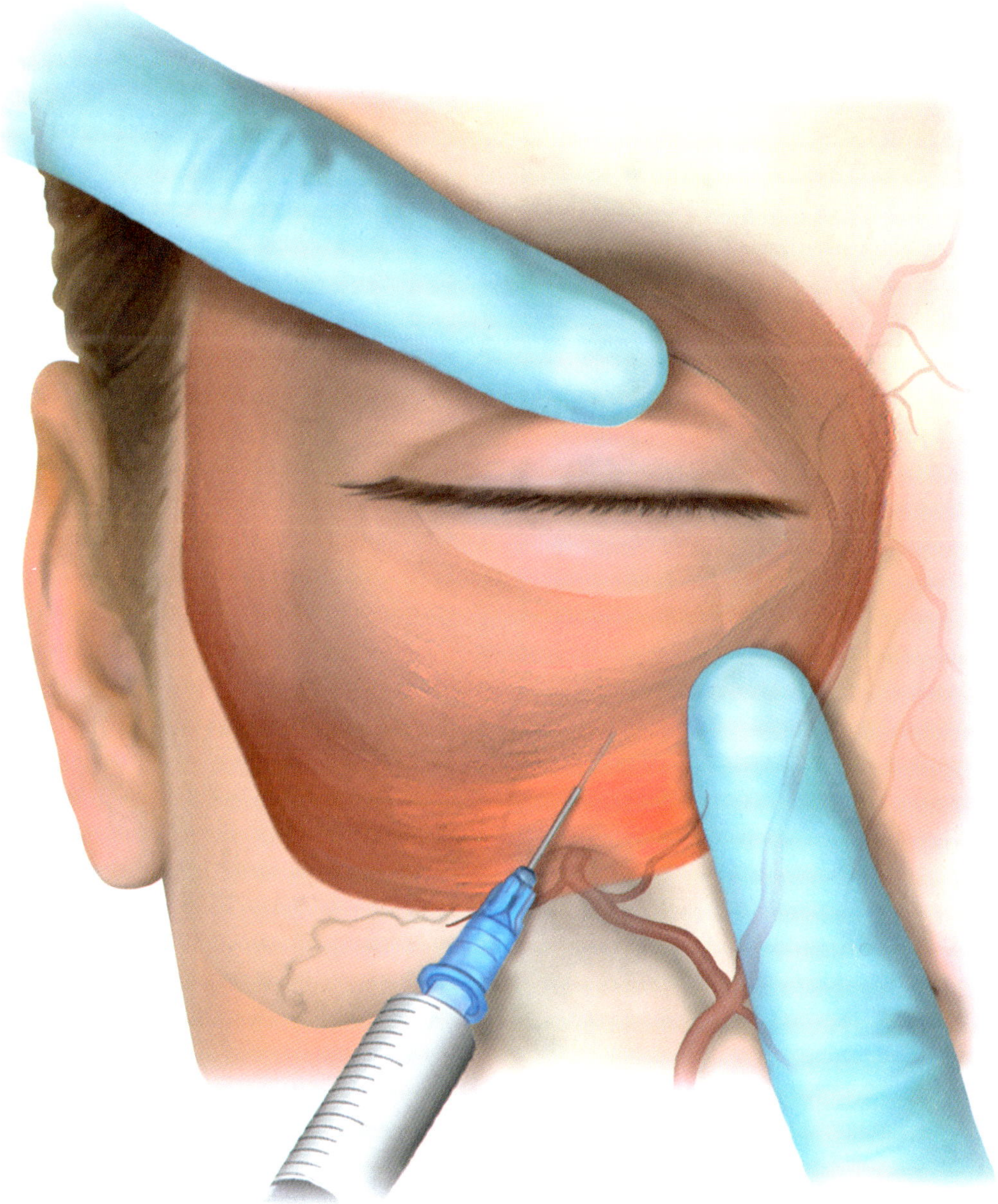

Figure 5 Tear trough treatment injection point

Immediate complications

Here are some of the most common immediate complications that might occur.

> Pain: alleviated thanks to the presence of lidocaine.

> Rash, swelling and bruising: alleviated by applying ice immediately before and after the procedure.

> Asymmetry: due to a technical error, usually overcorrection.

Delayed complications

Delayed complications include.

> Hemosiderin patches: the use of any type of filler in this area can be associated with the formation of bruises and the consequent formation of brown-orange patches of hemosiderin. This is more frequent with dark complexions.

> Swelling: this is due to overcorrection or poor choice of filler. Additional precautions should be taken in patients with malar bags, in which swelling is more likely to develop due to the hydrophilic nature of the filler. It can be treated with hyaluronidase.

> Infections: not very frequent. They are caused by *Staphylococcus epidermidis* or *Propionibacterum acnes*. Filler should not usually be injected if there is an infection in a neighbouring area.

> Tyndall effect: this is due to the injection of the product too close to the surface, tingeing the skin with a bluish colour.

> Blindness: although extremely rare, it is nevertheless mentioned in literature. According to Coleman, it is due to the retrograde migration of the filler towards the central artery of the retina. Once again, in order to avoid its onset, it is important to limit the amount of filler that is injected in a single session and inject the product slowly, without hurrying (21).

Bibliography

1. Bucay VW, Day D. Adjunctive skin care of the brow and periorbital region. Clin Plastic Surg. 2013;40:225–236.
2. Loeb R. Fat pad sliding and fat grafting for leveling lid depressions. Clin Plast Surg 1981; 8: 757-76.
3. Flowers RS. Tear trough implants for correction of tear trough deformity. Clin Plast Surg 1993; 20: 403-15.
4. Wong CH, Hsieh MK, Mendelson B. The tear trough ligament: anatomical basis for the tear trough deformity. Plast Reconstr Surg. 2012;129:1392-3402.
5. Wong CH, Mendelson B. Extended Transconjunctival Lower Eyelid Blepharoplasty with Release of the Tear Trough Ligament and Fat Redistribution. Plast Reconstr Surg. 2017 Aug;140(2):273-282.
6. Yang N, Qiu W, Wang Z, Su X, Jia H, Shi H. [Anatomical studying of the tear trough area]. Zhonghua Zheng Xing Wai Ke Za Zhi. 2014 Jan;30(1):50-3. Chinese.
7. Pessa JE. Discussion: The tear trough ligament: anatomical basis for the tear trough deformity. Plast Reconstr Surg. 2012 Jun;129(6):1403-4.
8. Wong CH, Hsieh MK, Mendelson B. The tear trough ligament: anatomical basis for the tear trough deformity. Plast Reconstr Surg. 2012 Jun;129(6):1392-402.
9. Hirmand H. Anatomy and nonsurgical correction of the tear trough deformity. Plast Reconstr Surg 2010; 125: 699-708.
10. Turkmani MG. New Classification System for Tear Trough Deformity. Dermatol Surg. 2017 Jun;43(6):836-840.
11. Willemsen JC, Mulder KM, Stevens HP. Lipofilling with minimal access cranial suspension lifting for enhanced rejuvena- tion. Aesthet Surg J

2011; 31: 759-69.
12. Liao SL, Wei YH. Fat repositioning via supraperiosteal dissection with internal fization for tear trough deformity in an Asian population. Graefes Arch Clin Exp Ophthalmol 2011; 249: 1735-41.
13. Kim HS, Choi CW, Kim BR, Youn SW. Effectiveness of Transconjunctival Fat Removal and Resected Fat Grafting for Lower Eye Bag and Tear Trough Deformity. JAMA Facial Plast Surg. 2019 Mar 1;21(2):118-124.
14. Chiu CY, Shen YC, Zhao QF, Hong FL, Xu JH. Treatment of Tear Trough Deformity: Fat Repositioning versus Autologous Fat Grafting. Aesthetic Plast Surg. 2017 Feb;41(1):73-80.
15. Wollina U. Improvement of tear trough by monophasic hyaluronic Acid and calcium hydroxylapatite. J Clin Aesthet Dermatol. 2014 Oct;7(10):38-43.
16. Bernardini FP, Cetinkaya A, Devoto MH, Zambelli A. Calcium hydroxylapatite (Radiesse) for the correction of periorbital hollows, dark circles, and lower eyelid bags. Ophthalmic Plast Reconstr Surg. 2014 Jan-Feb;30(1):34-9
17. Lee JH, Hong G. Definitions of groove and hollowness of the infraorbital region and clinical treatment using soft-tissue filler. Arch Plast Surg. 2018 May;45(3):214-221.
18. Berguiga M, Galatoire O. Tear trough rejuvenation: A safety evaluation of the treatment by a semi-cross-linked hyaluronic acid filler. Orbit. 2017 Feb;36(1):22-26.
19. Huber-Vorländer J, Kürten M. Correction of tear trough deformity with a cohesive polydensified matrix hyaluronic acid: a case series. Clin Cosmet Investig Dermatol. 2015 Jun 25;8:307-12.
20. Niforos F, Acquilla R, Ogilvie P, Safa M, Signorini M, Creutz L, Kerson G, Silberberg M. A Prospective, Open-Label Study of Hyaluronic Acid-Based Filler With Lidocaine (VYC-15L) Treatment for the Correction of Infraorbital Skin Depressions. Dermatol Surg. 2017 Oct;43(10):1271-1280.
21. Brown M, Gatherwright J, Katira K, Rowe D. Evaluation of blunt and sharp needle tips in correction of the tear trough deformity. J Plast Reconstr Aesthet Surg. 2014 Dec;67(12):e310-1.
22. Sharad J. Dermal Fillers for the Treatment of Tear Trough Deformity: A Review of Anatomy, Treatment Techniques, and their Outcomes. J Cutan Aesthet Surg. 2012 Oct;5(4):229-38.

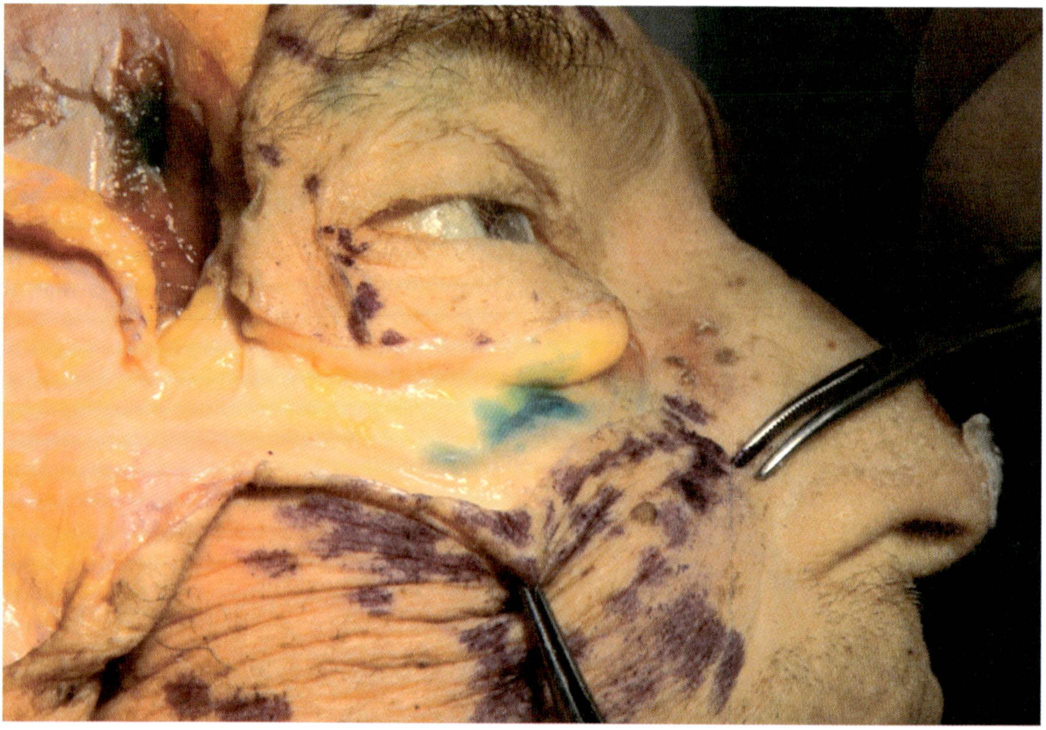

Tear trough and lower palpebral bag, one of the three usually present

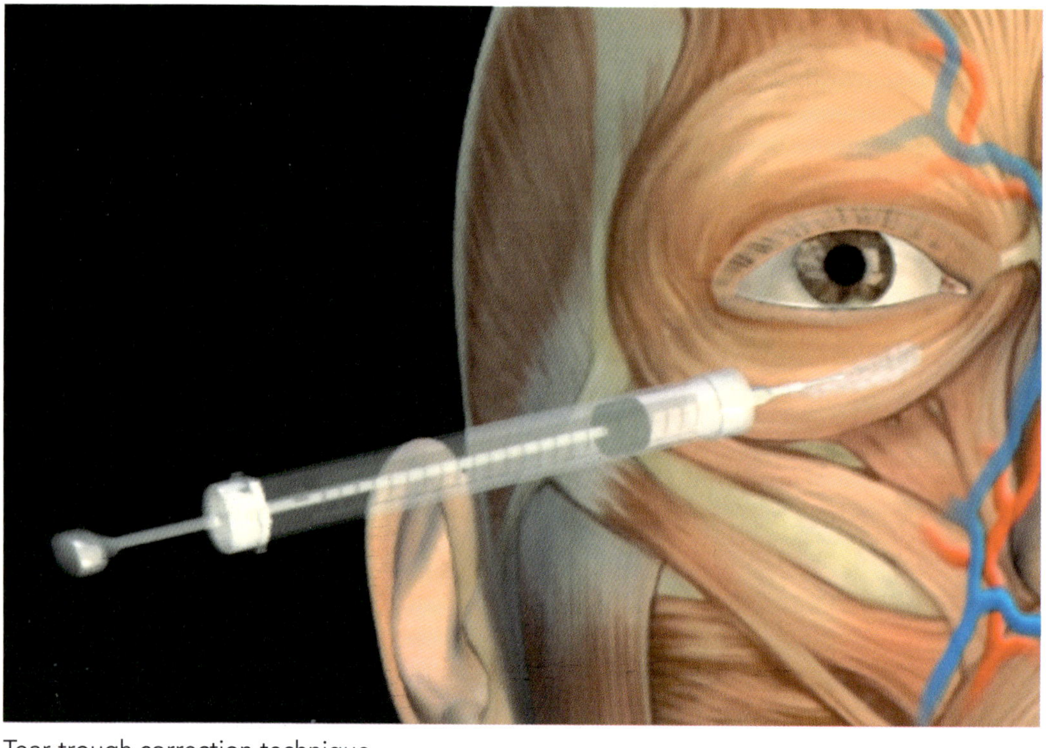

Tear trough correction technique

CLINICAL CASES

CLINICAL CASE 1

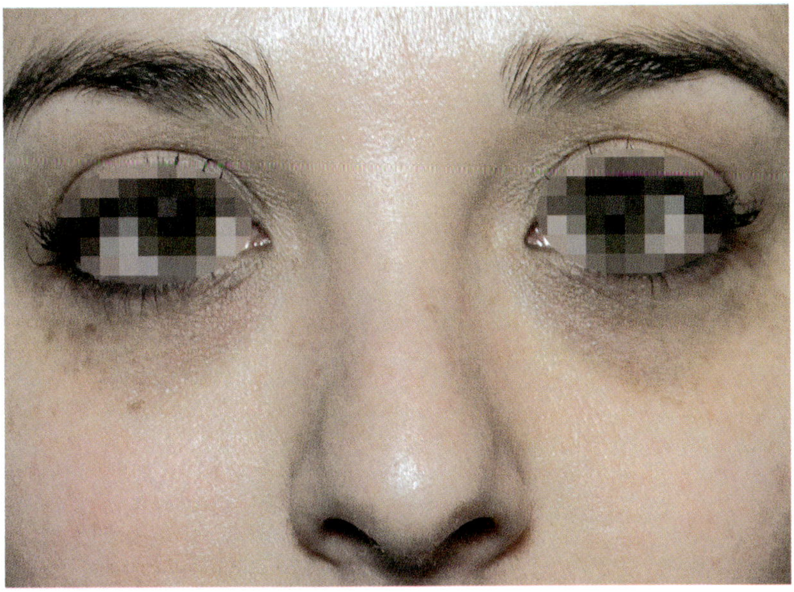

BEFORE

<

VIDEO 2

Tear trough: morphing before and after

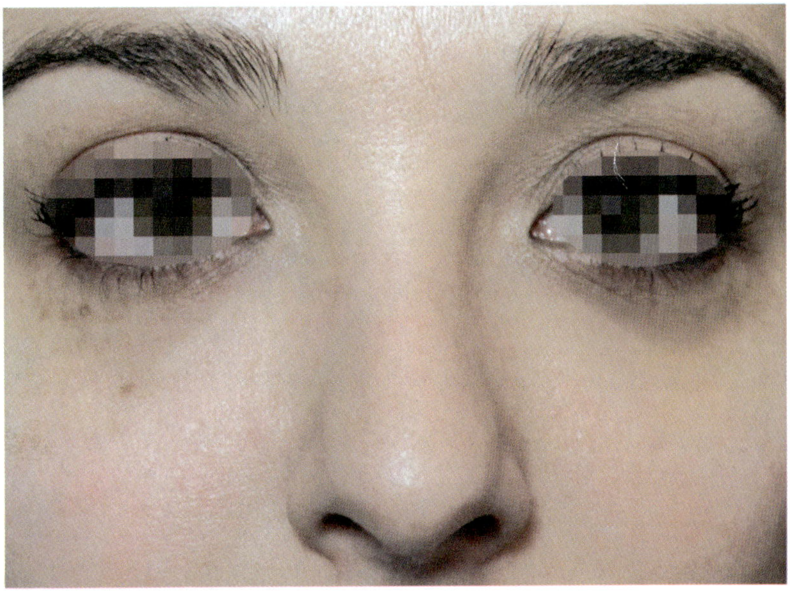

AFTER

>

28-year-old patient with a congenital tear trough. No indication of any pathology which might have caused it. Slight pigmentation of the defect which could lead to its definition as a "dark circle", which cannot be improved by injective treatment.

CLINICAL CASES

CLINICAL CASE 2

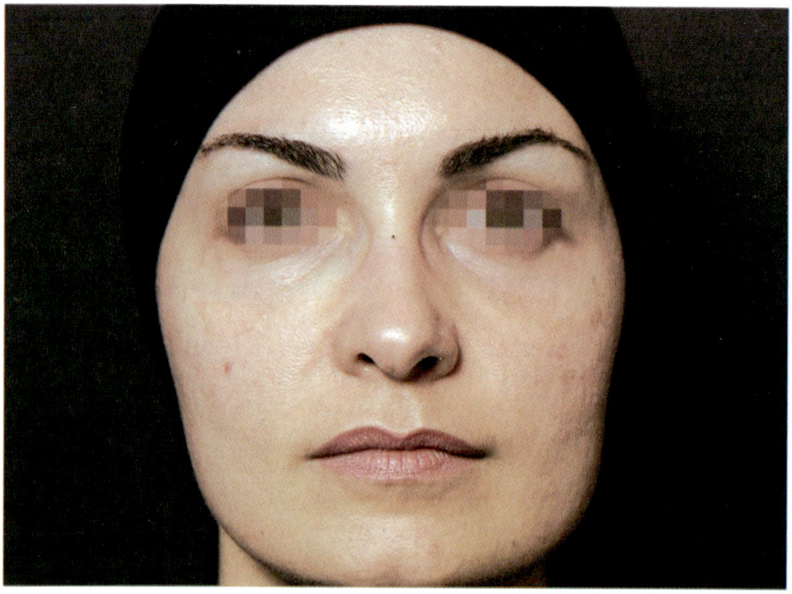

BEFORE

<

AFTER

>

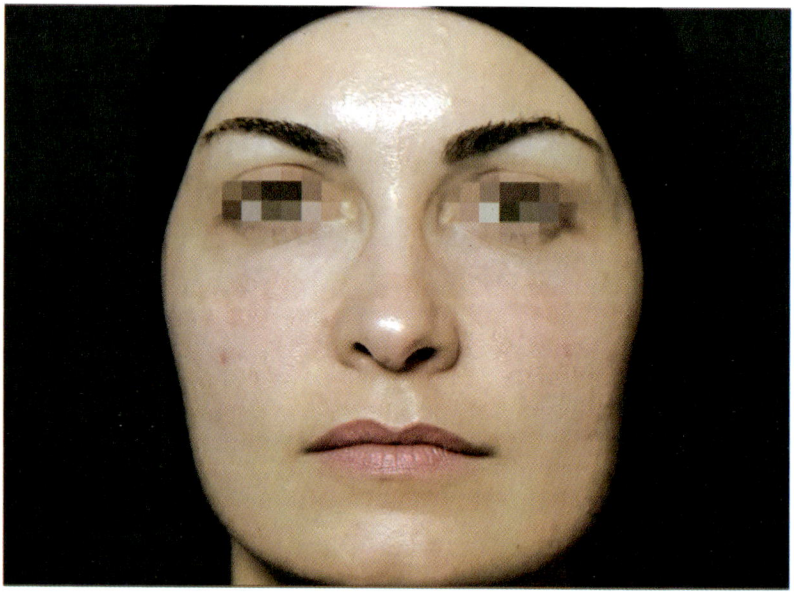

30-year-old patient with a recent pregnancy behind her. Says that she has always had tear troughs. Treated with HA filler with modest hypoplasia of the zygomatic region. Treated with non-hydrophilic dedicated HA, 0.3 ml per side. No complications. Very satisfied.

CLINICAL CASES

CLINICAL CASE 2

VIDEO 3

Semeiotic
of the tear trough

VIDEO 4

Tear trough
correction technique

VIDEO 5

Morphing
of clinical cases

VIDEO 6

Morphing
of clinical cases

CLINICAL CASES

CLINICAL CASE 3

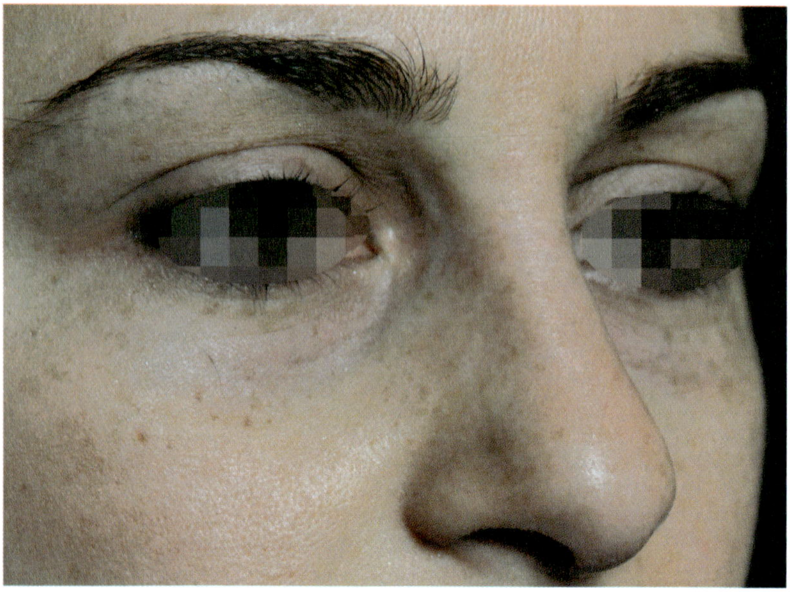

BEFORE

VIDEO 7

Tear trough correction technique

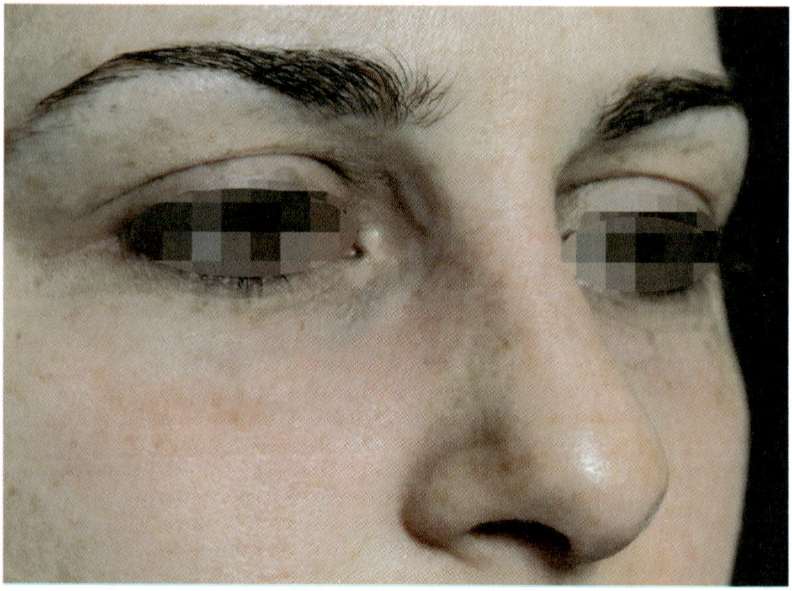

AFTER

35-year-old patient with no pathology. Tear trough occurring after a particularly difficult pregnancy. Various attempts at aesthetic treatment without success. Result, in the picture below, after appropriate treatment with dedicated hyaluronic acid.

CLINICAL CASES

CLINICAL CASE 4

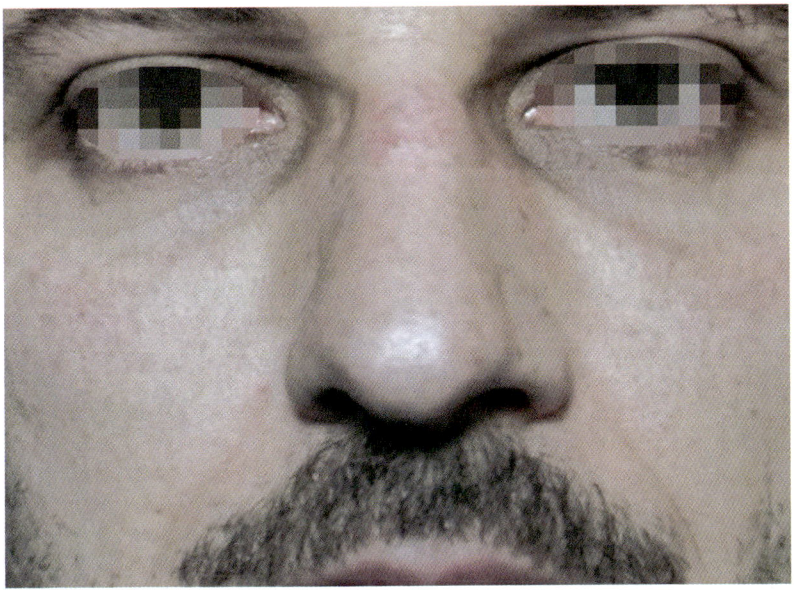

BEFORE

<

VIDEO 8

Tear trough: morphing before and after

AFTER

>

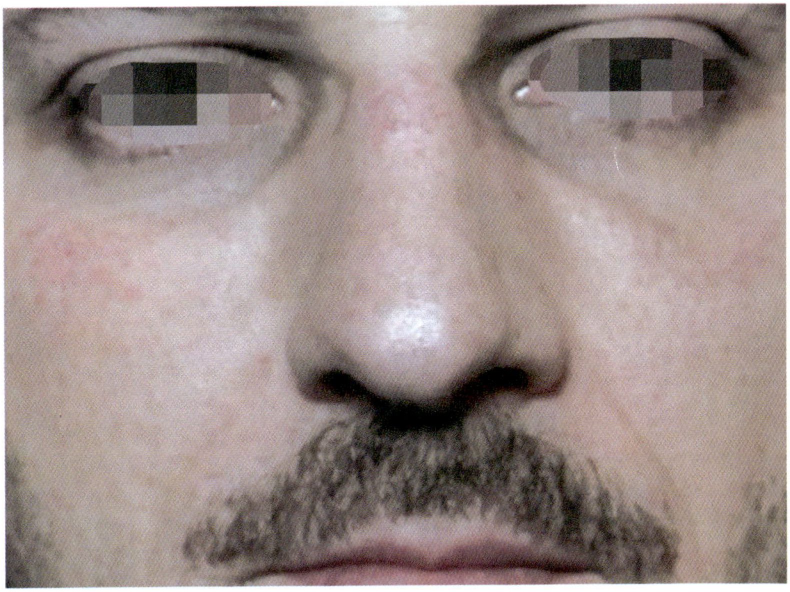

49-year-old man. Reports the appearance of the tear trough following military service over twenty years earlier. Correction of the tear trough with 0.6 cc of dedicated hyaluronic acid.

CLINICAL CASES

CLINICAL CASE 4

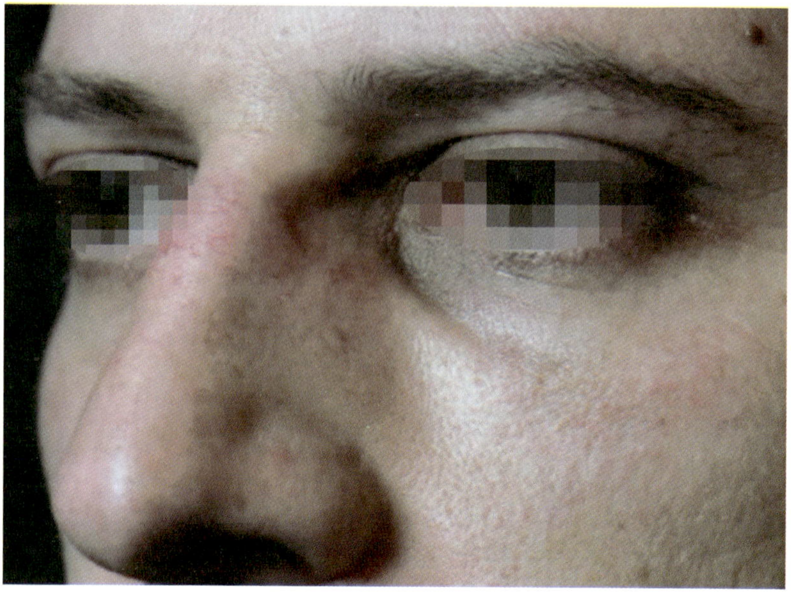

BEFORE

<

AFTER

>

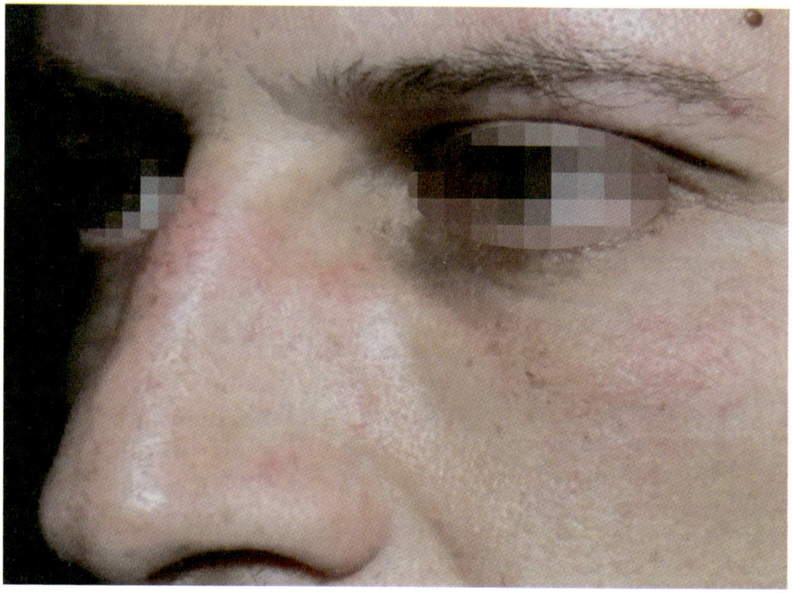

The same case, before and after correction.

4

CHEEKS

Anatomy of the cheeks

The cheeks, which are considered a focal point of beauty, are membranous muscle structures.

From an anatomical point of view, they are divided into an external or cutaneous surface and an internal or mucous membrane surface, both with an irregular quadrilateral shape and of different extension.

The external surface (fig. 1), which is more extensive than the internal one, has limits that are marked conventionally:

> cranially, by a plane that passes throu-

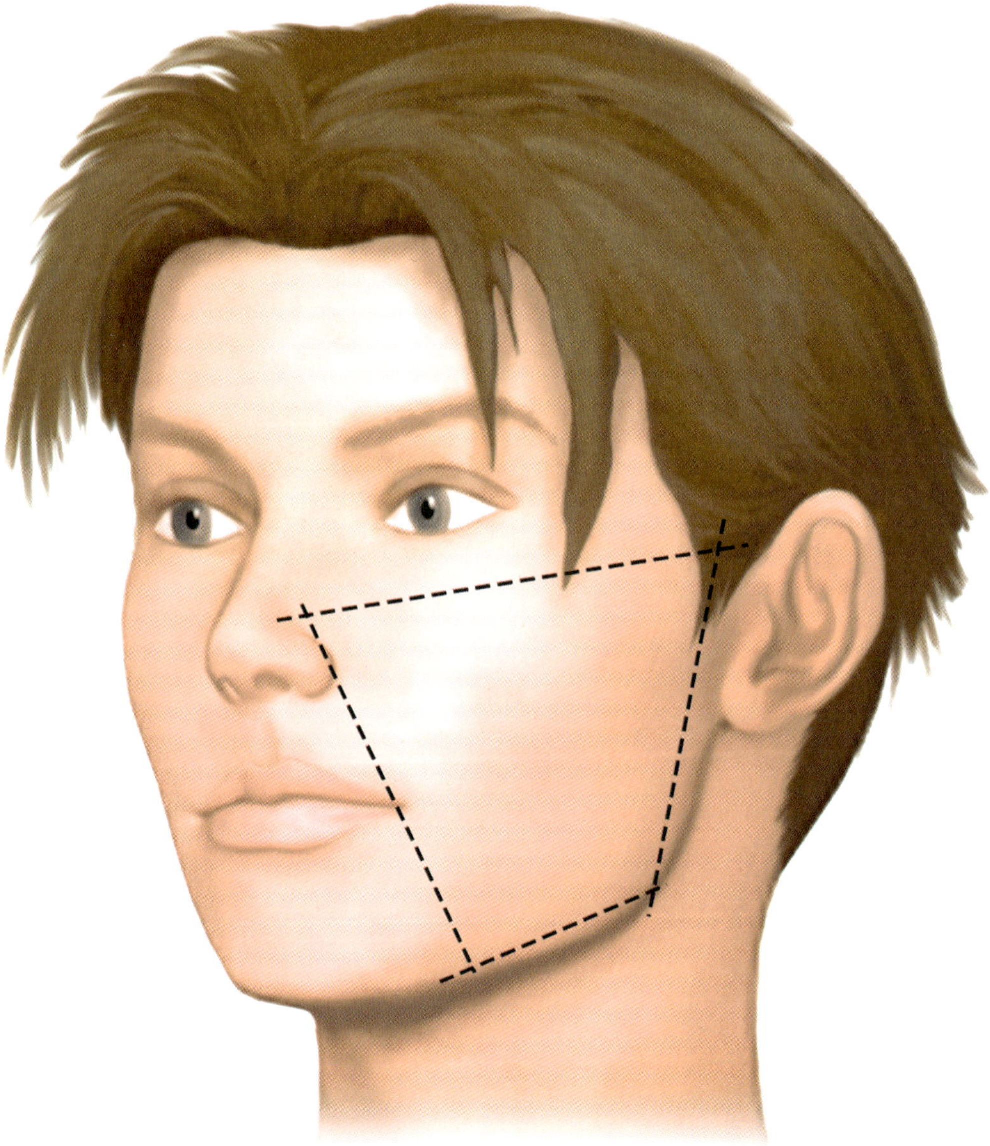

Figure 1 Anatomical limits of the cheek

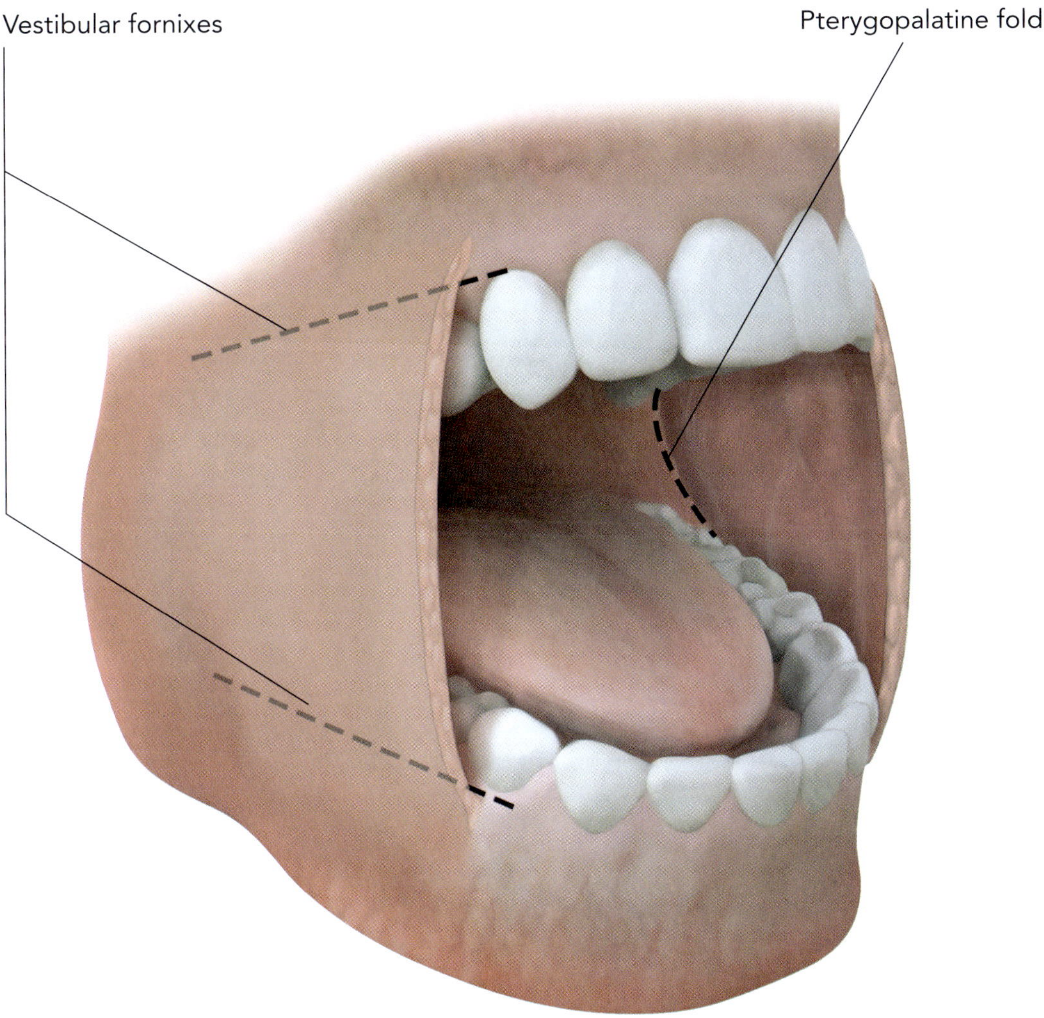

Figure 2 Limits of the cheek in the oral area

gh the floor of the orbital cavity;
- caudally, by a plane that passes through the lower edge of the mandible;
- posteriorly, by a plane tangent to the rear edge of the branch of the mandible;
- anteriorly, by a plane that passes through the nasal ala and the lip commissure.

The inner surface (fig. 2) has sharper limits:
- cranially and caudally, it is delimited by the vestibular fornixes;
- posteriorly, by a vertical fold, the pterygopalatine fold, which corresponds to the ridge of the pterygopalatine raphe;
- anteriorly, there are no demarcation limits of the lips.

On the inner surface, near the lip commissure, we can sometimes see the

Fordyce corpuscles, small yellowish bumps which are nothing more than ectopic sebaceous glands.
Due to the inexorable passage of time, in addition to the visible resorption of fat and tissue ptosis, linear wrinkles called crinkles, and wrinkles caused by sleeping in the same position all the time often appear.
Little can be done by fillers in either case and we often have to rely on surface techniques such as peeling or biorevitalization.
As we have already said, the shape of the cheeks is that of a quadrilateral with irregular contours, but still with very defined limits. The structure of the cheeks is made up of thick, richly vascularized skin with numerous sebaceous glands, hairy in men and hairless in women, and frequently affected more or less intensely by the signs of ageing.
The subcutaneous tissue (mainly represented by fat) is richly represented and subject, as we said, to the effects of atrophy as time goes by.
This anatomical region has no vascular or nerve structures of great importance requiring the alteration of the manoeuvres performed to inject facial fillers. It is, however, necessary to distinguish a few technical notes.

Methods for treating the cheeks

The cheeks can be affected by surface ageing with the formation of wrinkles of varying intensity, mainly due to photoaging or adipose involution, and in this case it is necessary to correct the volumes. It is evident that repairs of the defect are variable and, with the use of elastic fillers with low G′ and G″ and tan close to the unit, injected with a needle positioned at a minimal angle, almost tangential to the skin, it is possible for a highly skilled practitioner to remedy the deficiency in substance. On the contrary, even if we try to remain close to the surface, the use of a microcannula can be considered unsuitable, as it can result in the formation of unsightly mounds or even create a visible and unsightly abrasion of the hypodermis if we overdo our efforts to stay near the surface. In any case, it is advisable to use modest quantities of substance to avoid visible lumps on the surface (fig. 3).
This said, if you want to restore volume that has been lost over the years, it is advisable to use a microcannula, preferably a 25 G/40 mm, with a soft filler; shaping the cheeks with massage is almost impossible due to the absence of a valid supporting bone base. The fillers to be used must have a higher G′ and G″ and a lower tan, but the characteristic that should be carefully assessed is the filler's moulding capacity, i.e. its supposed biodynamics and the likelihood that it will easily adapt to such an irregular region.
The entry point of the microcannula, using a 21 G needle or a 23 G at most, will always be below the defect to be corrected, which must always be previously marked out with a pen. Once the needle or cannula has been introduced, it will be possible to inject 0.3 cc of lidocaine, which, thanks to its short half-life, will simplify the practitioner's task and reassure the patient, making the treatment more comfortable and painless.
Another recommendation is represen-

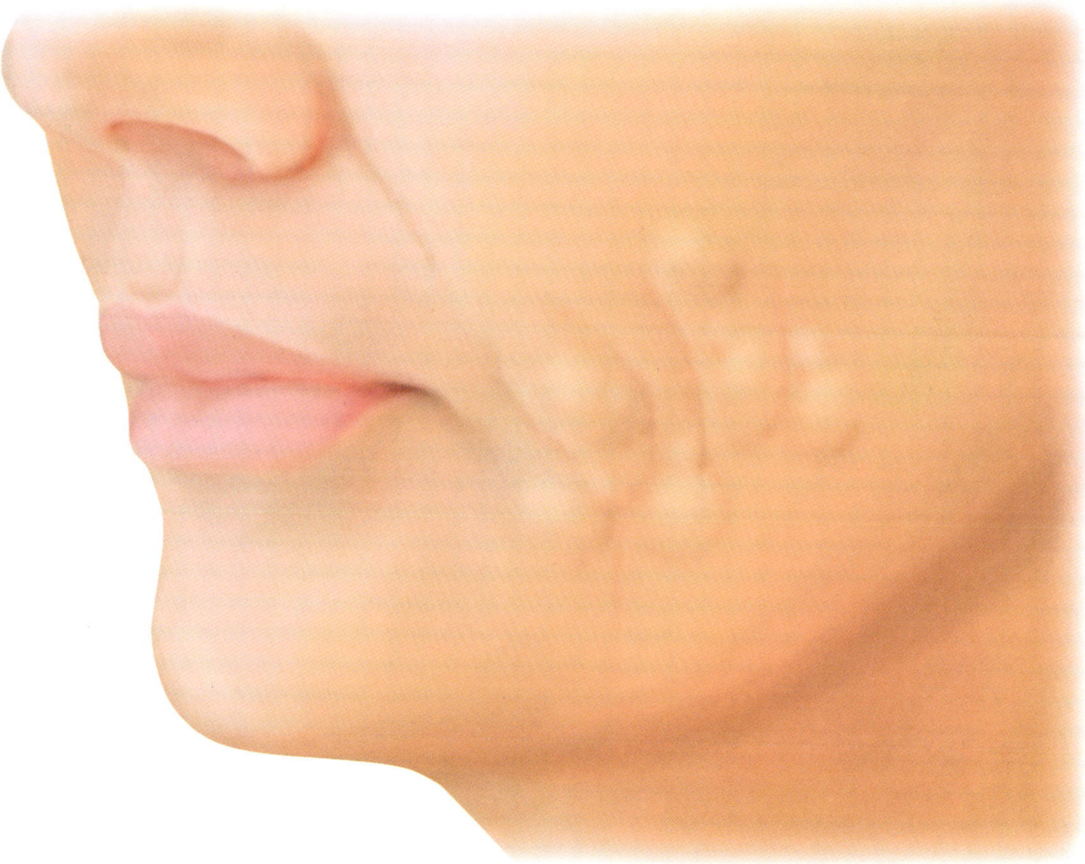

Figure 3 Macroscopic aspect of cheek correction. In actual fact, you should not see any lumps, which may have to be smoothed out with vigorous massage

VIDEO 1

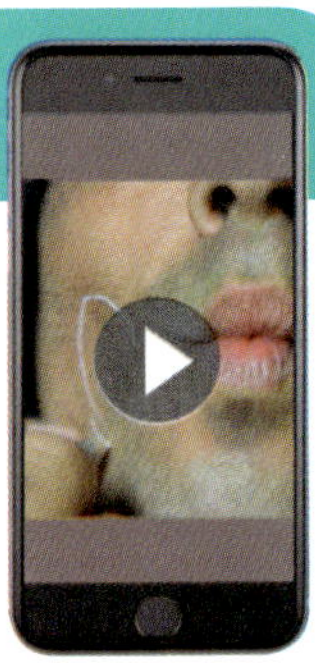

Cheek correction technique with cannula

ted by the possibility of first inserting the cannula on its own, without assembling it, and then connecting it to the syringe in order not to have a lever with too long an arm, which could be detrimental to precision. Once you have inserted the cannula, it is always a good idea to check the level reached, lifting it to make sure that it is not too shallow, and then start a series of to-and-fro movements in order to create small, fan-shaped spaces in which to

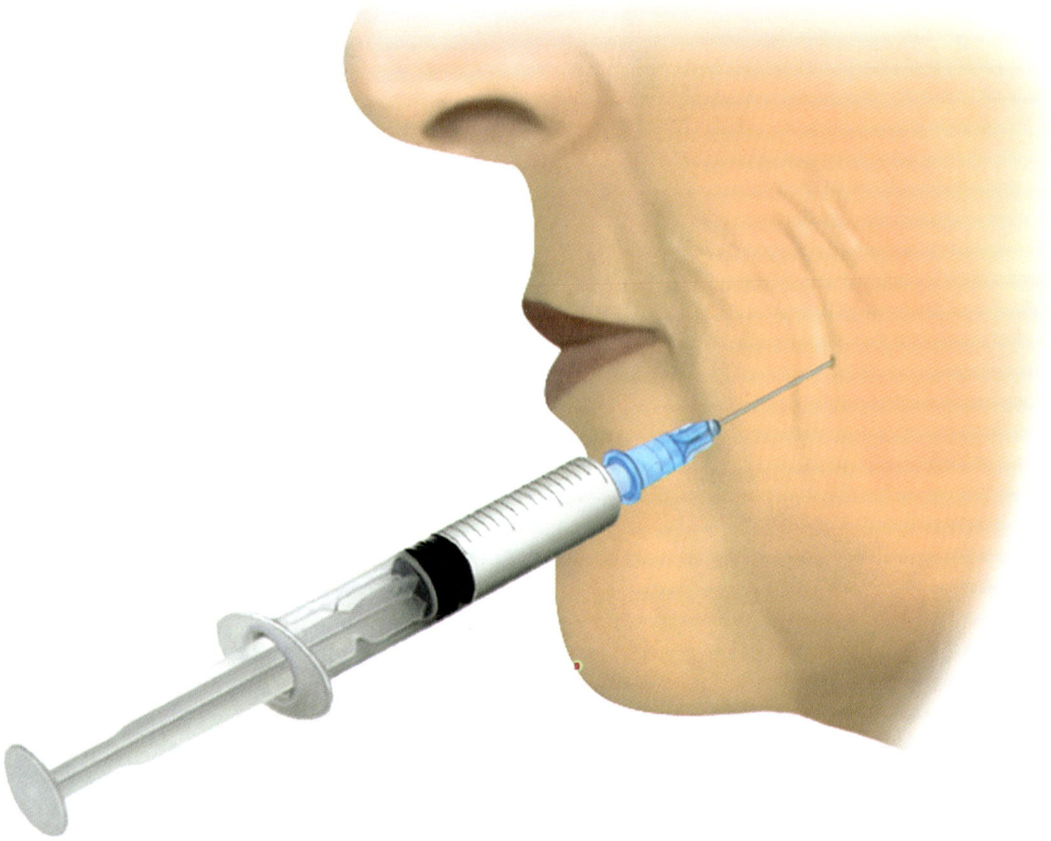

Figure 4 Cheek correction technique with needle

deposit microdroplets of about 0.10-0.20 cc of filler.

This will fill the target area evenly, with no steps or deformities that would be hard to correct later. Apart from small bruises that disappear in a few days or can be encouraged to reabsorb with the use of a topical preparation containing lactoferrin or vitamin K, there are usually no complications whatsoever. Infections are very rare, but a thin layer of antibiotic ointment can be applied before discharging the patient, as air pollution could contribute to etiopathogenesis in a wound which takes some time to heal. The clinical effect is always satisfactory and the average duration of the repair, which, if carried out with a microcannula, requires at least twice the amount of product used with a needle, is about 7-8 months, with a slow and gradual resorption of the product used.

Bibliography

1. Luciano Fonzi. Anatomia funzionale e clinica dello splancnocranio. Edi Ermes, 2000.
2. Kablik J, Monheit GD, Yu L, Chang

G, Gershkovich J. Comparative physical properties of hyaluronic acid dermal fillers. Dermatol Surg. 2009;35 Suppl 1:302-312.
3. Mowlds DS, Lambros V. Cheek Volumization and the Nasolabial Fold. Plast Reconstr Surg. 2018;141(5):1124-1129.
4. Whitehead DM, Schechter LS. Cheek Augmentation Techniques. Facial Plast Surg Clin North Am. 2019;27(2):199-206.
5. Ho D, Jagdeo J. Safety and Efficacy of a Volumizing Hyaluronic Acid Filler for Treatment of HIV-Associated Facial Lipoatrophy. JAMA Dermatol. 2017;153(1):61-65.
6. Shamban A, Clague MD, von Grote E, Nogueira A. A Novel and More Aesthetic Injection Pattern for Malar Cheek Volume Restoration. Aesthetic Plast Surg. 2018;42(1):197-200.

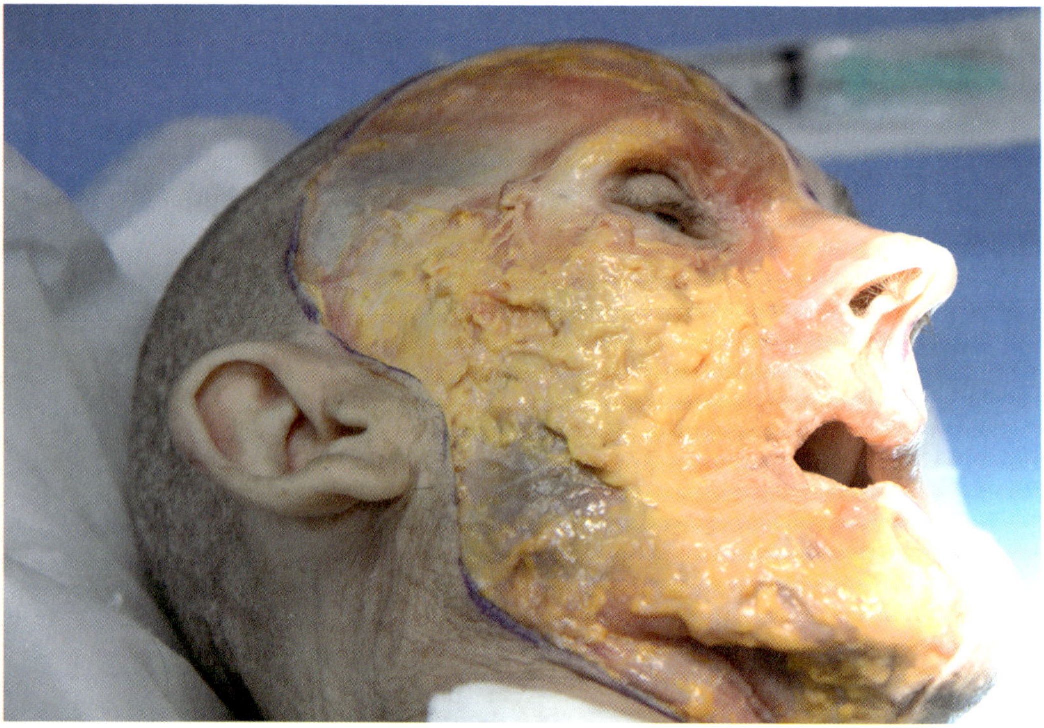

Superficial muscular aponeurotic system (SMAS) in an anatomical preparation

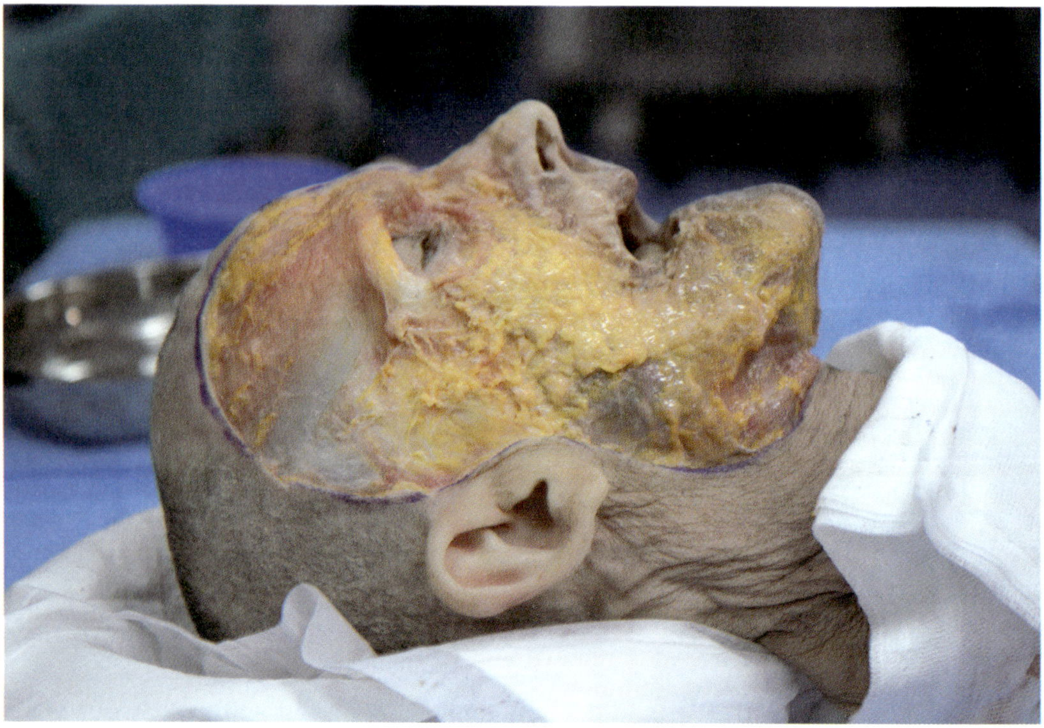

Superficial muscular aponeurotic system (SMAS) in an anatomical preparation

CLINICAL CASES

CLINICAL CASE 1

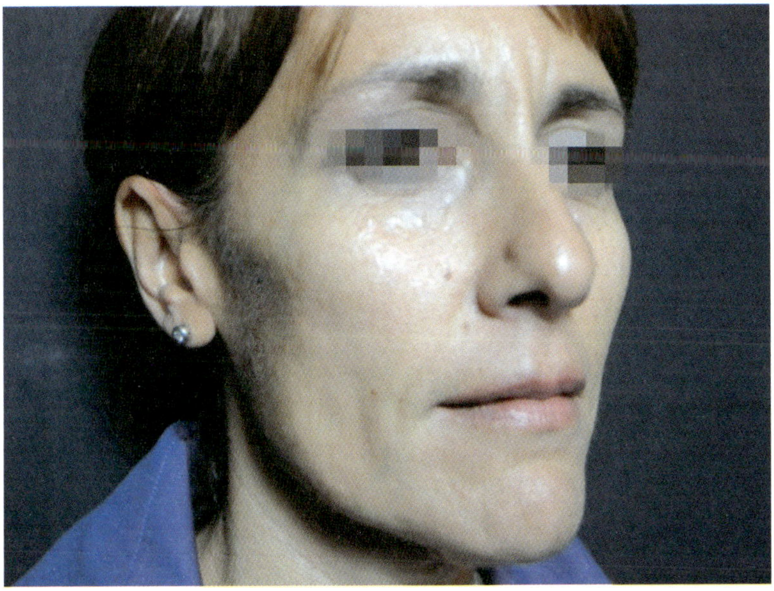

BEFORE

<

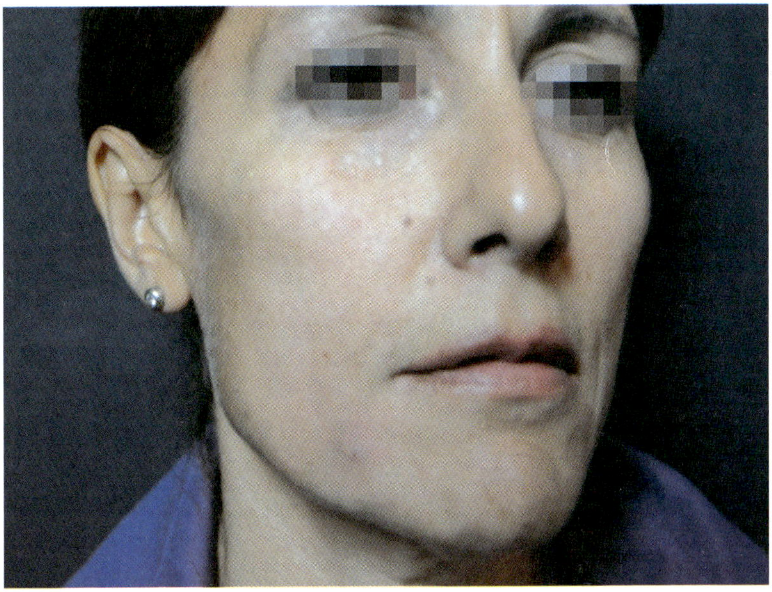

AFTER

>

38-year-old patient, pathologically thin with continuous alternation of bulimia and anorexia. Treated with 1.5 ml of medium density HA per side. In this case, a psychiatrist's opinion was sought to assess the appropriateness of the treatment. The psychiatrist was strongly in favour.

CLINICAL CASES

CLINICAL CASE 2

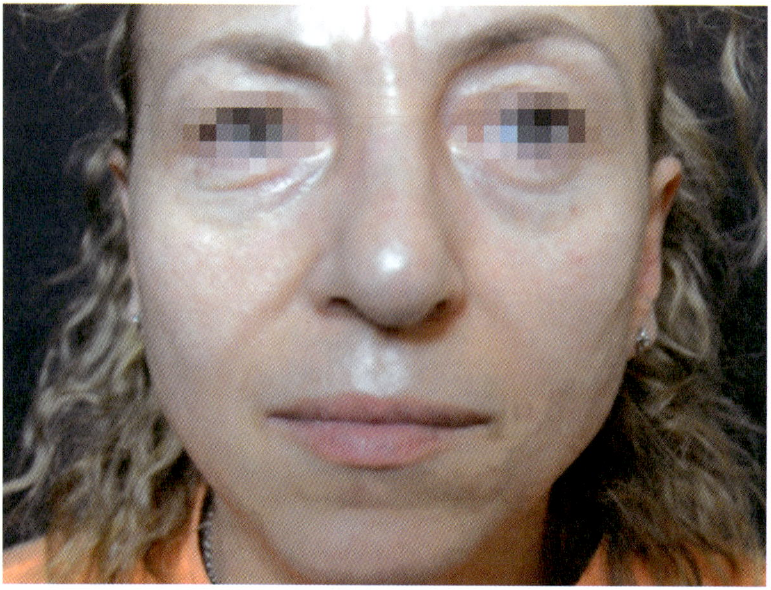

BEFORE

AFTER

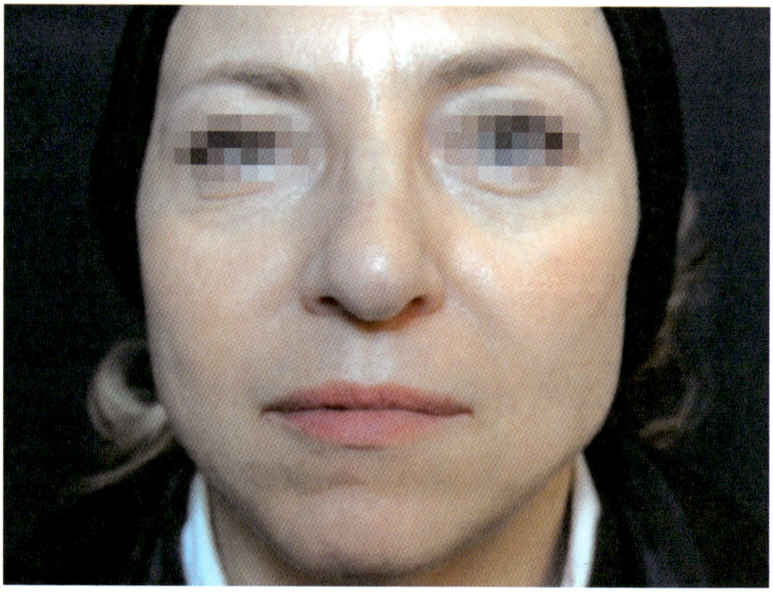

35-year-old patient, recently having undergone extensive surgery. Reconstruction of the cheek with cannula and medium density HA filler. No anaesthetic. 1 ml of HA was used for each cheek. The patient continues to repeat the treatment every 7/8 months.

CLINICAL CASES

CLINICAL CASE 3

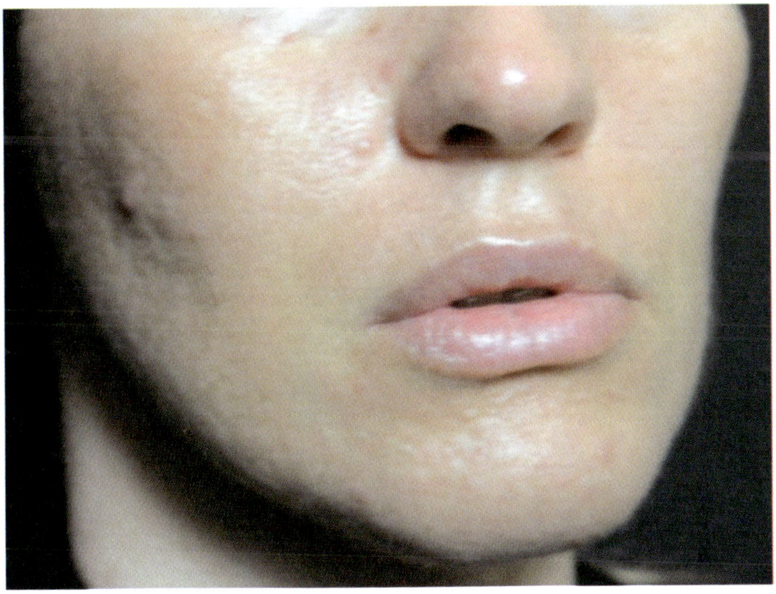

BEFORE

AFTER

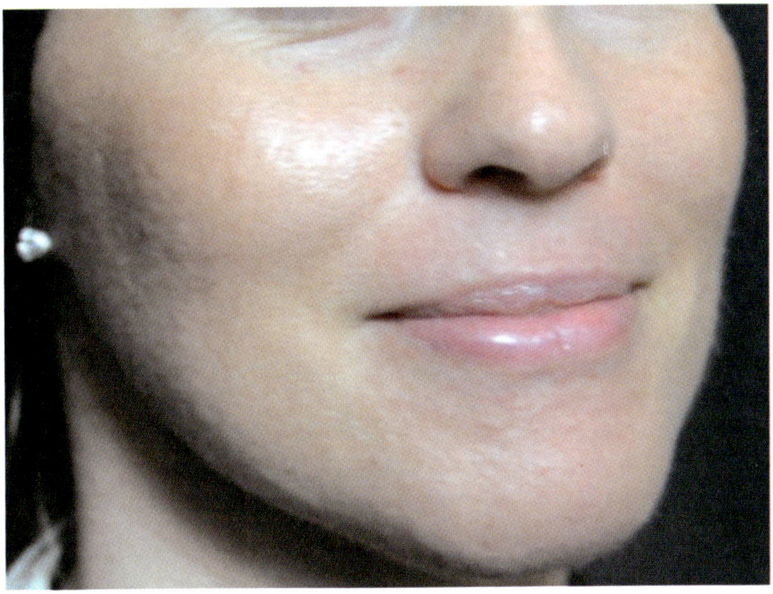

30-year-old patient. No particular problems but the desire to have a more harmonious face. Treated with 0.8 ml of medium density HA filler injected with a microcannula.

5

NOSE

Anatomy of the nose

The nose is an unpaired median facial organ, the primary purpose of which is breathing. In addition to its purpose, which must always be preserved, from an anatomical and topographical point of view it is made up of various sub-units, all of which are closely linked to each other.

In the cranio-caudal direction, we begin with the root of the nose, which is usually concave but is sometimes also occupied by the so-called nasal hump, the ridge of the nose. The straightness of this ridge is ensured, when present, by nasal cartilage and, from the conjunction on the midline, by the two nasal bones, which are jointed at the bottom with the ethmoid and jaw bones (fig.1). This area is frequently occupied by a bone hyperplasia known as a hump (fig. 2), which is the part of the nose usually corrected with the so-called liquid rhinoplasty technique. The nostrils, i.e. the openings of the nose towards the outer surface, lead to the nasal choanae; these are determined laterally by the alar cartilage and anteriorly by the outer surface, opening towards the nasopharynx posteriorly. Behind the alar cartilages there are two more small cartilages, known as triangular cartilages, which are essential to the nasal breathing mechanism: their lesion, or worse, their collapse, prevents correct breathing and can represent a major aesthetic problem. Together, these units form the nasal pyramid (fig. 3).

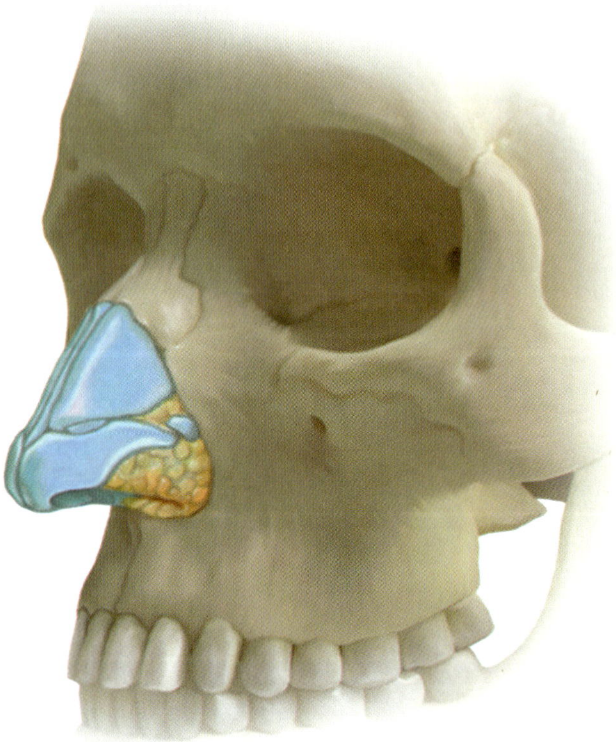

Figure 1 Osteo-cartilaginous nasal skeleton

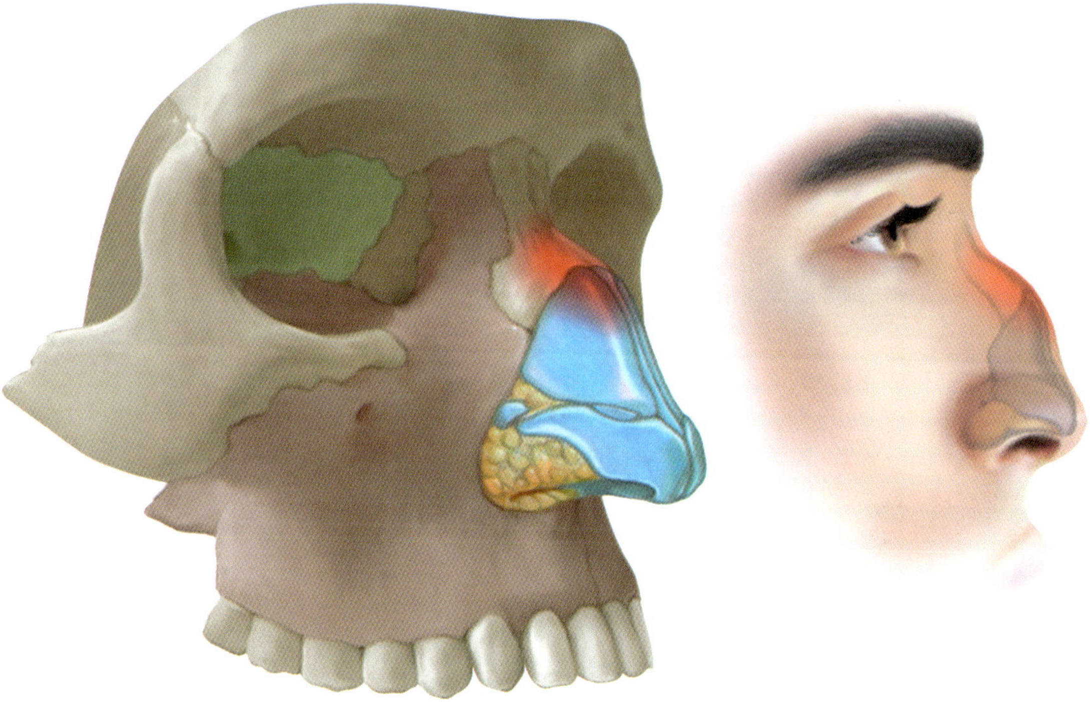

Figure 2 Bony hump

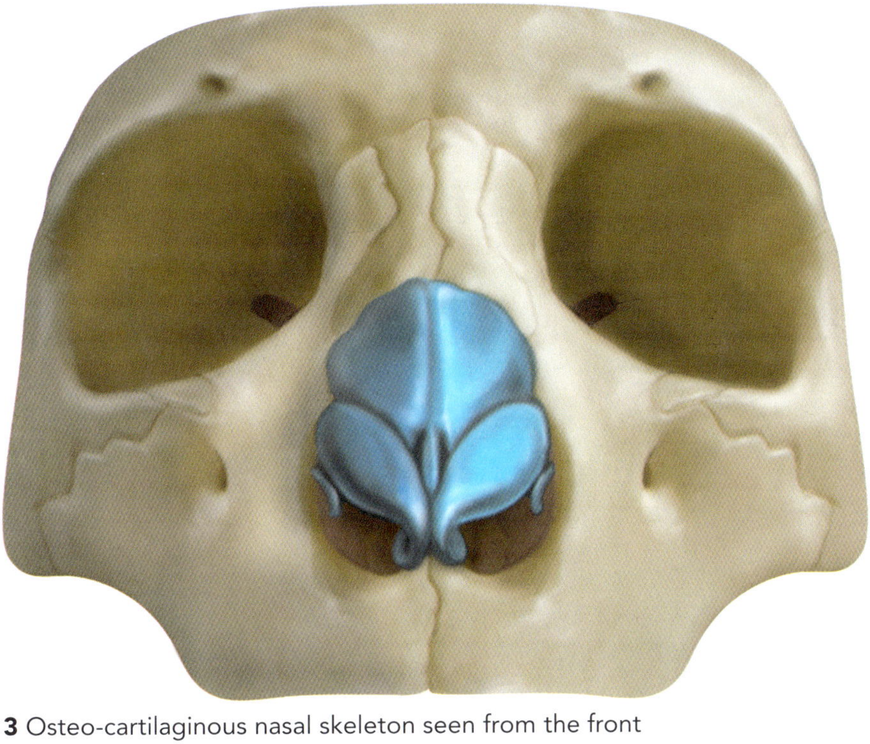

Figure 3 Osteo-cartilaginous nasal skeleton seen from the front

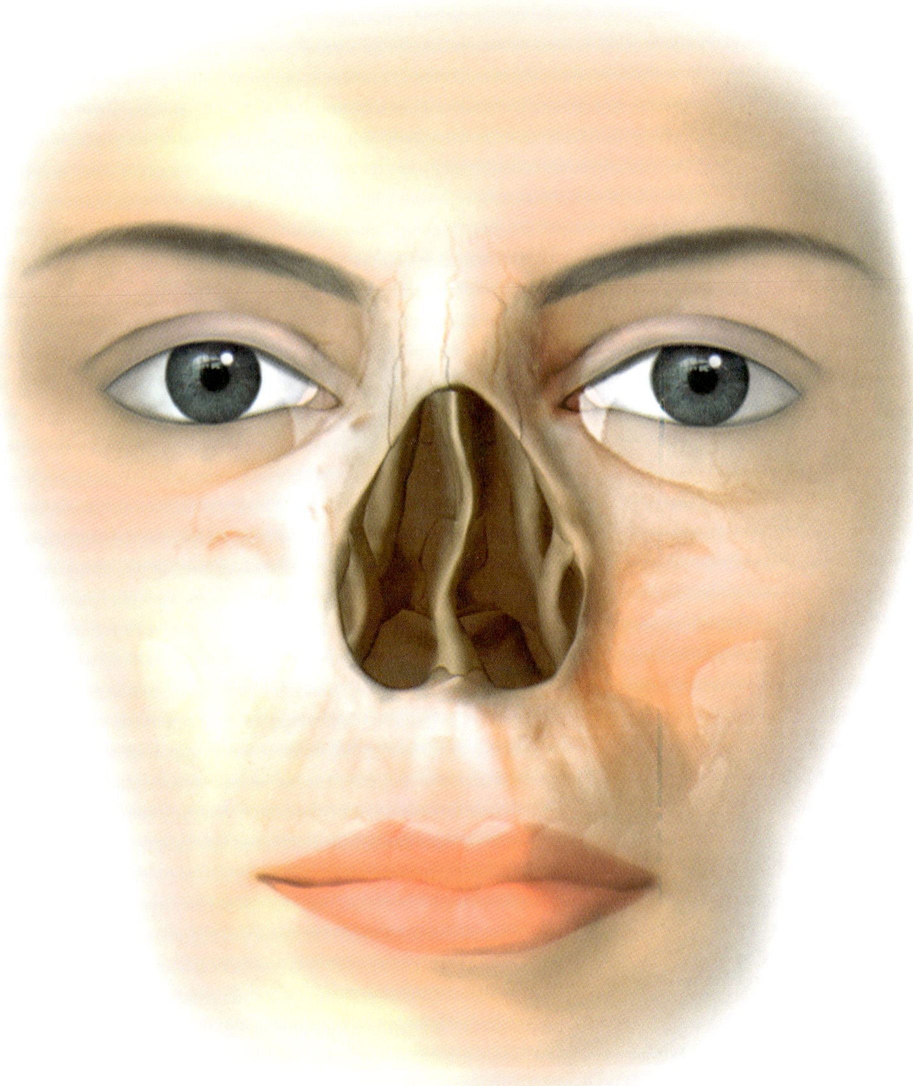

Figure 4 Nasal septum

The nasal units are rarely in perfect aesthetic balance, but most of the time they have been subjected to alterations that can be congenital or acquired, often as a result of trauma. Furthermore, the axis of the nose, which should theoretically separate the face into two symmetrical parts, can be deviated by the concomitant presence of a deviated septum (fig. 4) or of a cartilaginous hypertrophy, for congenital or acquired reasons, pushing it by a few degrees to be more prominent on one side of the face than the other. The nose, which should ensure the har-

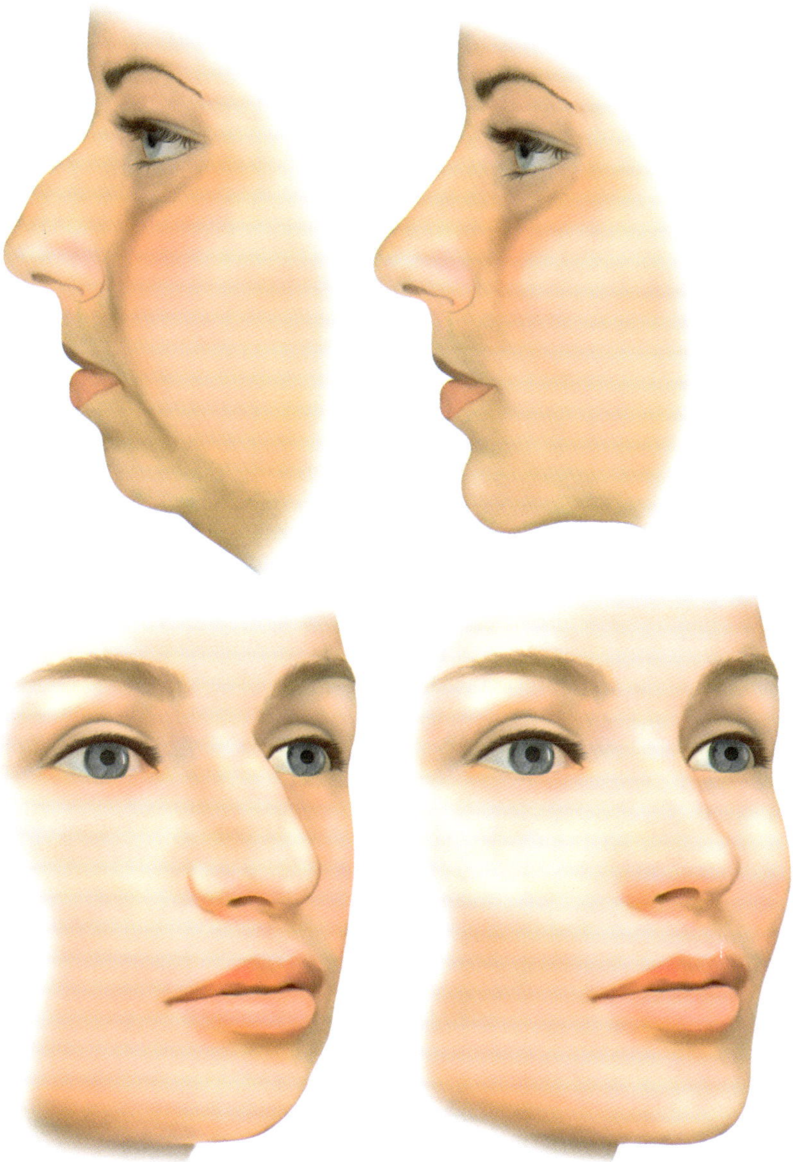

Figure 5 Importance of the nasal septum in nasal aesthetics and their correction

mony of the middle third of the face, must always be considered in relation to other prominences, such as lips, chin and cheekbones, and should, therefore, encourage the aesthetic doctor to consider corrections that also involve other aesthetic units of the face.

We have already said that the beauty of the face, as well as the balance of the aesthetic units, is created by the right combination of hollows and curves, and we are quite happy to say it again. In short, there is not much point in having a wonderful nose (fig. 5) if it is accompanied by

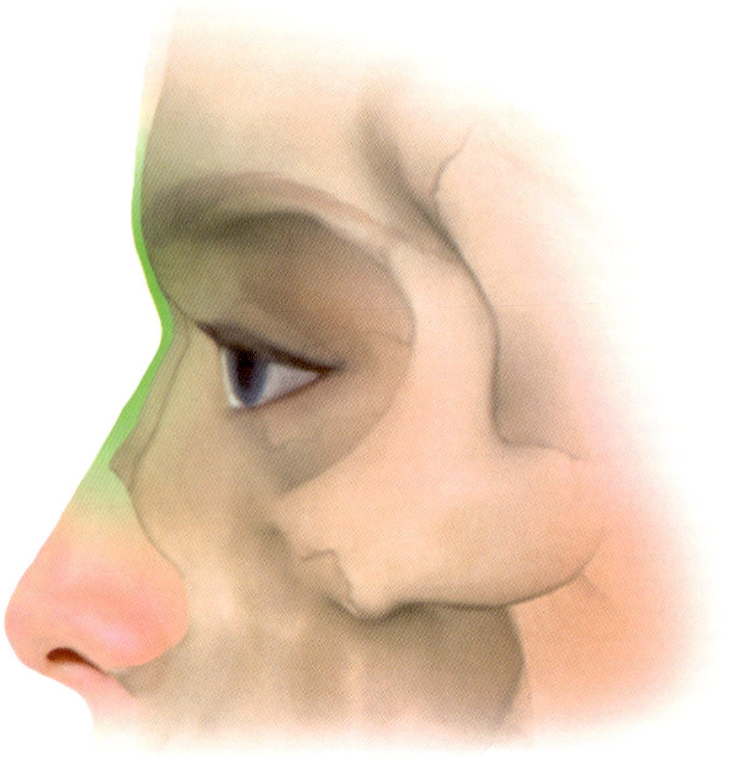

Figure 6 Root of the nose and frontonasal angle

a receding chin or flat cheekbones.
But if we examine the areas of the nose of cosmetic medical interest we have to consider the individual areas, even if the fact that they are so small can sometimes embarrass us.
The root of the nose is one of these; it extends from the forehead in a caudal direction for about one centimetre on average and connects to the forehead, forming the frontonasal angle (fig. 6).
This is a very important aesthetic unit and is also the area where we will insert the needle most in order to correct the nasal pyramid. Moreover, with the name of glabella (fig. 7), by which it is usually known in aesthetic medicine, it represents an area of vascular formations which, if injured or blocked, can lead to very serious complications, which we will talk about shortly.
The frontonasal angle is usually 120-130° wide but is wider in the so-called Greek nose and narrower in the aquiline nose (fig. 8).
Another measurement to be taken into consideration is the nasolabial angle, which can reach up to 110° in women, while in men it is closer to a right angle (fig. 9). Then there is the facial plane, a plane which, according to the classical rules of beauty, has to touch the forehead, nose and chin at the same time and is usually close to 30° (fig. 10).

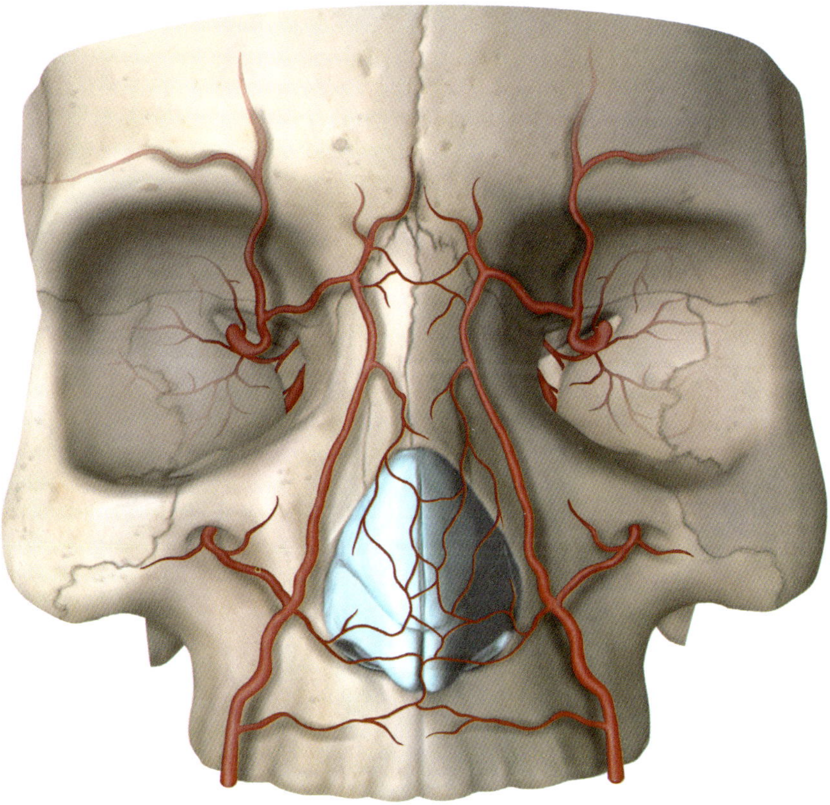

Figure 7 Arterial blood supply to the nose

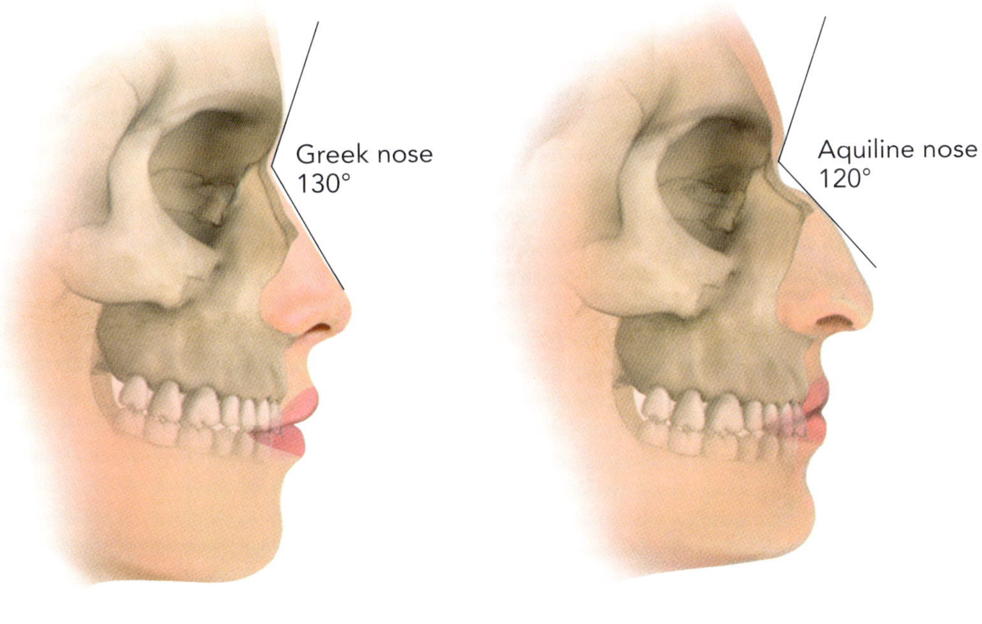

Figure 8 Differences in the frontonasal angle

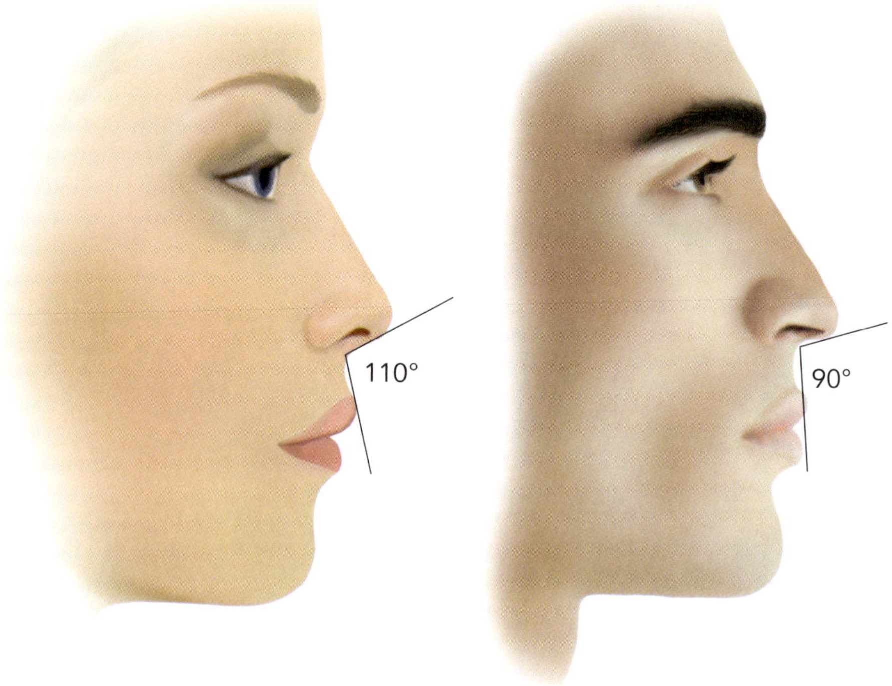

Figure 9 Nasolabial angle

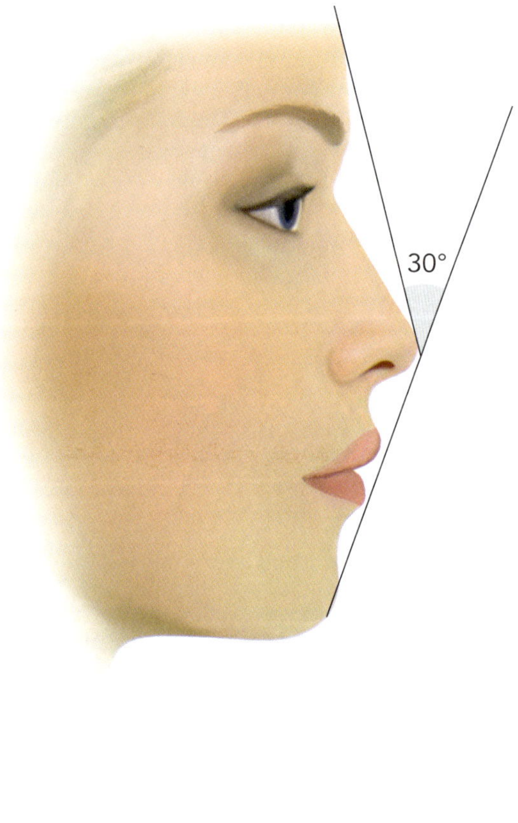

Figure 10 Facial plane

Vascularization of the nose

The vascularization of the nose is essential and a thorough knowledge of it prevents the onset of the most serious side effects.

Blood is supplied to the nasal pyramid mostly by the nasal ala artery, a branch of the facial artery, which runs along the profile of the pyramid and then becomes the nasal artery. This puts out branches which become the dorsal artery of the nose and then, decreasing

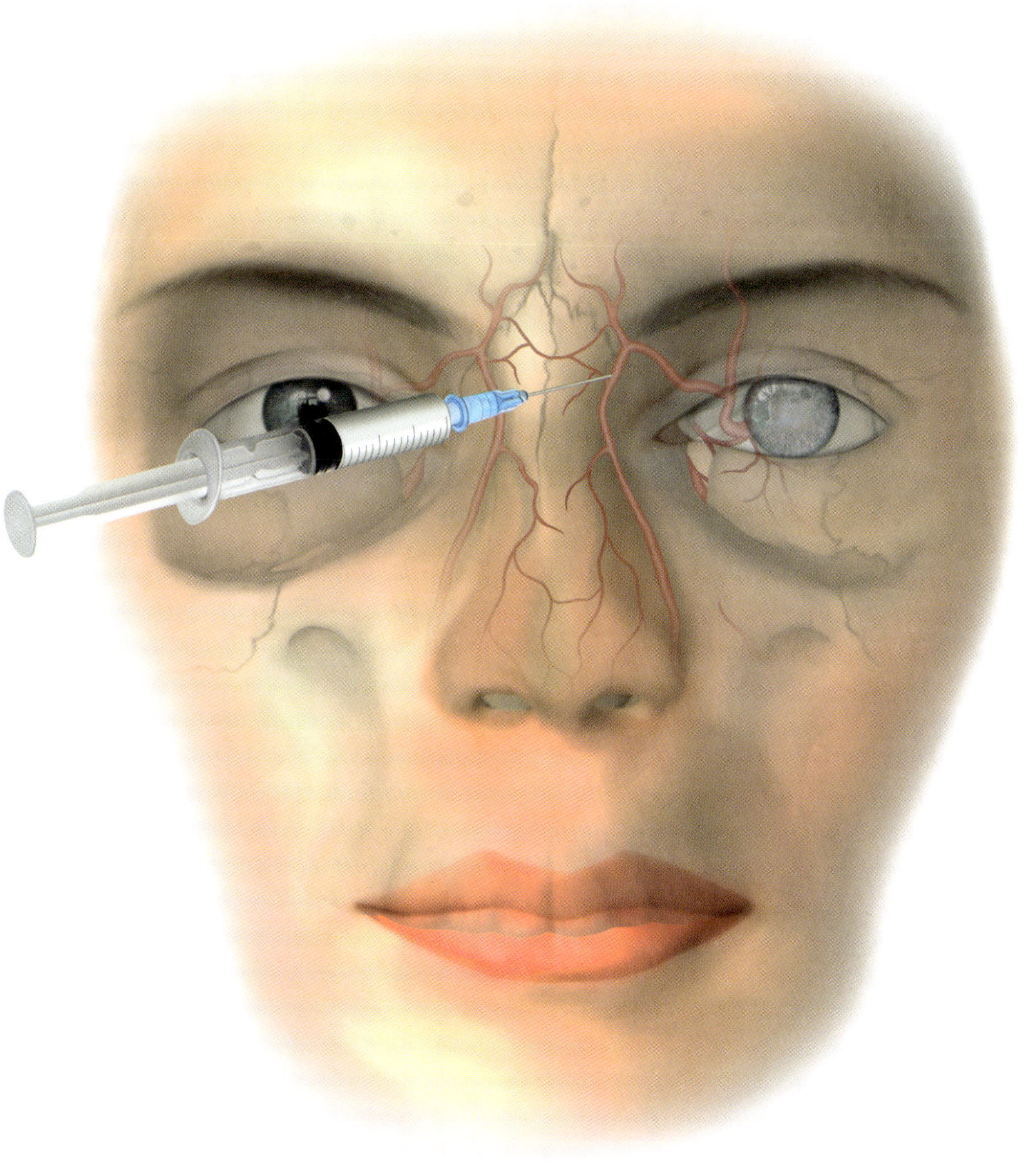

Figure 11 Accidental injection of the nasal artery, to be avoided at all costs

in size, anastomose with the terminal branches of the ophthalmic artery, which include the central artery of the retina. At this point, it is evident that the accidental injection of the nasal artery can cause arterial occlusion of the retinal artery, leading to permanent blindness. It is calculated that, after 10 minutes or slightly longer of occlusion, sight is irremediably impaired (fig. 11).

Nasal correction technique

Now, as we have seen, a few questions need to be asked when we are approaching medical rhinoplasty.

The first undoubtedly concerns the fact that our work may cause serious side effects. So, how much filler do I have to inject? Will I need more than the amount of 1 ml established to avoid vascular risks? Will the patient be able to avoid rubbing the area for at least 24 hours to prevent the filler from spreading?

The second question concerns the aesthetic effect. How big is the hump? Can I use filler above and below it without causing any side effects?

The third concerns straightening. A deviated septum will make it harder to correct, so will I be able to correct the area deviated by the septum from an aesthetic point of view only?

Now, assuming that the answer to all these questions is yes, I can proceed with the correction, using a quite dense high G′ filler, placing it above and below the bony hump, to create an apparent smoothness of the ridge (figs. 12 and 13). Obviously, this does not eliminate the hump but fills the dip

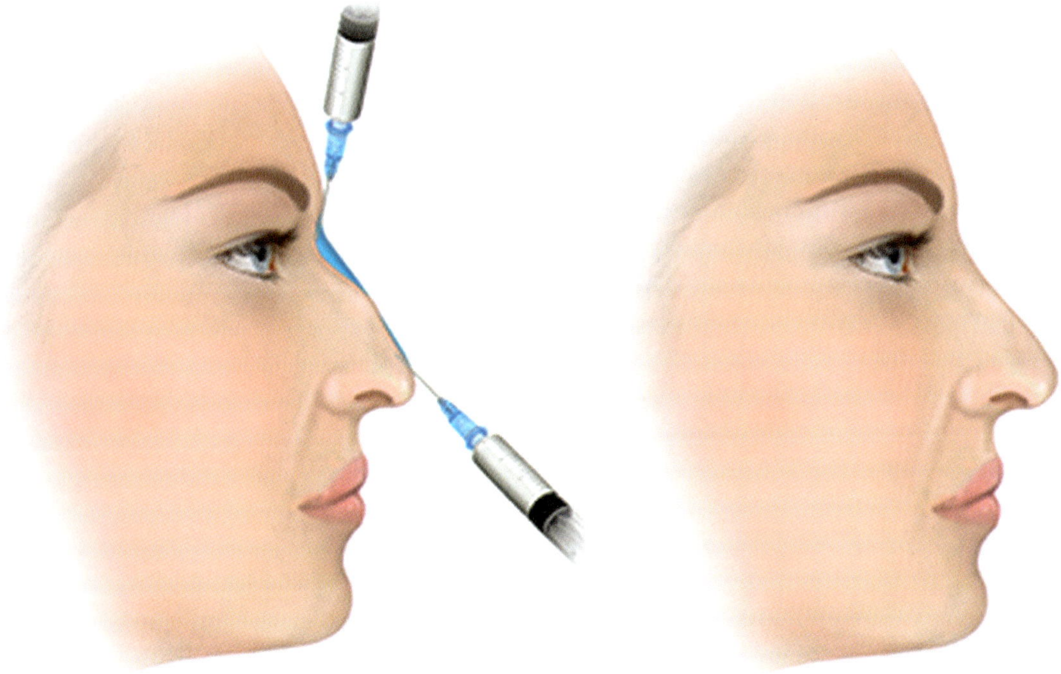

Figure 12 Nasal pyramid correction techniques

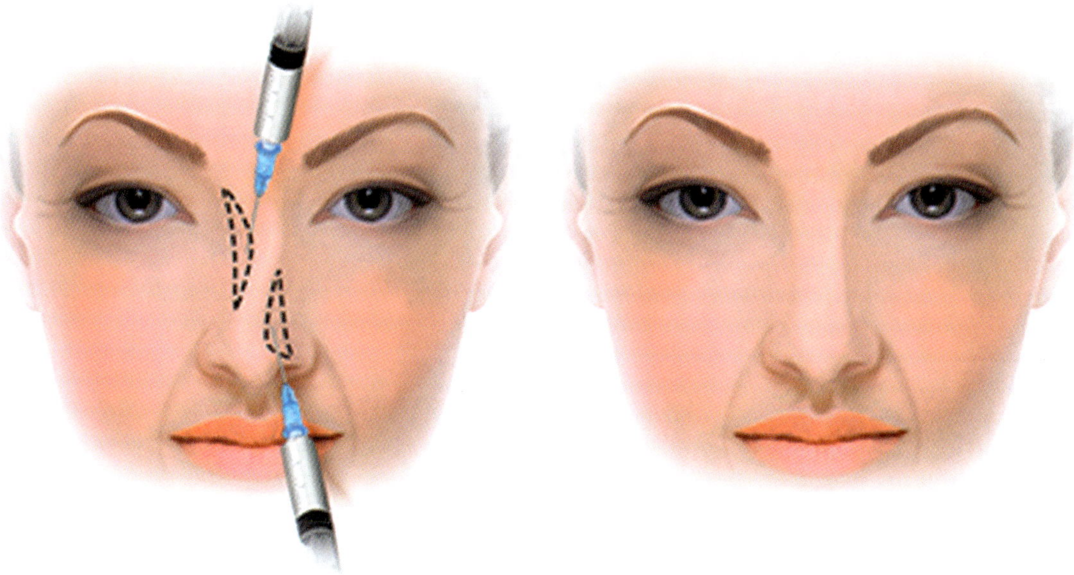

Figure 13 Deviated nose: correction techniques

above and below the hump.

Personally, I like to bend the needle to an angle of 45° and inject the filler slowly, following the midline of the nose, being very careful not to overdo things, and firmly squeezing the ridge of the nose between the fingers of my other hand in order to "set" the deposit.

After injecting the filler, I continue squeezing the ridge. I recommend telling the patient not to wear glasses or anything else that may deform the nasal ridge. The results are always satisfactory and never last less than eight months. It is also possible to use calcium hydroxyapatite.

Bibliography

1. Macneill P. Balancing bioethics by sensing the aesthetic. Bioethics. 2017;31(8):631-643.
2. Garritano FG, Quatela VC. Surgical Anatomy of the Upper Face and Forehead. Facial Plast Surg. 2018;34(2):109-113.
3. Corradi G, Chuquichambi EG, Barrada JR, Clemente A, Nadal M. A new conception of visual aesthetic sensitivity. Br J Psychol. 2019 Oct 6.
4. Hübner R, Fillinger MG. Comparison of Objective Measures for Predicting Perceptual Balance and Visual Aesthetic Preference. Front Psychol. 2016;7:335.
5. Helmy Y. Non-surgical rhinoplasty using filler, Botox, and thread remodeling: Retro analysis of 332 cases. J Cosmet Laser Ther. 2018;20(5):293-300.
6. Di Rosa L, Cerulli G, De Pasquale A. Psychological Analysis of Non-surgical Rhinoplasty. Aesthetic Plast Surg. 2020;44(1):131-138.
7. Jung GS, Chu SG, Lee JW, et al. A Safer Non-surgical Filler Augmentation Rhinoplasty Based on the Ana-

tomy of the Nose. Aesthetic Plast Surg. 2019;43(2):447-452.
8. Schelke LW, et al. Eenzijdige blindheid na een neuscorrectie met filler [Unilateral blindness following a non-surgical rhinoplasty with filler]. Ned Tijdschr Geneeskd. 2017;161:D1246.
9. Rivkin A. A prospective study of non-surgical primary rhinoplasty using a polymethylmethacrylate injectable implant. Dermatol Surg. 2014;40(3):305-313.
10. McKeown DJ. The risk of blindness following 'non-surgical rhinoplasty'. J Plast Reconstr Aesthet Surg. 2013;66(8):e238.
11. Sito G, Manzoni V, Sommariva R. Vascular Complications after Facial Filler Injection: A Literature Review and Meta-analysis. J Clin Aesthet Dermatol. 2019;12(6):E65-E72.

CLINICAL CASES

CLINICAL CASE 1

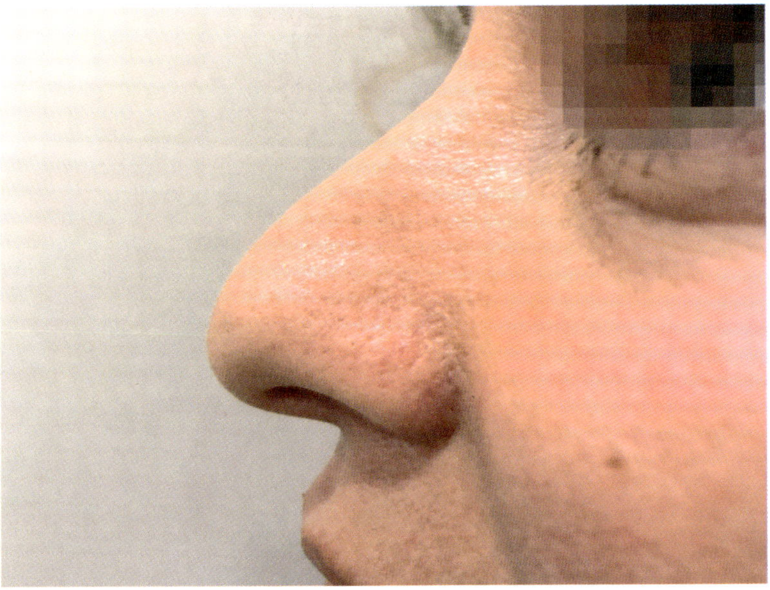

BEFORE

<

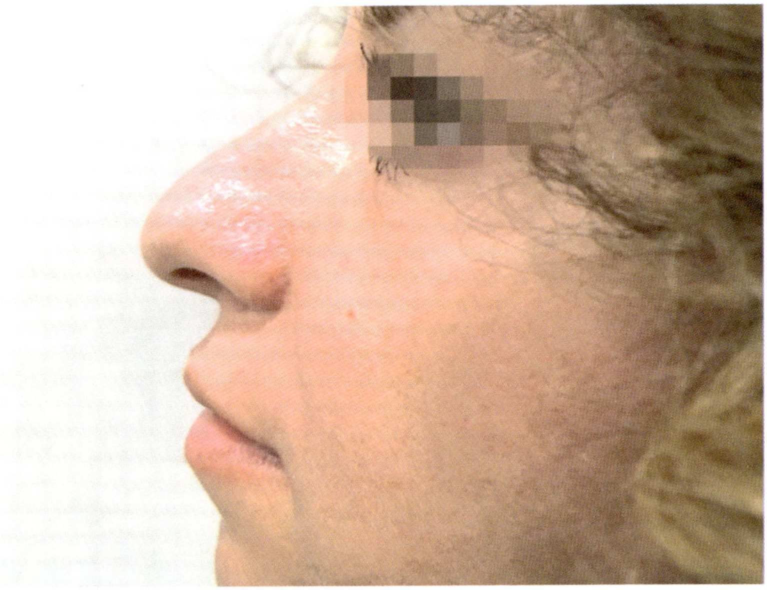

AFTER

>

A 34-year-old patient with a modest bone hump and drooping tip. Correction with high G′ biodynamic hyaluronic acid, injecting 0.5 cc along the midline and shaping manually, and injecting about 0.2 cc vertically into the columella. Shaping massage.

CLINICAL CASES

CLINICAL CASE 2

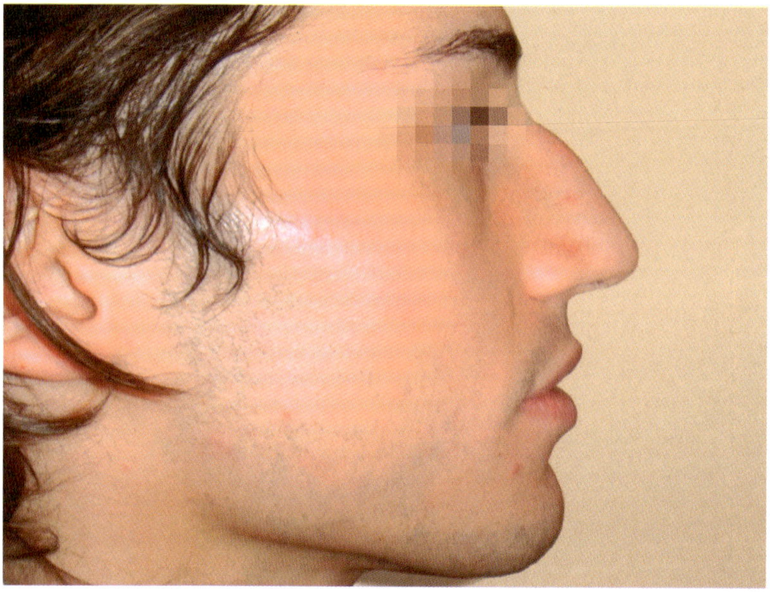

BEFORE

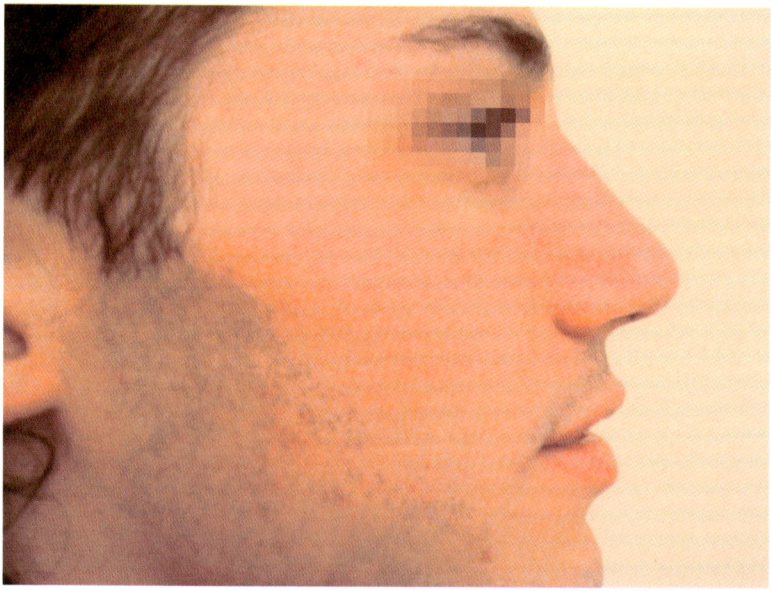

AFTER

A 32-year-old male patient with a large median osteo-cartilaginous hump. Correction with calcium hydroxyapatite, injecting 0.7 cc into the frontonasal angle and then below the hump.

CLINICAL CASES

CLINICAL CASE 2

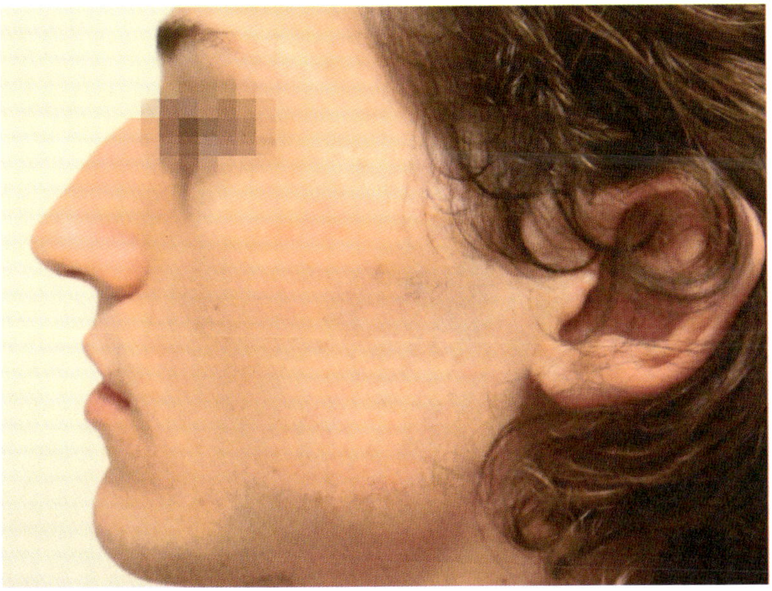

BEFORE

<

AFTER

>

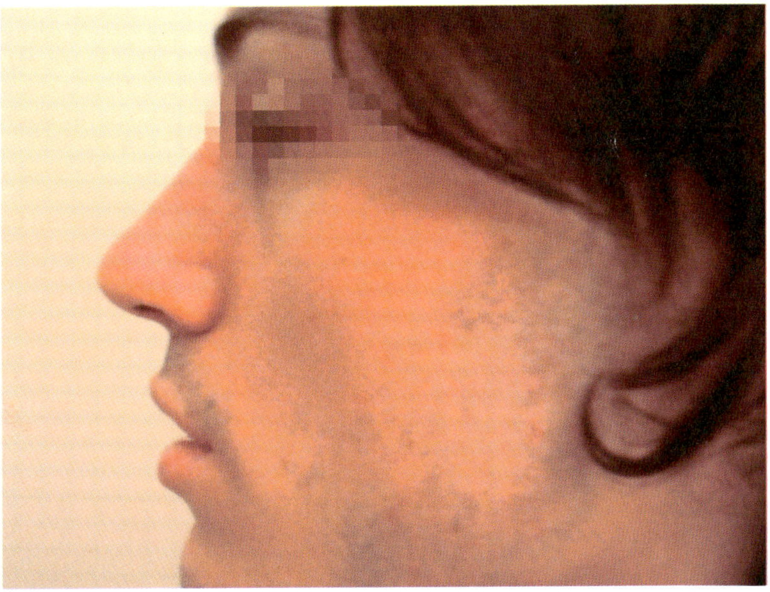

The same patient, left profile.

CLINICAL CASES

CLINICAL CASE 3

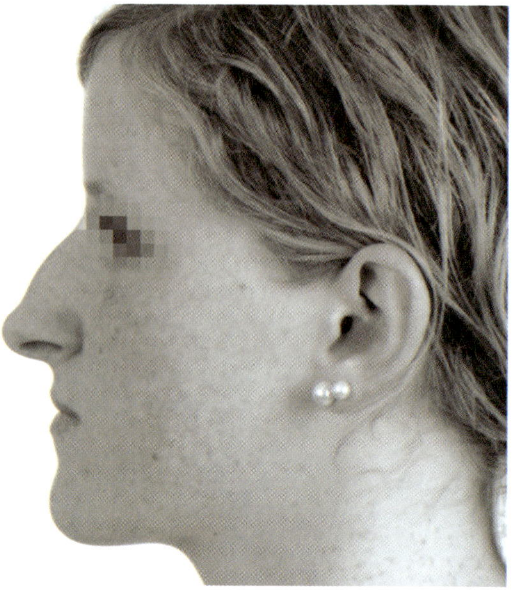

BEFORE

AFTER

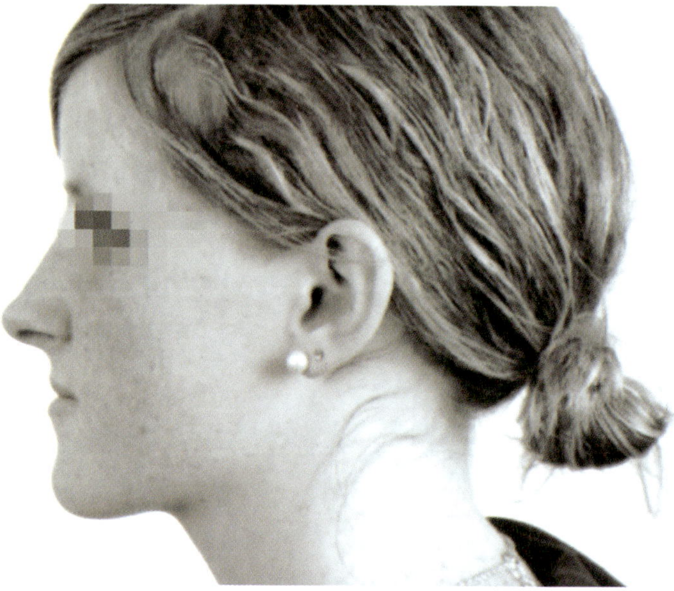

A 25-year-old woman afraid of surgery. Correctly aligned nose but with a large bony hump. Injection of 0.7 cc of high G' HA along the midline above and below the hump. Compression and shaping massage and application of steri-strip for seven days.

CLINICAL CASES

CLINICAL CASE 3

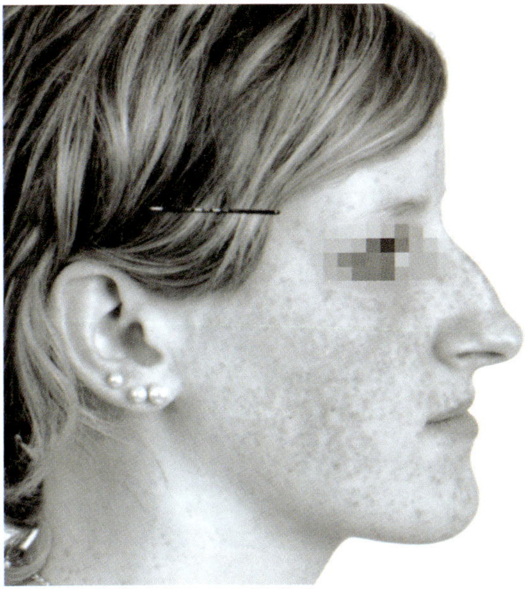

BEFORE

AFTER

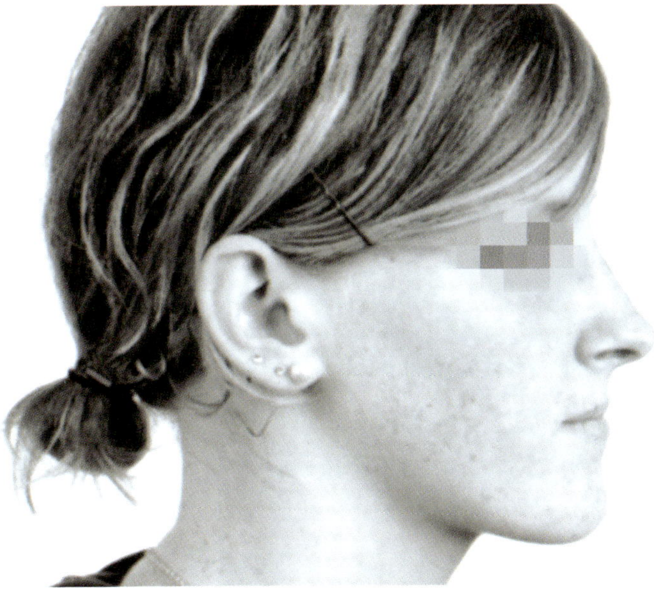

The same patient, opposite profile.

6

NASOLABIAL FOLDS

Anatomy of the nasolabial folds

The nasolabial folds are positioned at the corners of the mouth and run from the nasal alae to what are known as the labial commissures.

They are always present, in varying degrees depending on age or facial conformation, and are most noticeable when we smile. Nasolabial folds are never found in infants or people affected by mono or bilateral facial paresis. The folds, which are usually made up of strong fibrous tissue fibres, tend to become more prominent with age and are present even at a younger age in individuals with long, tapering faces. They are known as static formations because, unlike dynamic formations, we cannot stimulate them in any way.

Patients usually begin to notice them when the skin tends to start sagging and during particular but physiological moments in life, such as after pregnancy or losing weight. The nasolabial folds are a completely physiological area of our anatomy and not necessarily a symptom of old age, but they do become deeper as we age and make us look older.

With advancing age, some people de-

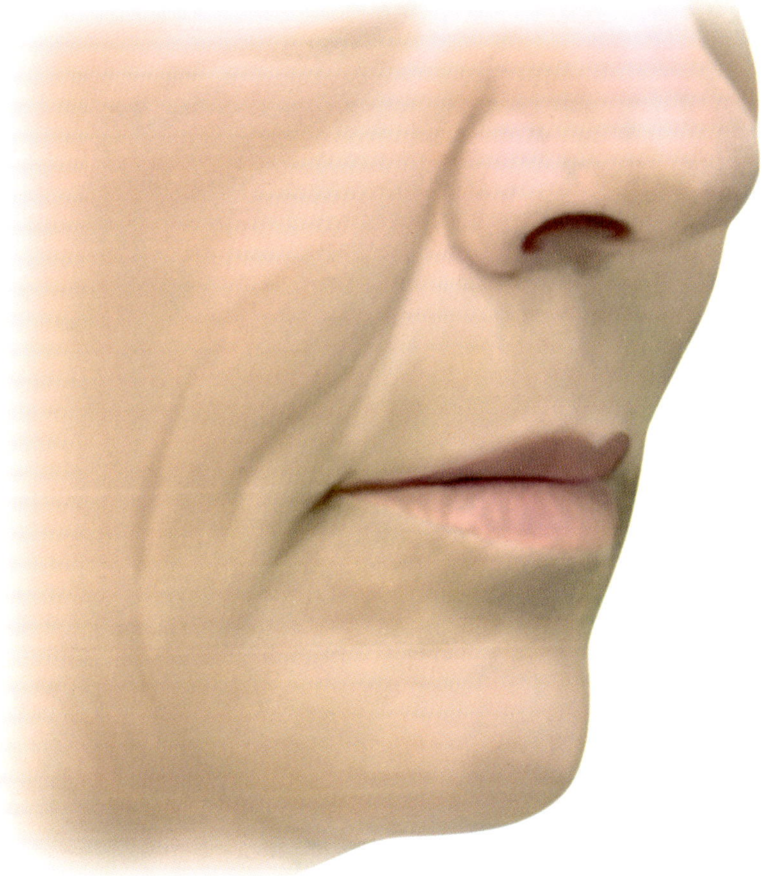

Figure 1 Nasolabial folds

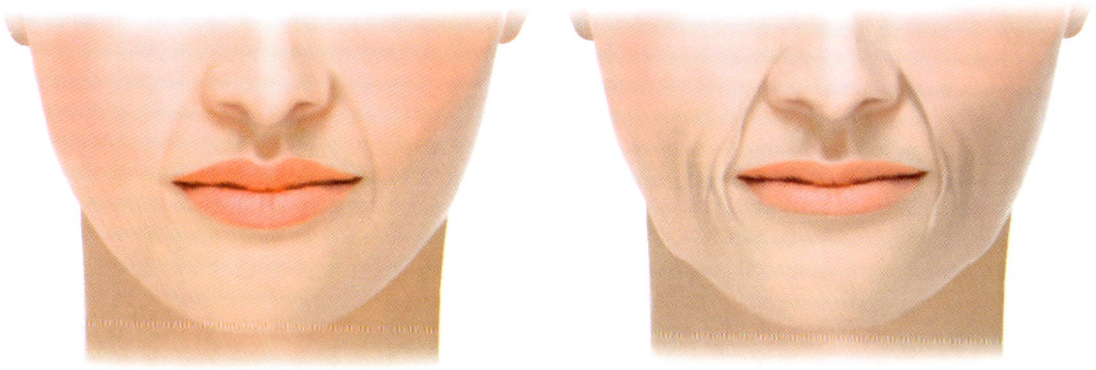

Figure 2 Different levels of severity of the nasolabial folds

velop parallel wrinkles, which usually start from the lip commissure and develop in an oblique direction, converging towards the chin; these lines are known as marionette lines.

The nasolabial folds become more evident due to a series of factors, such as:

> loss of collagen due to ageing, which makes the skin weaker and thinner;
> loss of fat, particularly the buccal fat pad, which makes the cheeks ptosic and worsens the appearance of the nasolabial folds, which are no longer supported by zygomatic fat;
> sun exposure, which damages the skin and causes changes in tissue morphology and the formation of wrinkles;
> other factors may be smoking, exposure to polluted environments, rapid weight loss or frequent yo-yoing between different weights.

Correction of the nasolabial folds

The nasolabial nose folds never pose a health concern, but they definitely generate aesthetic distress. Consequently, the correction of nasolabial lines or folds is one of the main reasons why patients turn to aesthetic doctors, who use facial fillers as their first remedy.

These substances, preferably hyaluronic acid, can range from denser fillers with a fairly high G'' and low, but not too low, tan delta, so as to maintain sufficient elasticity and a viscosity suitable for the area to be treated. Other good choices are biodynamic fillers, which do not cause excessive swelling, and the use of an electronic pen to increase precision and patient compliance.

It is clear, from that stated above, that the best treatment is with dermal fillers which, once injected under the epidermis, have the ability to lift it with an effect that depends partly on the type of filler used and partly on a dose-dependent mechanical effect, making the area "smoother" in relation to the surrounding areas.

The technique involves intradermal introduction, or almost, as the dermis is very thin, with a mainly retrograde technique, i.e. insertion of the needle, which can be 27 G or 30 G in diameter and 13 mm long, depending on the type of

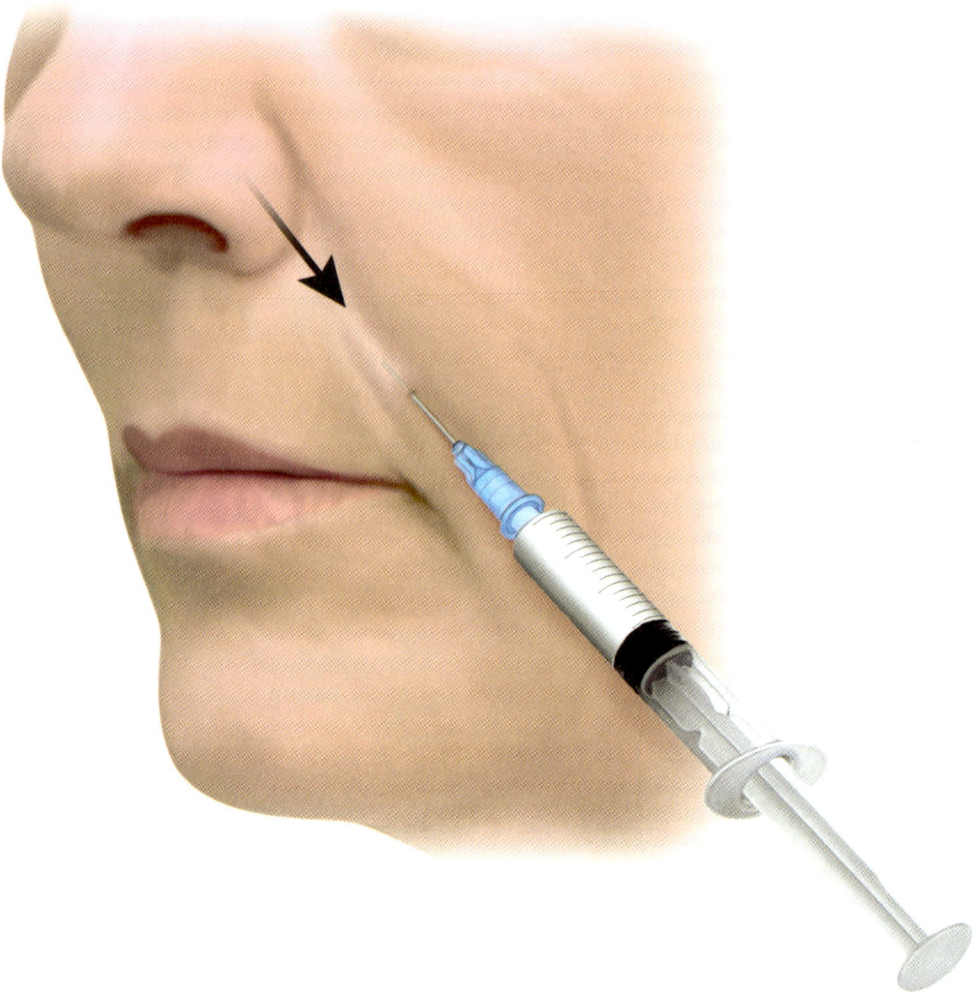

Figure 3 Nasolabial fold correction technique

filler used, and release of the substance during withdrawal.

Another possibility, complementary to the latter, is represented by cheekbone augmentation, which may or may not be simultaneous, making the face look healthier and firmer, with a slight lifting of the folds.

Literature presents many other systems for the treatment of nasolabial folds, such as the grafting of fat, which does, however, involve minor surgery, the use of growth factors, which are hard to prepare and very expensive, and even facial exercises.

In actual fact, the wide variety of facial fillers available offer a safe, low-maintenance way of achieving satisfactory and long-lasting results.

Naturally, the technique must be applied with care due to the deep presence of the facial artery, which runs along

the nasolabial folds and must be avoided at all costs (keeping the needle parallel or almost parallel to the skin), also avoiding compression with large boluses of filler. Ischemia occurs quite frequently in the area or in the nasal alae and requires thorough knowledge of solutions, such as the use of hyaluronidases, hot thermotherapy for vasodilation and nitro-glycerine patches.
Of course, the sooner action is taken, the better the results will be.

Bibliography

1. Mowlds DS, Lambros V. Cheek Volumization and the Nasolabial Fold. Plast Reconstr Surg. 2018;141(5):1124-1129.
2. Snider CC, Amalfi AN, Hutchinson LE, Sommer NZ. New Insights into the Anatomy of the Midface Musculature and its Implications on the Nasolabial Fold. Aesthetic Plast Surg. 2017;41(5):1083-1090.
3. Choi YJ, Kim HS, Min JH, Nam JH, Lee GY, Kim WS. A clinical study on the usefulness of autologous plasma filler in the treatment of nasolabial fold wrinkles. J Cosmet Laser Ther. 2017;19(3):174-180.
4. Suh JH, Oh CT, Im SI, Lim JS, Kim BJ, Lee JH. A multicenter, randomized, double-blind clinical study to evaluate the efficacy and safety of a new monophasic hyaluronic acid filler with lidocaine 0.3% in the correction of nasolabial fold. J Cosmet Dermatol. 2017;16(3):327-332.
5. Davila AA, Buck DW 2nd, Chopp D, et al. A novel prospective three-dimensional analysis of nasolabial fold augmentation. Aesthet Surg J. 2012;32(4):488-494.

CLINICAL CASES

CLINICAL CASE 1

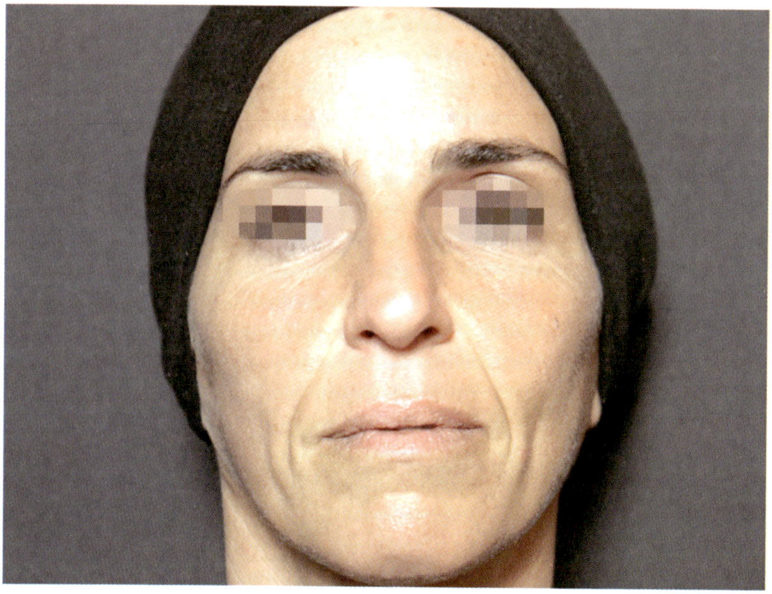

BEFORE

<

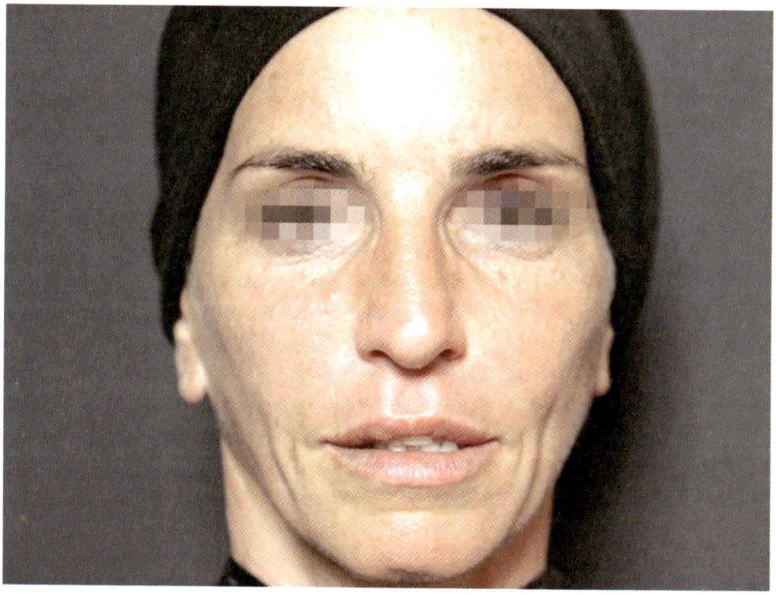

AFTER

>

46-year-old patient, marathon runner. As is often the case with these patients, the face looks "wasted", devoid of fat pads. In this patient in particular, the face is long and has almost no buccal fat pad. It was corrected with a linear technique using very elastic medium G' biodynamic hyaluronic acid, with 1 ml on each side.

CLINICAL CASES

CLINICAL CASE 1

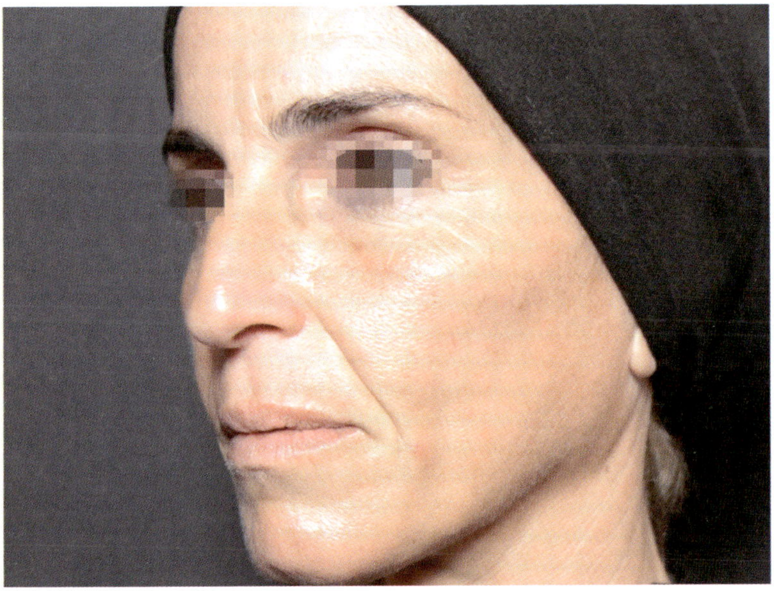

BEFORE
<

AFTER
>

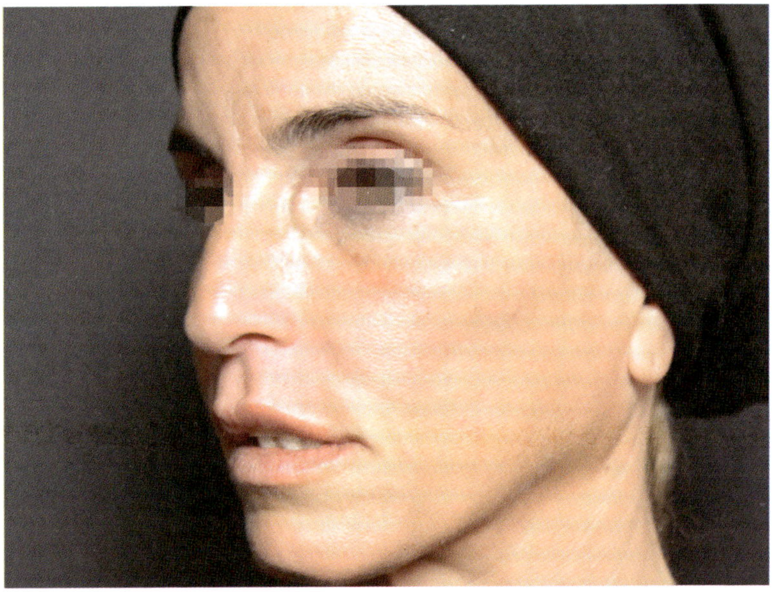

The same patient, seen from the left.

CLINICAL CASES

CLINICAL CASE 2

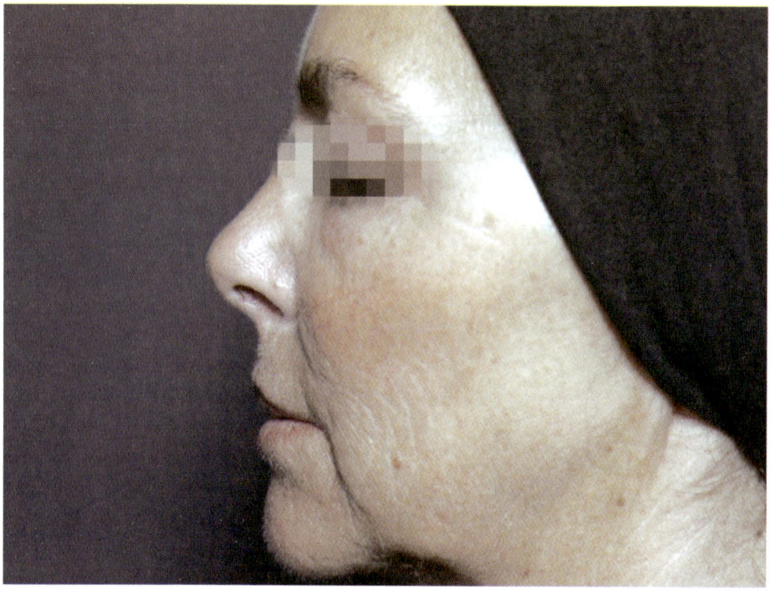

BEFORE

AFTER

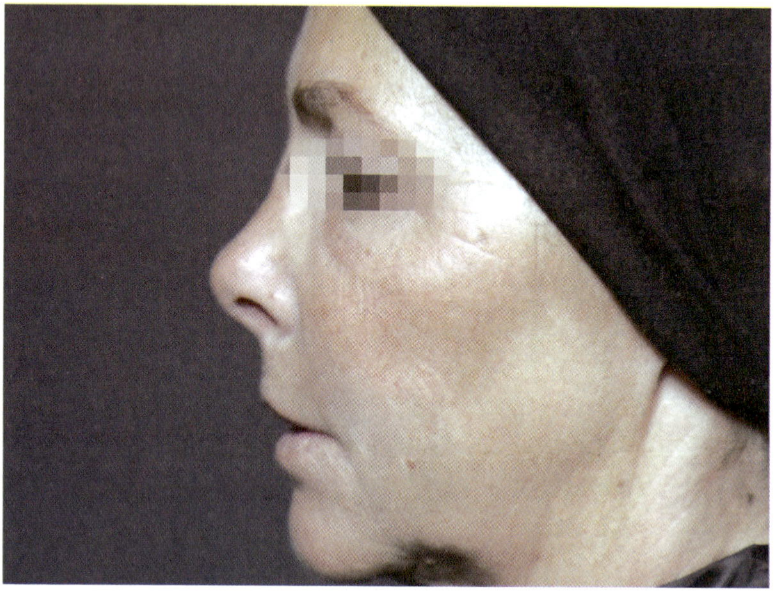

56-year-old patient, smoker. Note the sagging cheek, treated with correction of the cheekbones and nasolabial folds: 1 ml of medium G' hyaluronic acid on each side.

CLINICAL CASES

CLINICAL CASE 3

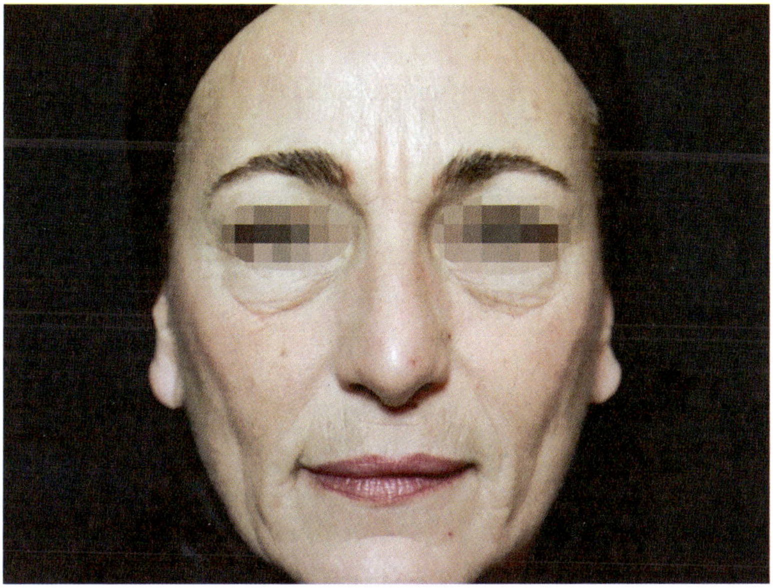

BEFORE

VIDEO 1

Nasolabial fold correction technique

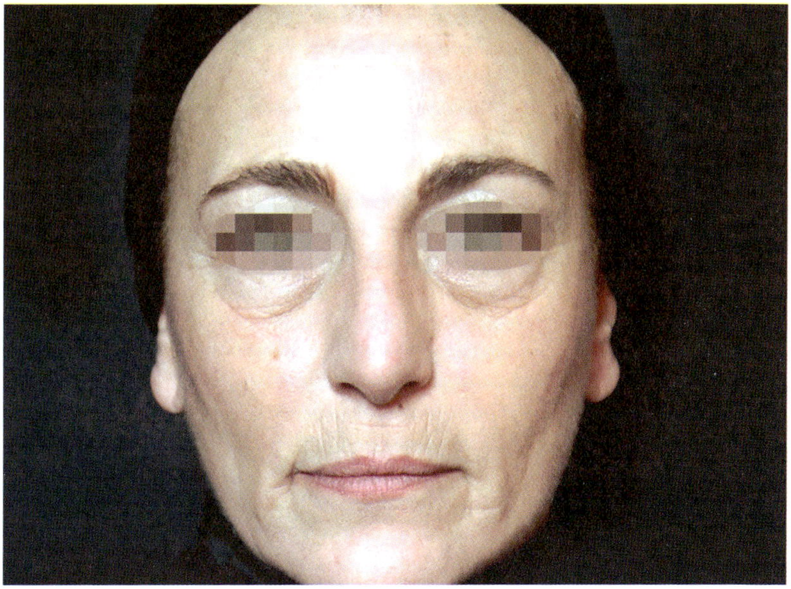

AFTER

56-year-old patient, smoker, with a long face. Correction of the nasolabial folds with medium density hyaluronic acid followed by biovitalization with hyaluronic acid and redensifying complex.

CLINICAL CASES

CLINICAL CASE 3

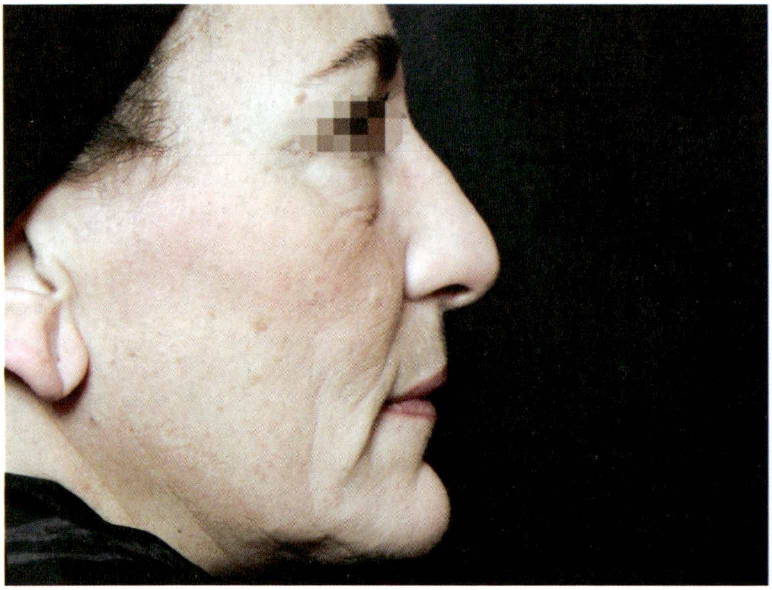

BEFORE
<

AFTER
>

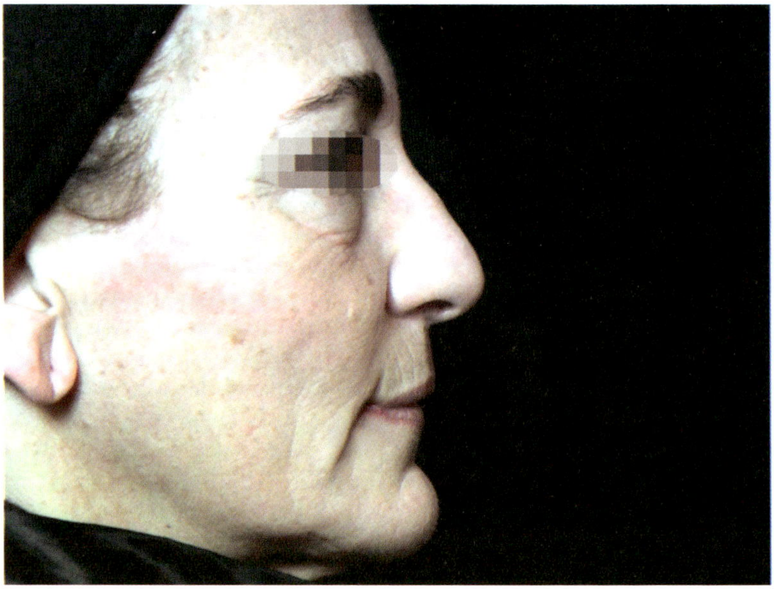

The same patient, seen from the side.

7

FACIAL WRINKLES

Wrinkles as an expression of age

These days it is almost seriously offensive to talk about wrinkles on a woman's face. The wrinkle, in its most common form, is synonymous with old age or looking old, so we prefer to talk about the redistribution of facial volumes, another key element of ageing but not so evident as wrinkles or correction of ptosis.

Wrinkles are actually a very well-defined histopathological phenomenon. They are commonly seen as the expression of ageing. Ageing is classified as intrinsic, due mainly to all the phenomena of organic ageing, and affects all our organs equally but in varying degrees, and extrinsic, caused by factors resulting from photodamage and air pollution. As you might guess, this second type of ageing, which some people call photoaging, mainly affects the areas that are most exposed, such as the face and hands.

From a histological point of view, wrinkles develop as a result of the intrinsic loss of elasticity caused by the decline in the production of collagen and elastin that occurs as time goes by, and the change in spatial direction of the collagen fibres, which are very evident under an electron microscope. Instead of maintaining their original parallelism, the fibres tend to cross over with each other, altering the skin texture.

On the contrary, there seems to be no quantitative difference in the distribution of collagen, elastin and glycosaminoglycans.

VIDEO 1

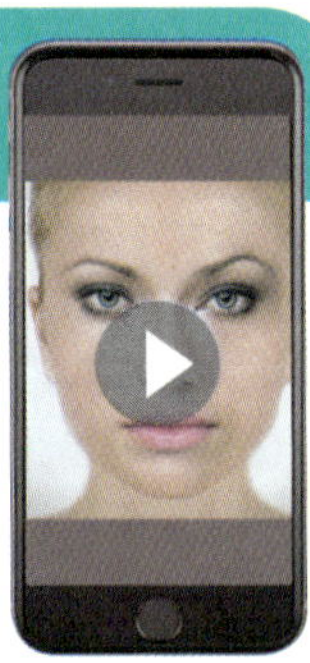

Signs of ageing

Classification of wrinkles

Many authors have also developed classifications of various kinds, and observations in order to group wrinkles into specific types. Listing them all seems pointless as they are very well known, but the most famous and also the most complete are by Fitzpatrick (tab. 1) and Glogau (tab. 2), and these still represent the foundation of all subsequent classifications.

Of course, it is necessary to distinguish static wrinkles from so-called dynamic wrinkles. A typical example of a static wrinkle is the nasolabial fold, while a dynamic wrinkle, one that we can somehow control, is the glabella line. But why do we need to distinguish them? Here's why.

For static wrinkles, i.e. wrinkles that are always present in the face, whether moving or immobile, we use fillers, while for dynamic wrinkles, without disregarding the role of fillers, which can also be used in combination, we use mostly Botox.

The synergistic action of filler and toxin undoubtedly produces more stable and brilliant results.

Now let's see look at the different types of wrinkle and how they are divided ac-

TABLE 1 - FITZPATRICK SKIN PHOTOTYPE CLASSIFICATION

	Characteristics	Reaction to sun	Exposure range
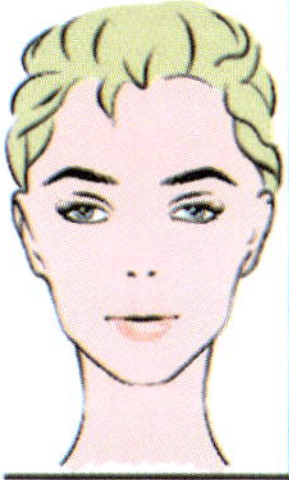	Blonde-red hair and very pale skin, light-coloured eyes	Very sensitive, usually develops a sun rash	Very high
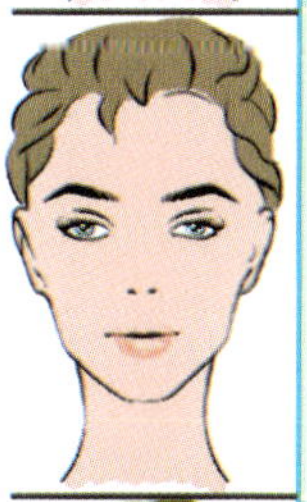	Blonde to light brown hair, fair skin and light-coloured eyes	Very sensitive, burns easily	Very high, high
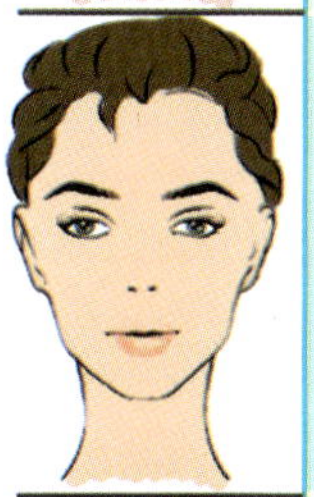	Dark hair and normal skin	Sensitive, sometimes burns	High, average
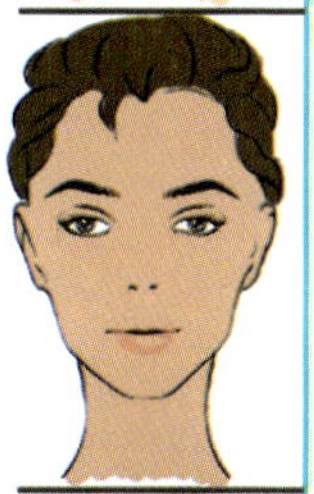	Dark hair and light brown skin	Fairly sensitive, rarely burns	High, average
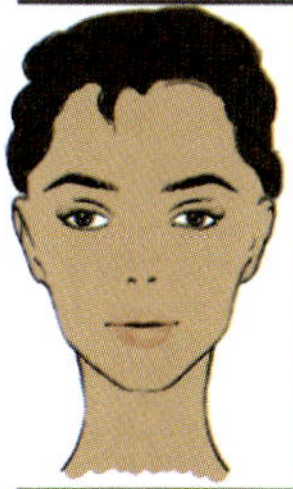	Dark hair, brown/olive skin and dark-coloured eyes	Not very sensitive, very rarely burns	Average
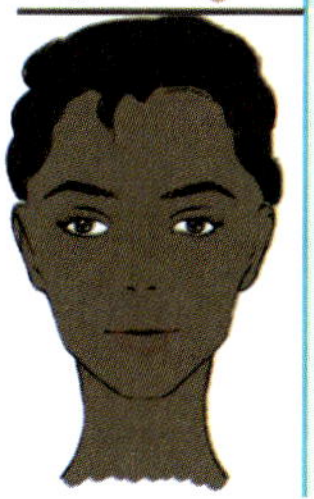	Dark hair, dark skin and dark-coloured eyes	Insensitive, never burns	Average, low

TABLE 2 - GLOGAU PHOTOAGING CLASSIFICATION

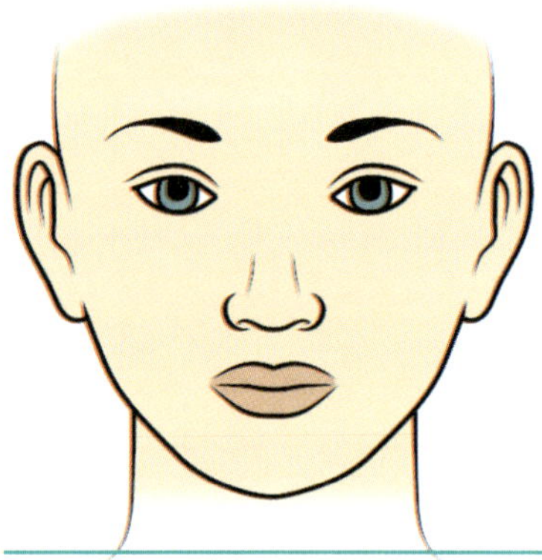

TYPE I, "no wrinkles"
- age of patient: 20-30
- early signs of photoaging
- mild pigment changes
- no keratosis
- minimal wrinkles

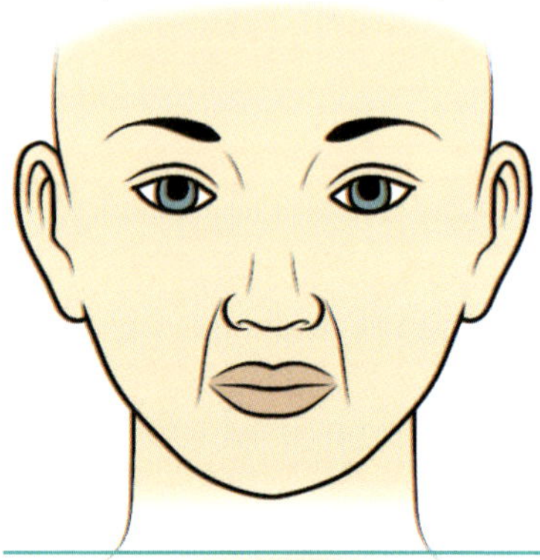

TYPE II, "wrinkles in motion"
- age of patient: 35-45
- light to moderate signs of photoaging
- first visibility of brown spots
- keratosis palpable but not visible
- the first "smile lines" start to appear

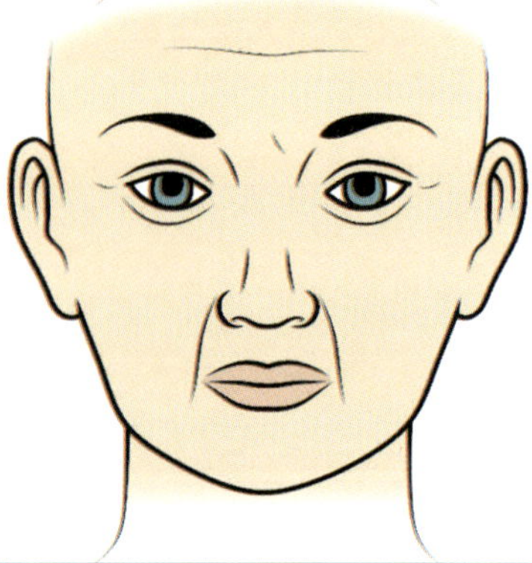

TYPE III, "wrinkles at rest"
- age of patient: 50 and over
- advanced signs of photoaging
- obvious discolourations, visible capillaries (telangiectasias),
- visible keratosis
- visible wrinkles even when the face is resting

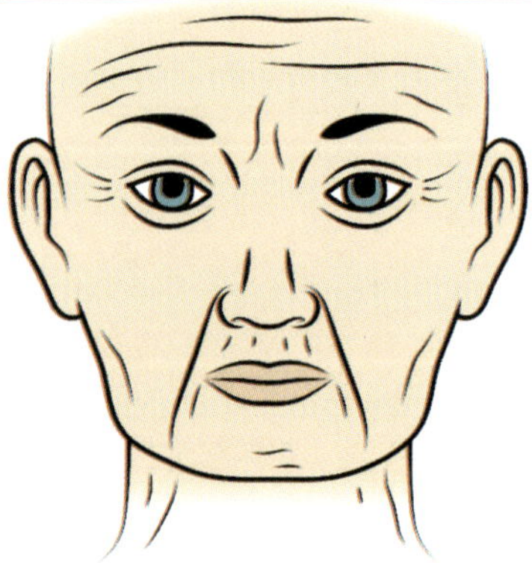

TYPE IV, "only wrinkles"
- age of patient: 60-70
- severe signs of photoaging
- grey skin colour
- prior skin malignancies
- wrinkles throughout, no normal skin

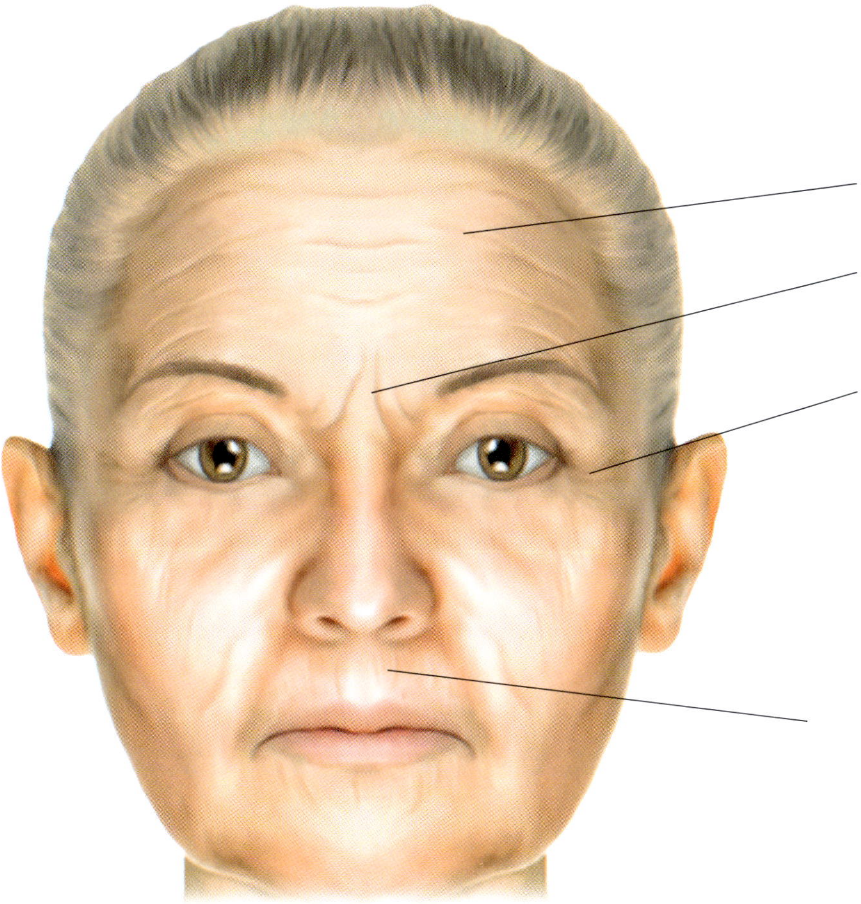

Figure 1 Lines

cording to position.
Wrinkles are divided into:
> lines;
> glyphic wrinkles;
> creases;
> crinkles;
> nasolabial folds.
Lines (fig. 1) include:
> forehead lines;
> crow's feet;
> glabella lines;
> vertical lip lines.
Glyphic wrinkles are caused by the accentuation of the skin texture, with its furrows becoming wider and deeper. Actinic damage plays an important role in their formation and they occur most typically In the lower cheek area (fig. 2).
Creases are asymmetric wrinkles that run in an oblique direction, developing typically as a result of how we sleep. They are most commonly found on the forehead and cheeks.
Crinkles are the result of an imbalance between supporting structure and the outer covering, together with the effects of gravity. They also develop in areas which are not photoexposed, primarily on cheeks, arms, thighs, hips and buttocks (fig. 3).

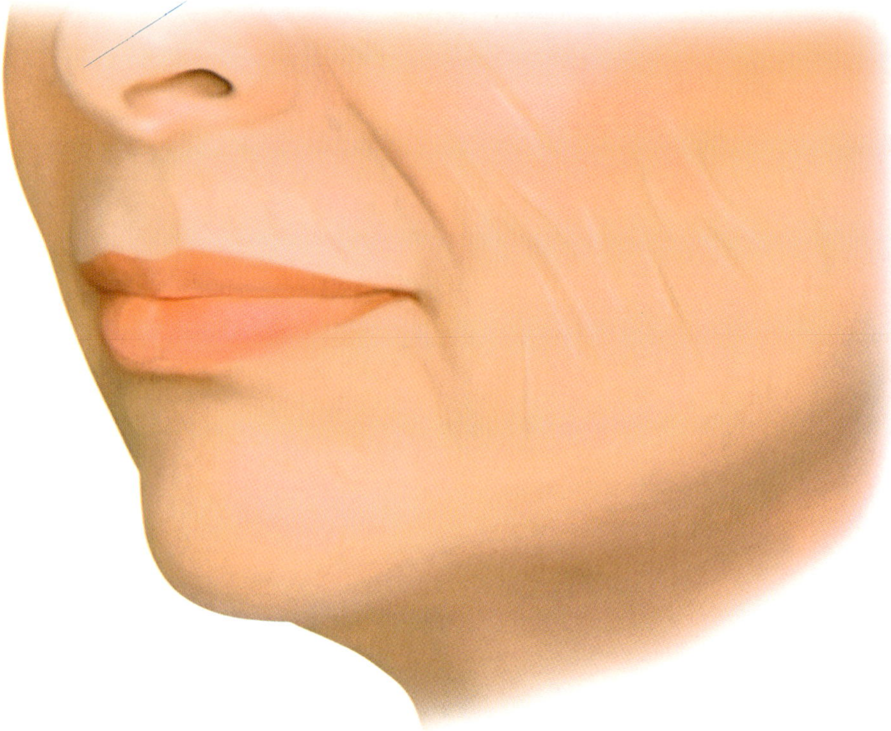

Figure 2 Glyphic wrinkles

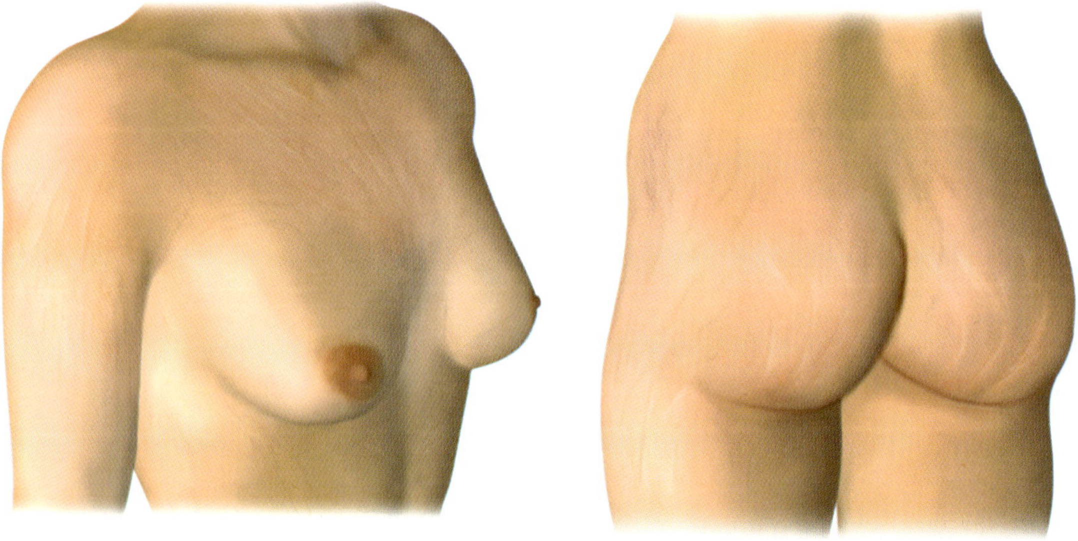

Figure 3 Crinkles

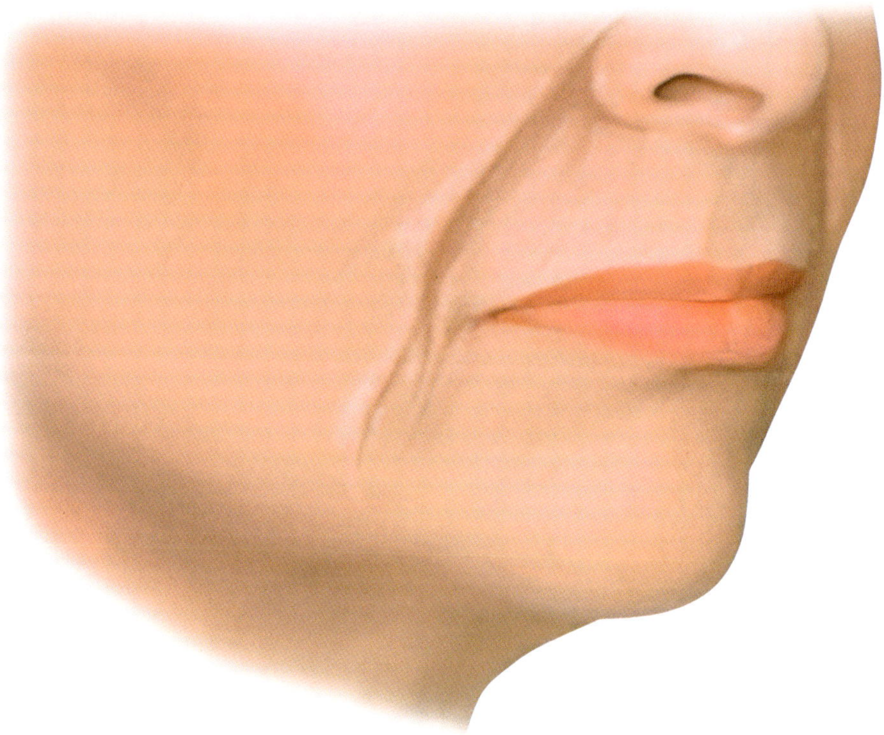

Figure 4 Nasolabial folds

Nasolabial folds are highlighted by the effect of gravity on lax tissues which remain anchored to the underlying structures near the perioral and masseter muscles (Smas) (fig. 4).

Bibliography

1. Fenske NA, Lober CW. Skin changes of aging: pathological implications. Geriatrics. 1990 Mar;45(3):27-35.
2. Zhang S, Duan E. Fighting against Skin Aging: The Way from Bench to Bedside. Cell Transplant. 2018 May;27(5):729-738.
3. Limbert G, Kuhl E. On skin microrelief and the emergence of expression micro-wrinkles. Soft Matter. 2018 Feb 21;14(8):1292-1300.
4. Samuel M, Brooke R, Griffiths C. Wrinkles. Clin Evid. 2005 Dec;(14):2104-16.
5. Puizina-Ivić N. Skin aging. Acta Dermatovenerol Alp Pannonica Adriat. 2008 Jun;17(2):47-54.
6. El-Domyati M, et al. Forehead wrinkles: a histological and immunohistochemical evaluation. J Cosmet Dermatol. 2014 Sep;13(3):188-94.
7. Khavkin J, Ellis DA. Aging skin: histology, physiology, and pathology. Facial Plast Surg Clin North Am. 2011 May;19(2):229-34.
8. Gilchrest BA. Photoaging. J Invest Dermatol. 2013 Jul 1;133(E1):E2-6.
9. Samuel M, Brooke R, Griffiths C. Wrinkles. Clin Evid. 2003 Jun;(9):1882-95.

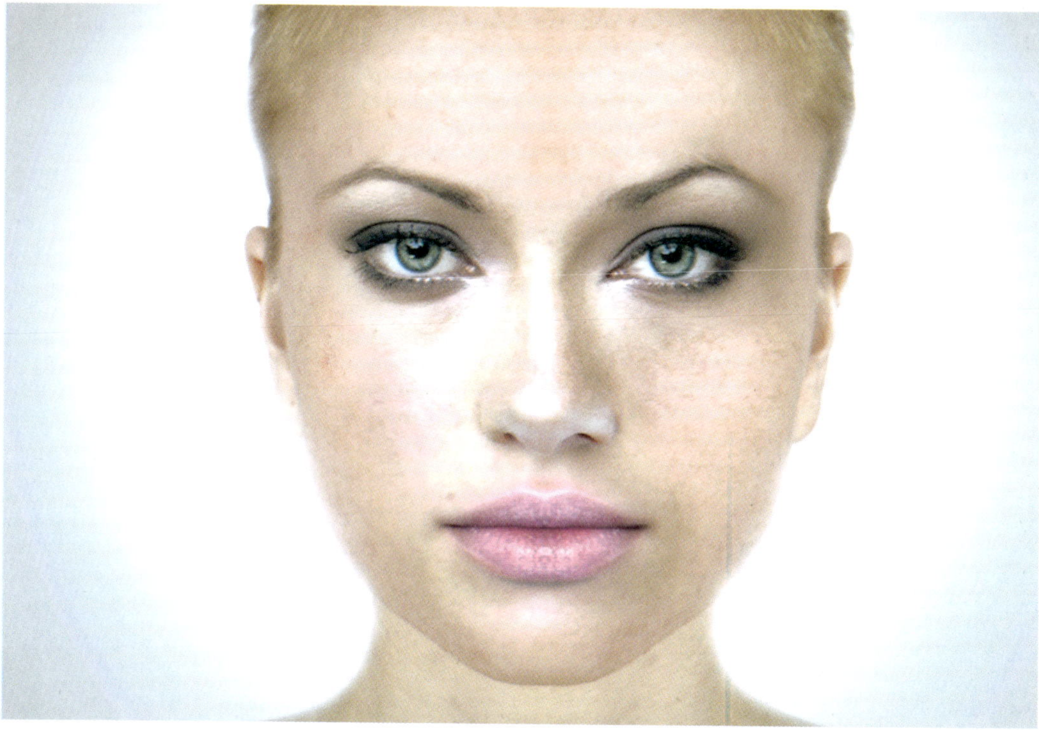

Signs of ageing: youthful face, fine lines

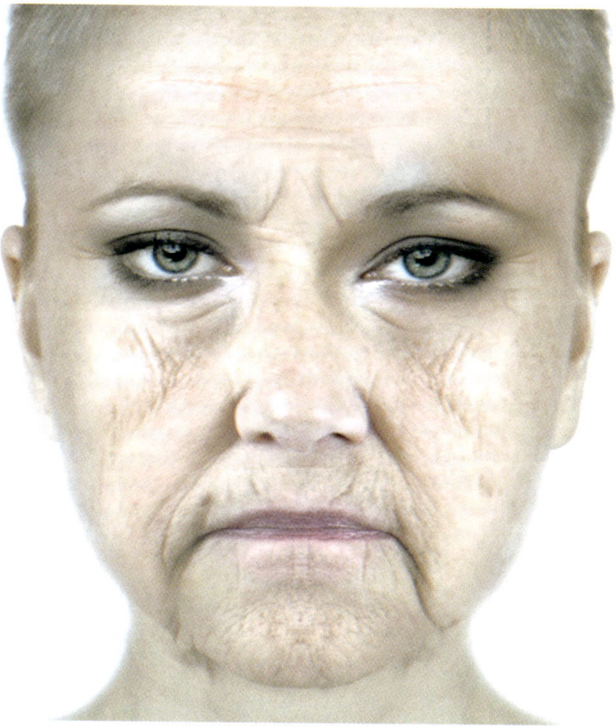

Signs of ageing: severe signs of photoaging

8

JAWLINE

Lucia Calvisi and Giuseppe Sito

Anatomy of the jawbone

It really is strange to think that the study of such an apparently small and almost insignificant bone led to the discovery of a new ancestor. Hexian man, whose fossil, found in Taiwan, dates back 190,000 years, and who appears to be more robust than *Homo erectus*, who was discovered earlier. This would mean that, in the Pleistocene, there seems to have been a population with characteristics different from those found on the Asian continent. The mandible was found in the sea, in an area that would have fallen within the so-called emerged areas during the Pleistocene.
This very recent news tells us just how important the jaw is, not only due to its aesthetic or functional appearance, but also, and above all, because it somehow identifies the face.

The mandibular bone is an unpaired median bone, which occupies the central part of the face (fig. 1). It has a vague horseshoe shape and contains the dental alveoli with the lower dental arch. The morphological anatomy of the mandible is not complex, but we must remember that important muscles are attached to it and it houses significant anatomical landmarks. The mandibular bone extends frontally downwards, ending in the mental protuberance and tubercle, indicating the symphysis between the two halves of the mandibular bone. In the centre, just above the tubercle, there is usually a chin dimple, another important anatomical landmark.
There are also numerous other tubercles and muscle insertions in the front and back of the face, forming the flo-

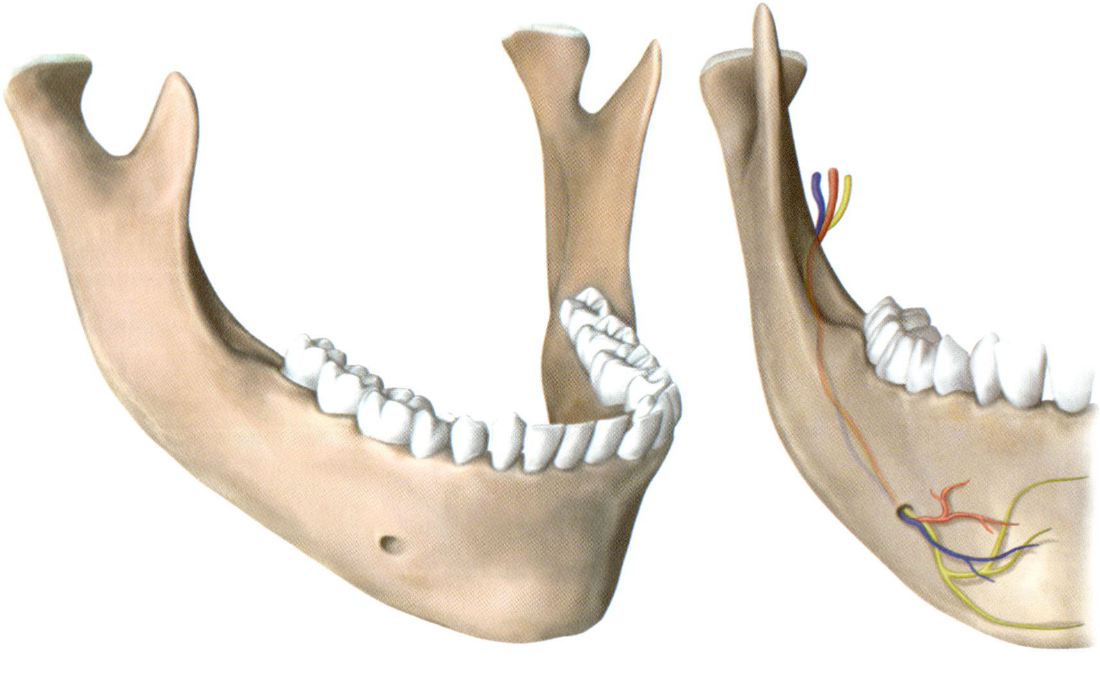

Figure 1 Jawbone

or of the mouth, but these are not so relevant, while the posterior border, forming the craniometric gonion point, on the other hand is important. It occurs where the angle of the mandible and the ascending ramus, which houses the stylomandibular ligament, meet and is in relation to the parotid.
The temporal, masseter, external and internal pterygoid, genioglossus, mylohyoid, geniohyoid and digastric muscles are attached to the mandible and are all of great importance. The inferior alveolar nerve is contained in the mandibular canal right to the end, at the mental foramen in the premolar area. Here it exits the body of the mandible and splits into three branches: the first one conveys sensitivity to the skin on the chin, while the other two reach the skin, the lip mucous membrane and the mucous membrane of the inferior alveolar surface. The buccal gingiva and dental elements are innervated by the dental plexus or inferior alveolar plexus, made up of ramifications that branch off from the inferior alveolar nerve along its intraosseous route. The nerve in the mandibular canal is accompanied by the neurovascular bundle. Their mutual position has not yet been standardised, but cadaveric studies suggest that the veins are positioned more cranially than the lower alveolar nerve, while the artery is found in a more lingual position than the nerve. This region also contains important neurovascular structures, such as the facial artery and vein and branches of the facial nerve (fig. 2). The facial artery is situated approximately 27 mm in front of the apex of the mandible. It crosses the masseter muscle and is embedded in deep subcutaneous fat. It then runs along the platysma towards the modiolus at the corner of the mouth where it forms the inferior and superior labial artery branches, continuing as an angular artery. It rises closer to the surface in the nasolabial fold.
This clearly indicates how the area of the so-called jawline runs from the mandibular ramus to the temporomandibular joint and to the mental symphysis with the mental tubercle. It has an elongated "t" shape, covered by muscles and then by subcutaneous tissue and skin. In men, the skin is covered by thick hair.
The jawline represents the transition between face and neck and, as time goes by, the ptosis of the soft tissues causes the face and neck to merge into a single area, blurring the two and causing them to look distorted.
The jawline and chin are an integral part of the perception of the attractiveness and youthfulness of a face, both in men and women, with the appropriate differences depending on sex. In women, a well-defined jaw with gentle, feminine contours is preferred, while in men, a more powerful, square jaw is a sign of virility.
A "strong" jawline is always appreciated in actors and politicians.
As time goes by, there is a loss of volume in this region as well, and this is due to several factors: bone resorption, repositioning of subcutaneous fat, muscle fatigue and skin laxity are among the main factors that contribute to the ageing of this region. Age-related re-

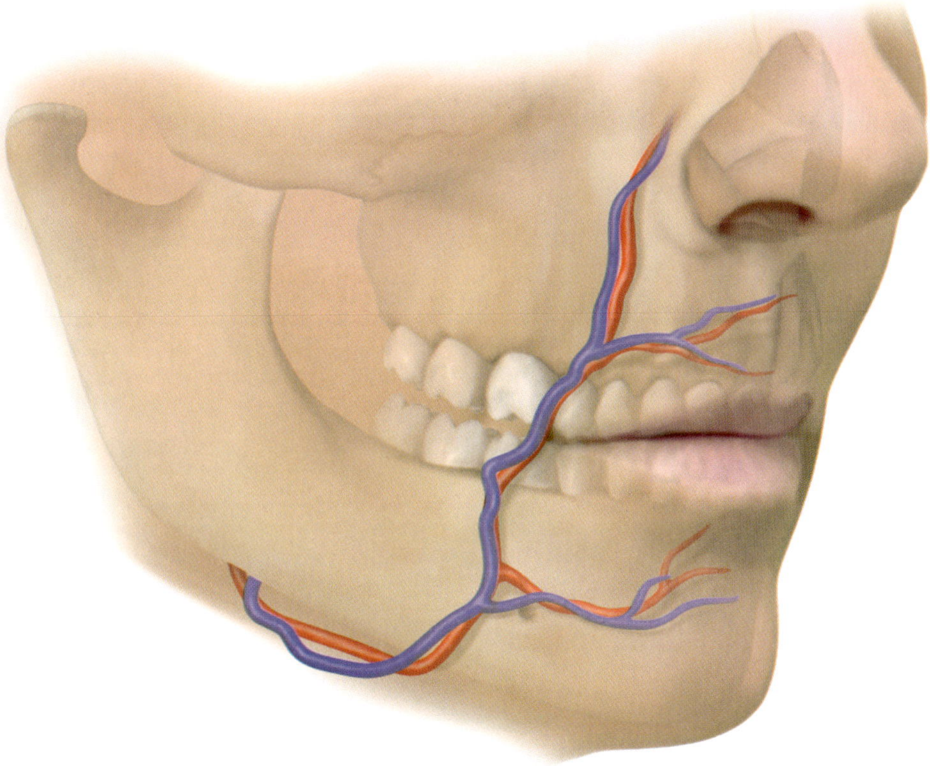

Figure 2 Facial artery and vein. Note the progression and division of the upper and lower labial arteries and veins

sorption of the mandibular bone, skin ptosis and loss of tone of the lower lip depressor muscle in particular lead to the formation of marionette wrinkles.

Preparing the patient

As with all aesthetic procedures, when treating the mandibular region and chin it is essential to carefully evaluate the patient before injecting the filler. Particular attention should be paid to the mandibular angle, mandibular profile, chin, pre-jowl and marionette lines.
The patient should be examined in static and dynamic conditions and photographed in anterior, oblique and posterior positions.
The aim of the treatment is to make the jawline straighter and more defined, to soften the transition between chin and jowl and to elongate the jowl anteriorly. The aesthetic endpoint in men is different from that in women because in men we seek a squarer, more prominent jaw, also working on the vertical branch, and a wider chin than in women.

Injection technique

The fillers used to treat this area are hyaluronic acid, calcium hydroxyapatite and polylactic acid, with high G′ hyaluronic acid being preferred as it allows safer and longer lasting shaping, thanks to the rheological properties which are also evident in the stretch and strength tests. It is essential to disinfect the area using antiseptic and then deposit a small 0.5 cc bolus of product at the mandibular angle, after aspiration, in order to make the profile of the mandible straighter (fig. 3). Alternatively, a 25 G cannula can be used to trace the mandibular angle, entering from the highest part of the lower angle of the mastoid, just below the projection on the skin.

As far as the front is concerned, enter the jowl with a 25 G cannula, trace the chin and then proceed along the remainder of the jawline (fig. 4).
As already mentioned, the use of a finer cannula, which would be the equivalent of a sharp needle, is never recommended.

Complications

The most common complications when using filler along the jawline are redness, bruising and swelling.

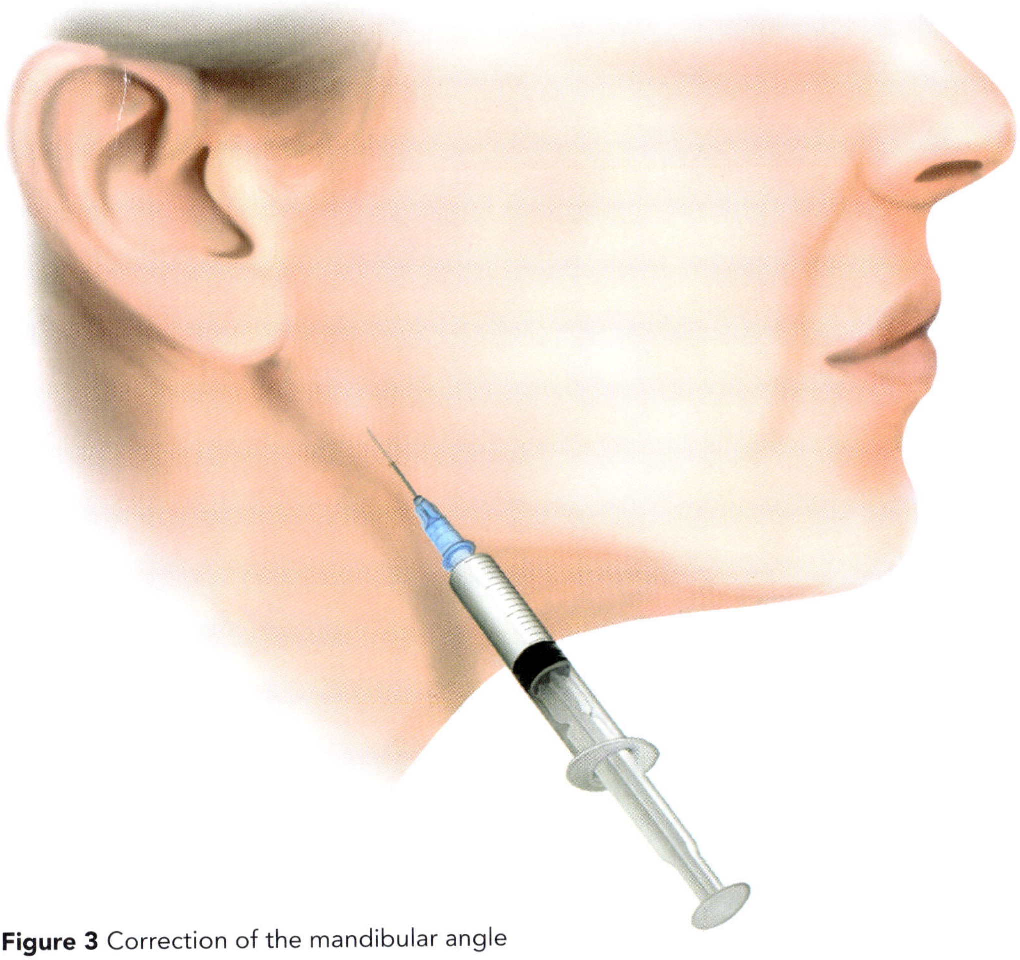

Figure 3 Correction of the mandibular angle

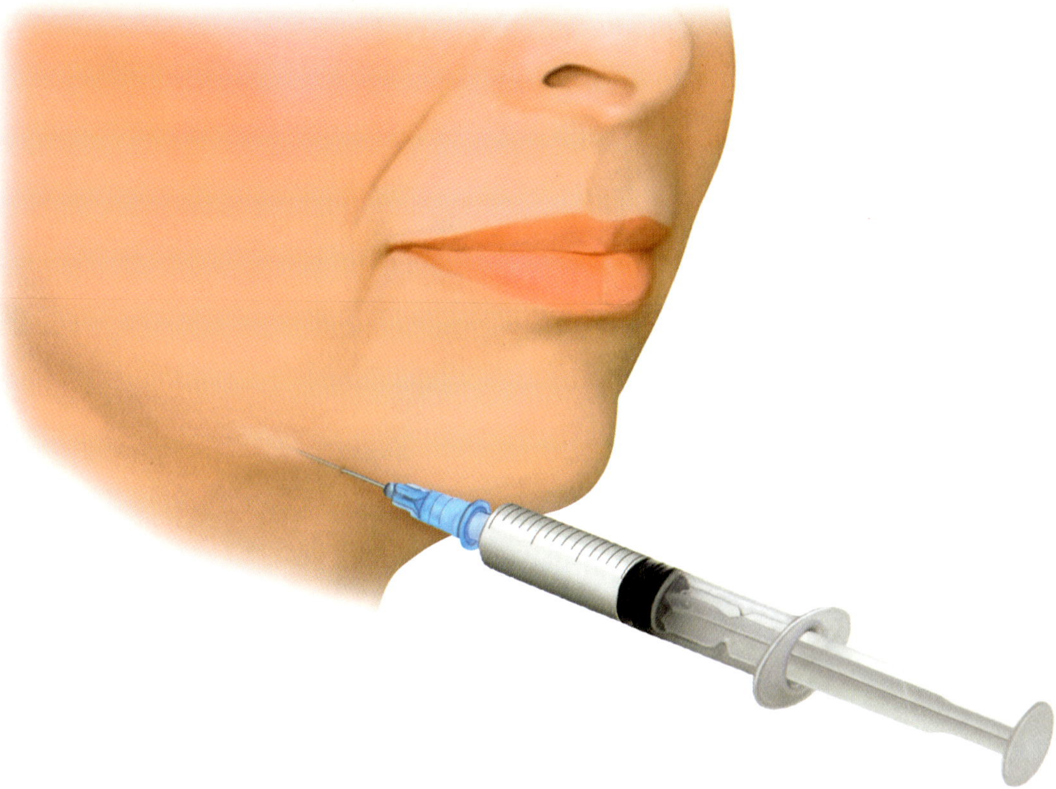

Figure 4 Correction of the mandibular arch

Other rare complications are infection and formation of foreign body granuloma.
The results are always exceptional, with the formation of a jawline that regains its role as the line of transition between face and neck, losing its sagginess with an overabundance of skin.

Bibliography

1. Weinstein T, Deflorian M, Parenti A, Fumagalli L, Mandelli F, Rossi M, Cattalini C, Testori T. (2011). Il nervo alveolare inferiore, il forame mentoniero e il canale incisale anatomia e variabilità anatomica ed esami strumentali per evidenziare lesioni neurologiche. Quintessence international. Anno 27. Numero 4. 48-57.
2. Naini FB, Garagiola U, Wertheim D. Analysing chin prominence in relation to the lower lip: The lower lip-chin prominence angle. J Craniomaxillofac Surg. 2019 Aug;47(8):1310-1316.
3. Saponaro G, Gasparini G, Boniello R, Pelo S, Doneddu P, Todaro M, et al. The Rules of Attractiveness: A Study on the Lower Facial Third. J Craniofac Surg. 2018 Oct;29(7):1945-1946.
4. Mommaerts MY. The ideal male jaw angle - An Internet survey.

J Craniomaxillofac Surg. 2016 Apr;44(4):381-91.
5. Juhász MLW, Marmur ES. Examining the Efficacy of Calcium Hydroxylapatite Filler With Integral Lidocaine in Correcting Volume Loss of the Jawline-A Pilot Study. Dermatol Surg. 2018 Aug;44(8):1084-1093.
6. Moradi A, Watson J. Current Concepts in Filler Injection. Facial Plast Surg Clin North Am. 2015 Nov;23(4):489-94.

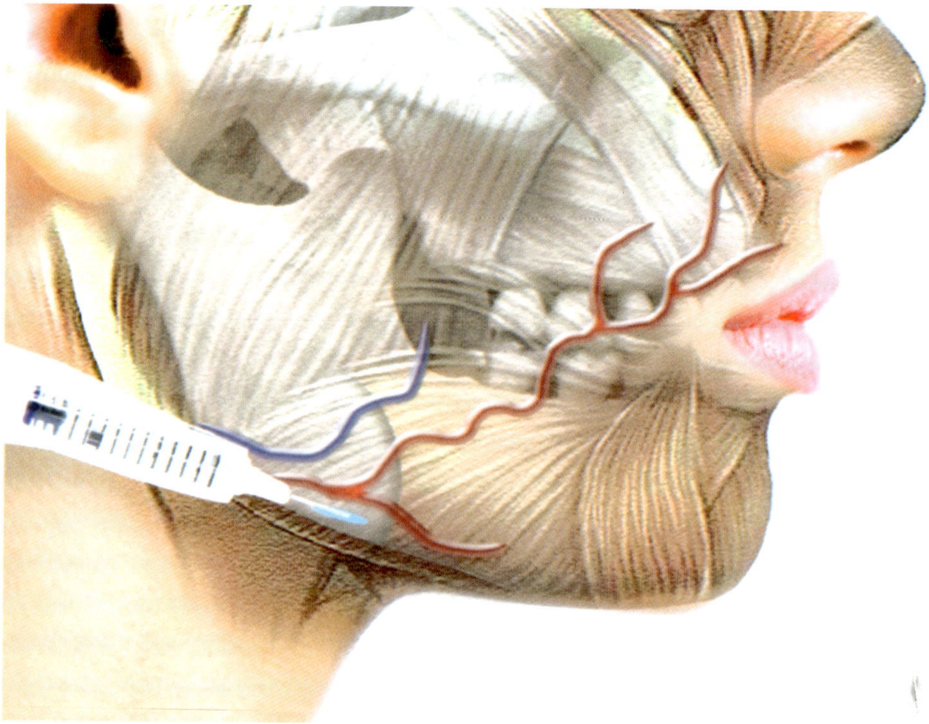

Graphic anatomy of the mandibular region and injection technique

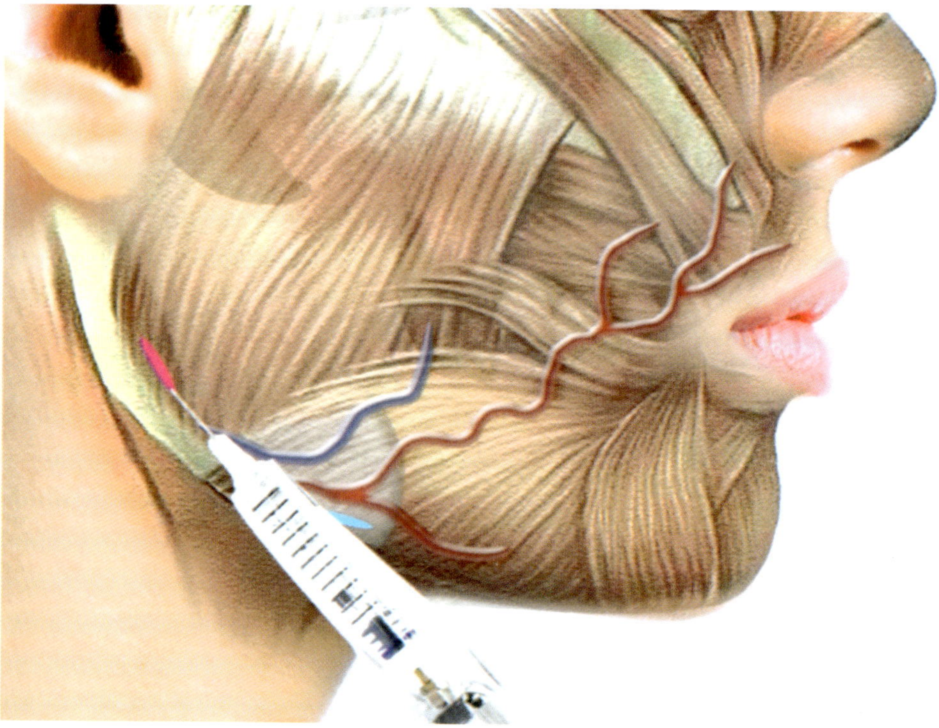

Graphic anatomy of the mandibular region and injection technique

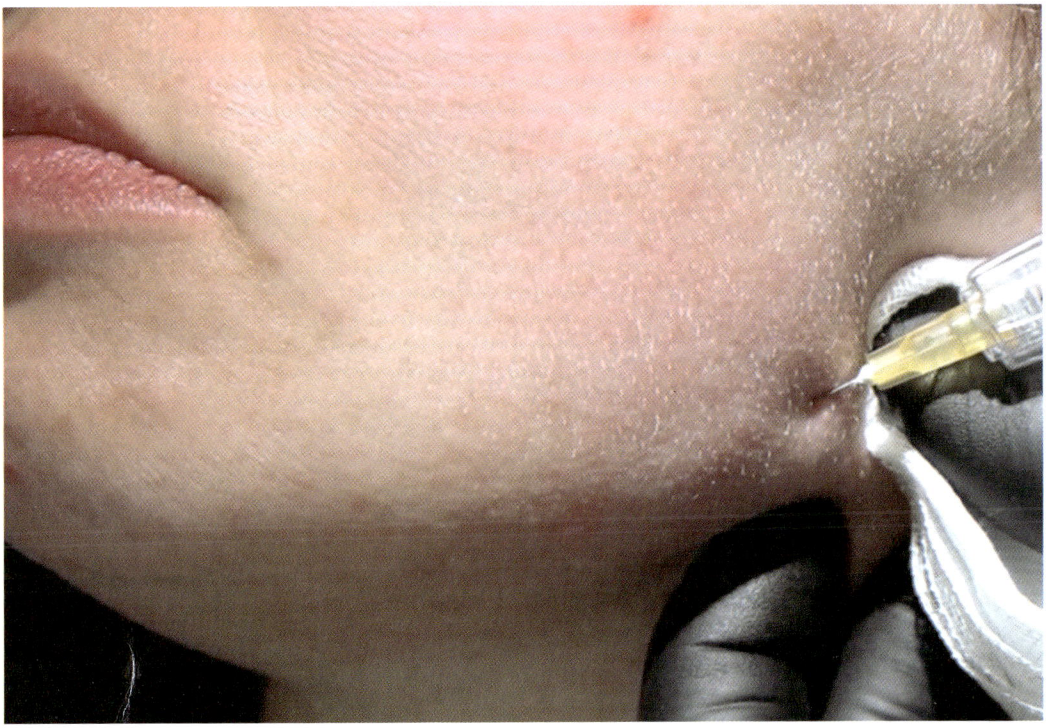

Injective treatment of the jawline using the multilayer technique: supra-muscular plane

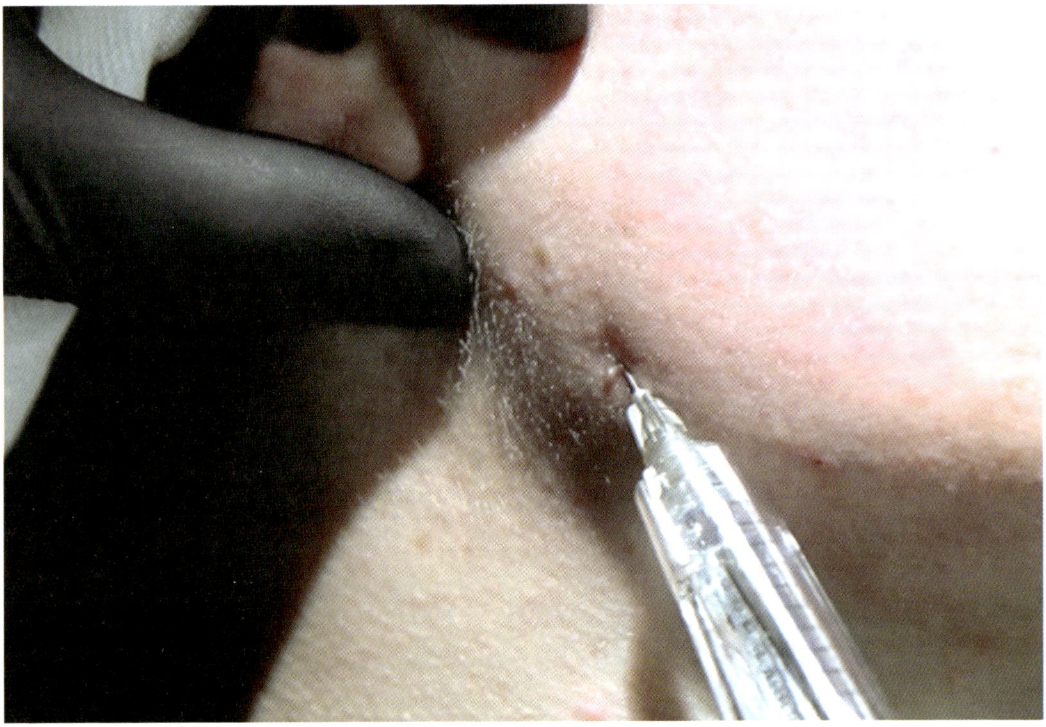

Injective treatment of the jawline using the multilayer technique: supra-periosteal plane

CLINICAL CASES

CLINICAL CASE 1

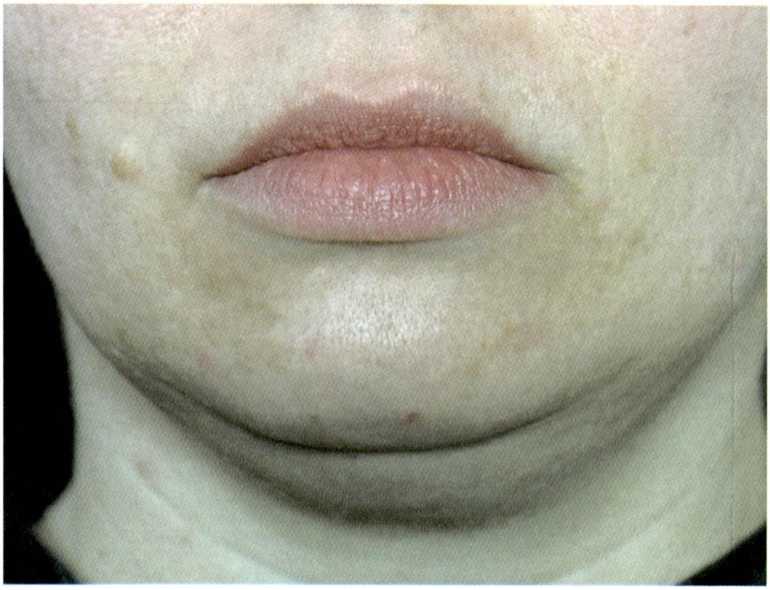

BEFORE

VIDEO 1

Injective treatment of the jawline using the multilayer technique

AFTER

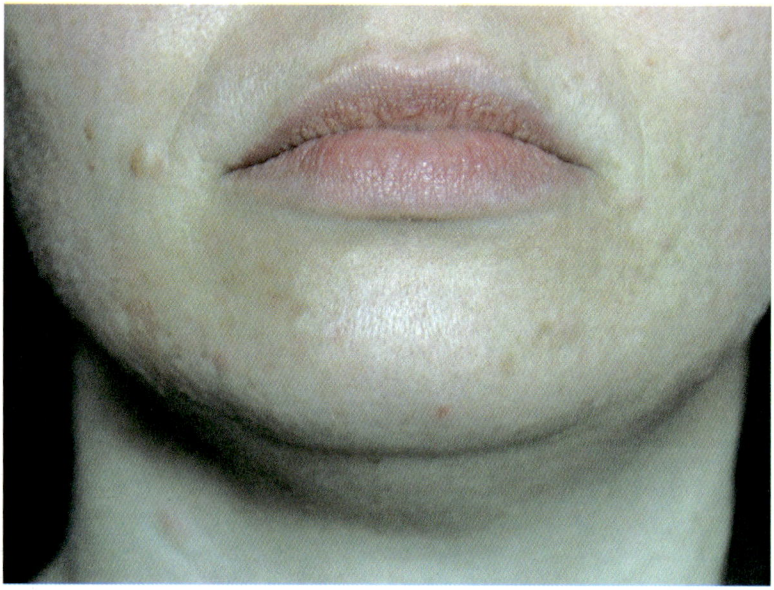

40-year-old female patient. Slight excess of skin along the jawline and submental region. Subperiosteal correction with 1 ml of high G' resilient HA on each side. No analgesia, retrograde linear technique.

CLINICAL CASES

CLINICAL CASE 1

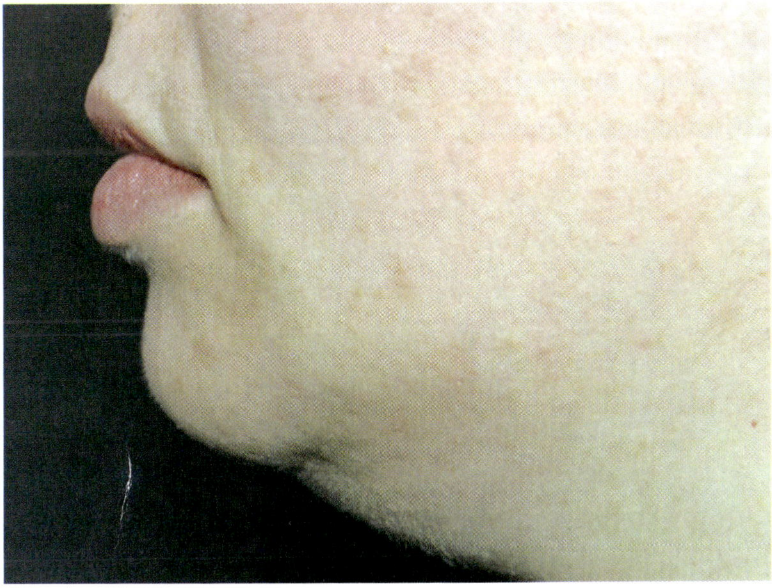

BEFORE

<

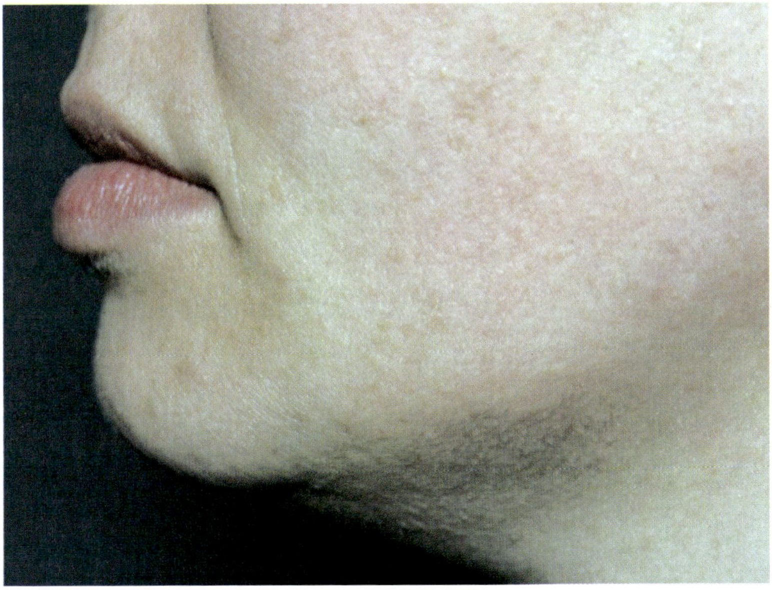

AFTER

>

Same patient, seen from the side.

CLINICAL CASES

CLINICAL CASE 1

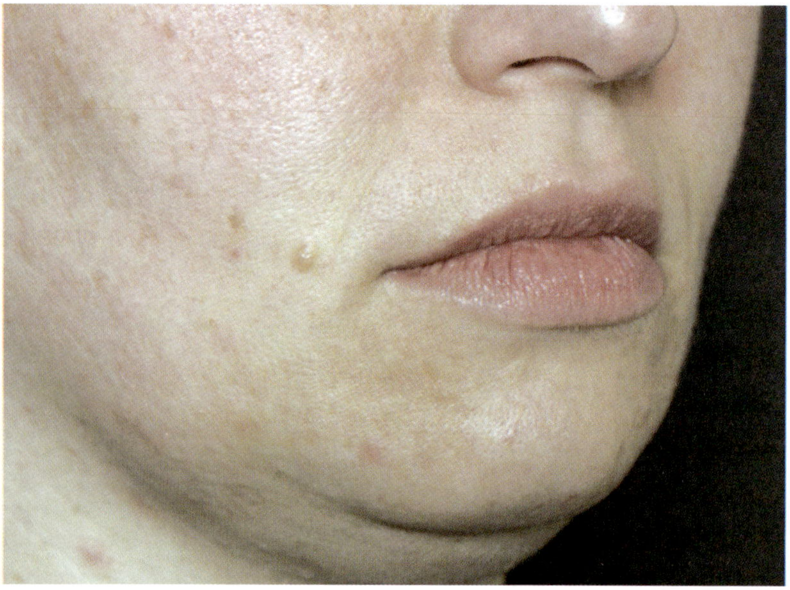

BEFORE

AFTER

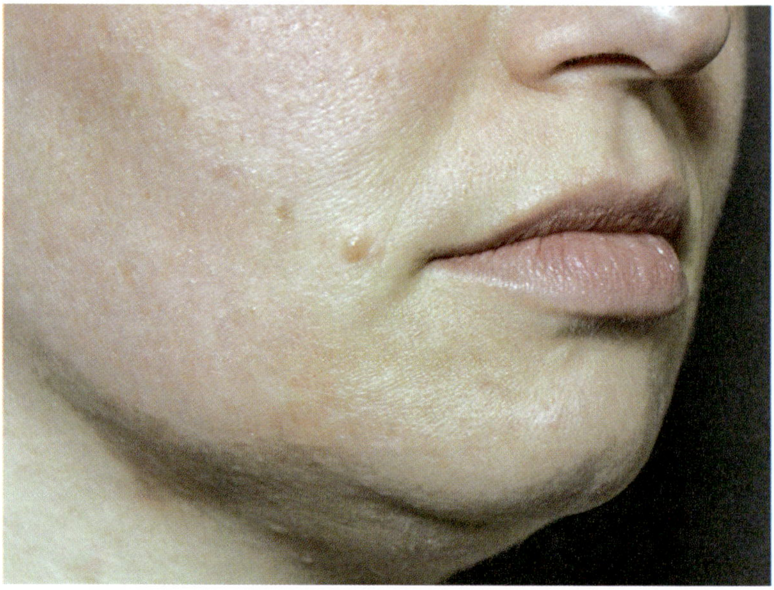

Same patient, in detail.

9

CHIN

«The chin is not an important part of the face,
less important than the nose and eyes,
but if it is missing, for some unknown reason,
people take you for an idiot»

Alberto Moravia

Anatomy of the chin

From an anatomical point of view, the chin is an unpaired region of the face, resulting, in terms of its bony plane, from the union of the two mandibular bones which create the mental dimple at midline level. A fibroelastic lamella then departs from the dimple and travels to the skin, ideally dividing the chin into two identical and symmetrical halves.

The soft parts, on the other hand, are divided into three planes, the most superficial of which consists of the skin, which is remarkably thick, covered with hair in men and almost smooth in women. The second is made up of the fatty muscle layer and the third, deeper plane consists of the periosteum. The muscular portion consists of three muscles, the triangular lip muscle, the square lower lip muscle, or lower lip depressor, and the mental muscle. There are also some thin fascia of the cutaneous muscles of the neck (figs. 1 and 2).

In anatomical topography, the chin falls within the lower third of the face. Like the rest of the face, this area is affected by sagging as we age, due to the resorption of fatty tissue and bone. The chin, like the other components of the lower third, is not exempt from these changes and therefore requires treatment aimed at "aesthetic rehabilitation" just like the rest of the face (fig. 3).

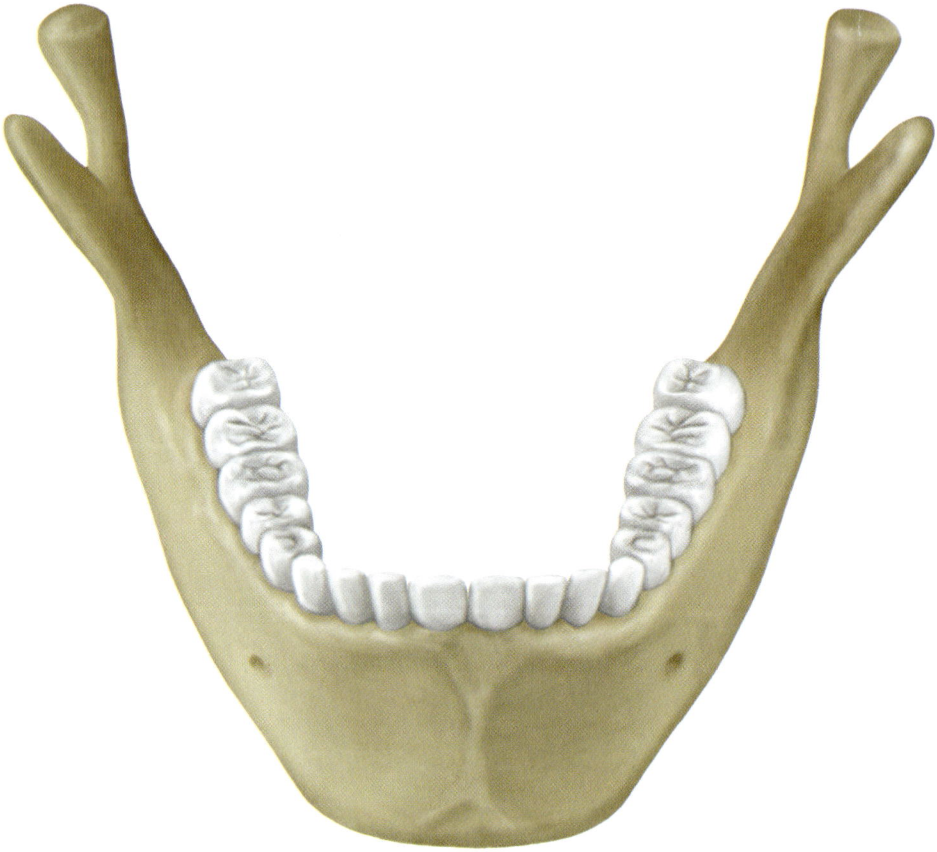

Figure 1 Mandibular arch with mental symphysis

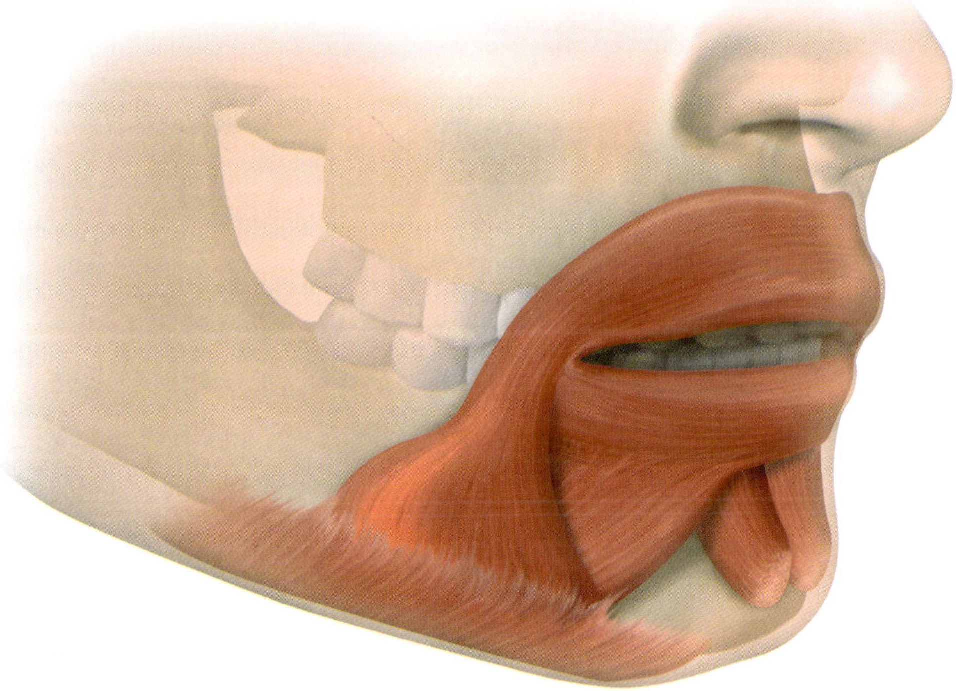

Figure 2 Muscles in the chin region

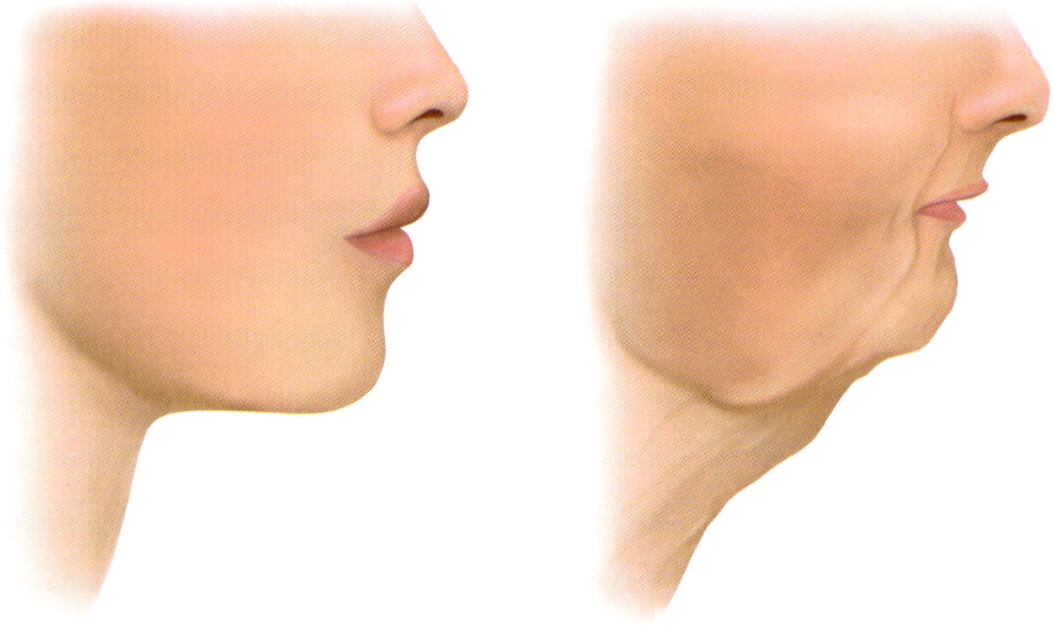

Figure 3 Normal chin and enognatism (hypoplasia of the chin)

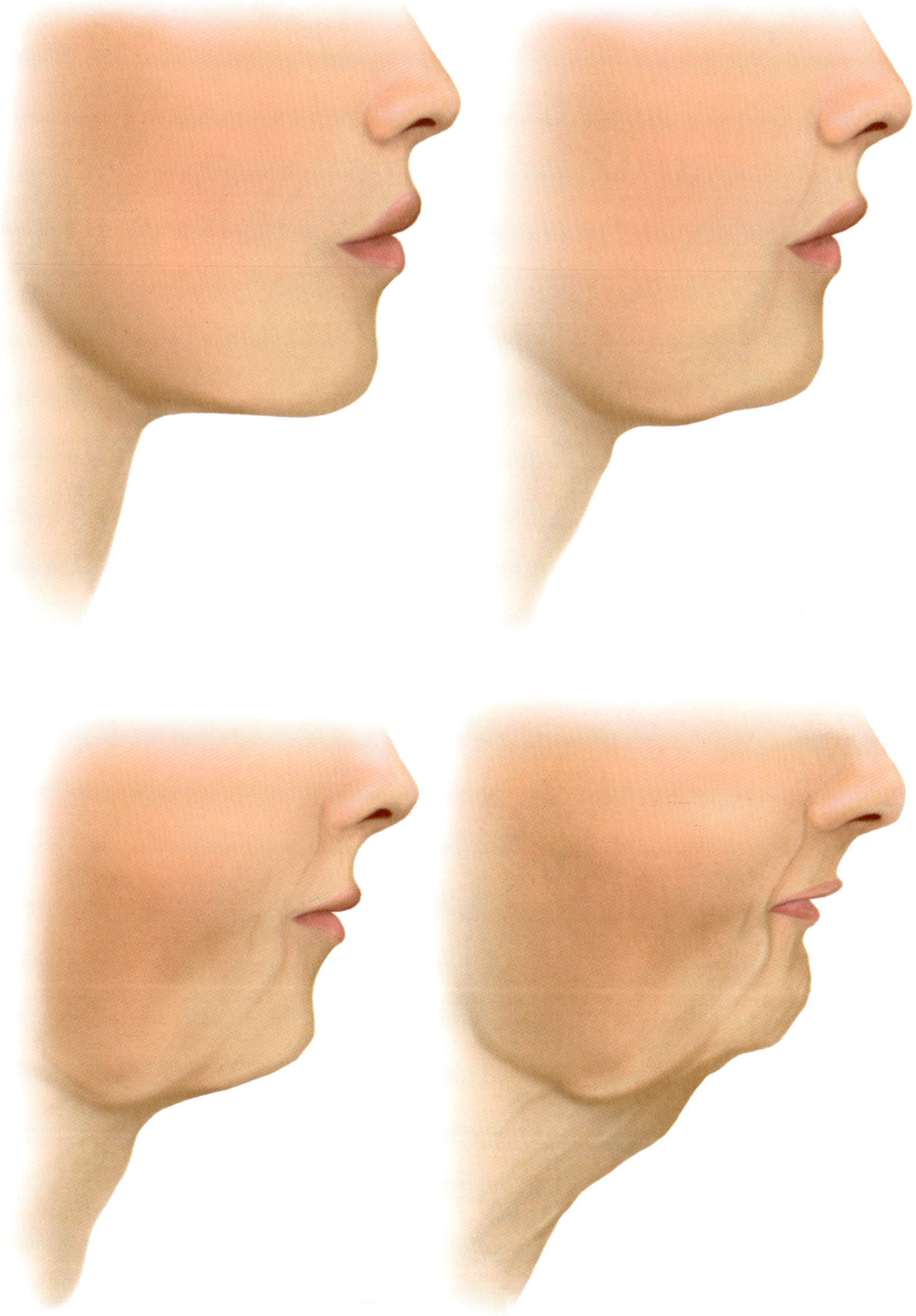

Figure 4 The chin and its alterations as we age

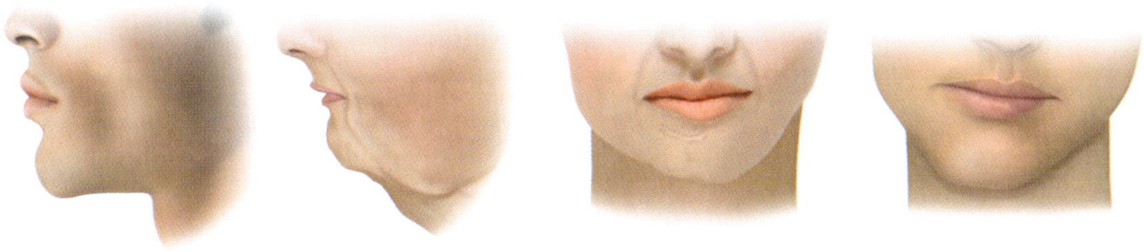

Figure 5 Various aspects of the chin region

All this causes obvious alterations as time goes by, as the mental dimple may slip further inwards and downwards when we are older. The sagging of the chin can depend both on the drooping of the skin and on muscular and ligament ptosis, for which there is little we can do (fig. 4).

From an aesthetic point of view, the chin, along with the cheekbones, represents one of the focal points of beauty, always considered as one of its so-called highlights. Facial beauty is expressed through a series of hollows and curves and a harmonious chin is undoubtedly an aesthetic feature of considerable importance, especially as far as the facial profile is concerned.

The chin is always a convex region and the extent of its convexity is determined by numerous factors: sex, age, race, past traumas and dental defects (fig. 5).

Correction of the chin

Now, bearing in mind that mentoplasty is usually offered to the patient, who tends not to ask for it, focusing attention on the nose rather than the chin, it is necessary to offer some advice on assessing the correction of this region.

First of all, the examination should ideally be carried out with the help of a three-panel mirror, so that even the smallest details that the patient wishes to correct can be shown, and always in an upright position, as the force of gravity exerts an action on the soft tissues.

Mentoplasty can be offered within the broader framework of a prophyloplasty or even on its own, to make the chin protuberance more prominent. Non-surgical or "medical" mentoplasty can be legitimately recommended for reshaping a small chin (microgenia of uncertain surgical interest), for reshaping the contour and redefining the oval of the face and also to offer a preview of the outcome of surgery to patients who are afraid of surgical procedures.

Microgenia is a pathology which, if mild (so-called first class), is very common. It occurs due to the underdevelopment of the mandibular symphysis or malocclusion. It can also develop as a result of bone tissue resorption, particularly in women of menopausal age, or due to a loss of dental elements or involutive soft tissue atrophy.

It is evident that the relationship between mouth, chin and nose needs to be re-harmonised, increasing the projection, which is always possible,

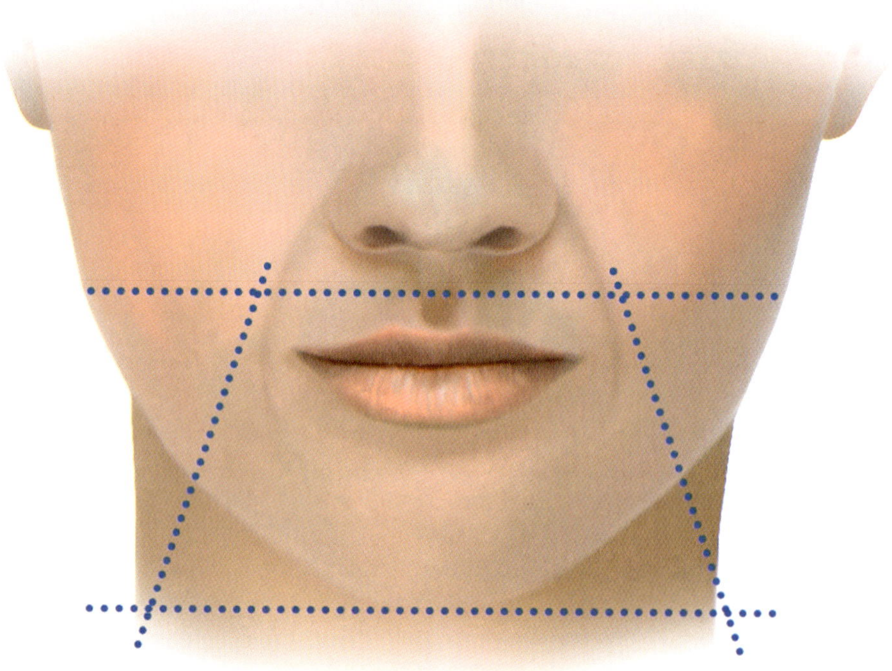

Figure 6 Limits of the chin region

and reshaping the contour, which is not always necessary.

The chin region has a vaguely quadrilateral shape limited at the top by a horizontal line, identified by the nasal lip groove, which distinguishes it from the lower lip and includes the cutaneous insertion of the superficial fibres of the mental muscle; laterally, the chin region is bordered by a vertical line, raised by the medial limit of the cheeks, which is identified by the nasolabial folds just to the side of the labial commissures; the lower limit coincides with the lower margin of the mandible, positioned above the suprahyoid region (fig. 6).

Sometimes the chin is withdrawn from its "normal" anatomical position, not only due to an alteration of the tissues, but also due to a generally involuntary contracture of the mental muscle, the terminal fascia of which are located at cutaneous level, and leads to the formation of what is known as a golf ball or orange peel chin. Before injecting filler to restore volume, it is a good idea to offer treatment with botulinum toxin to relax the muscle so that you can perform a more precise assessment of the actual conformation of the chin and then continue to enhance its volume using filler (fig. 7).

From a technical point of view, the correction of the chin with filler and specifically with hyaluronic acid or, as I often suggest for this region, with calcium hydroxyapatite, rightfully joins the list of deep, shaping corrections. In

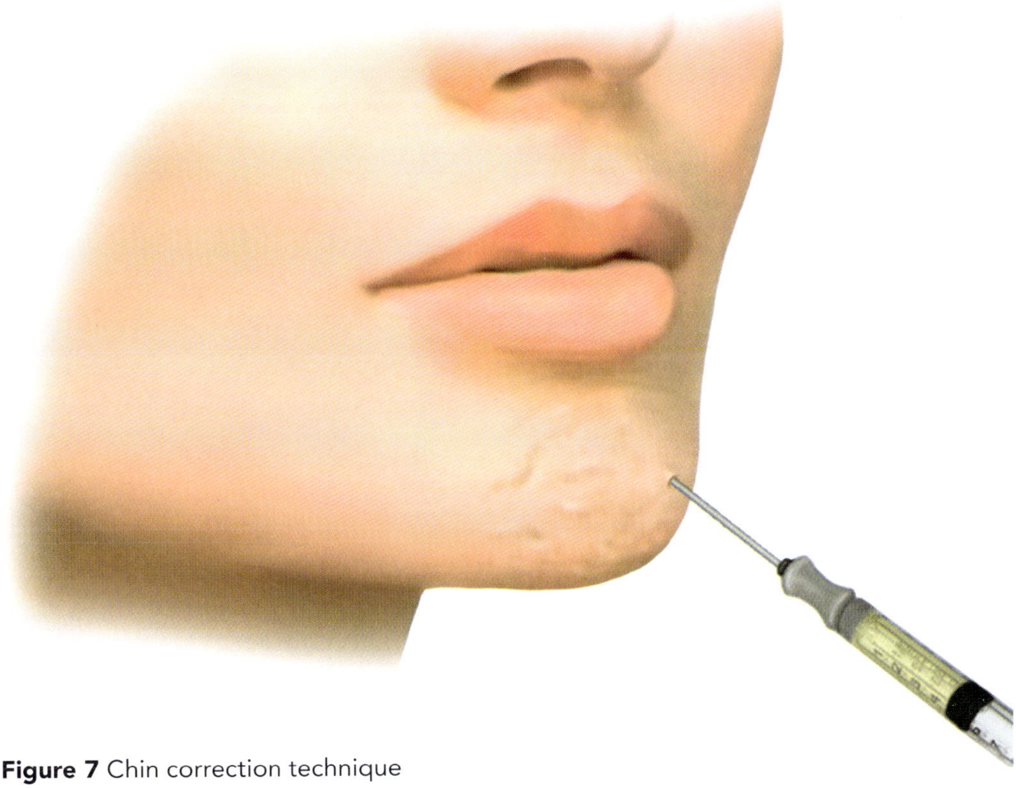

Figure 7 Chin correction technique

my opinion, calcium hydroxyapatite is very well suited to the volumetric correction of bones such as the chin and cheekbones, for example, while it is infrequently used, and rightly so, in the soft tissues.

The injection must go right the way through, until the tip of the needle touches the periosteum, with multiple boluses (usually two or three), then proceeding with a vigorous shaping massage (fig. 8).

The correction may only affect the chin protuberance, if you just want to move the chin forward, or both the front and the side, if you want to redefine a squarer, stronger, more masculine chin.

Mentoplasty can be rightfully considered within the correction of the jawline because, by bringing the chin forward, we obtain a relaxation of the line which, while slight, is nevertheless significant (fig. 9).

For the volumetric correction of the

VIDEO 1

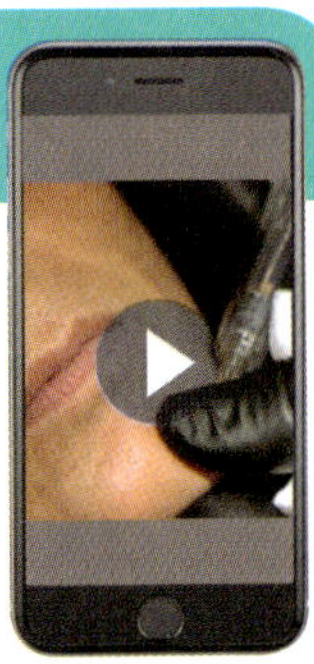

Correction of the chin using an electronic syringe

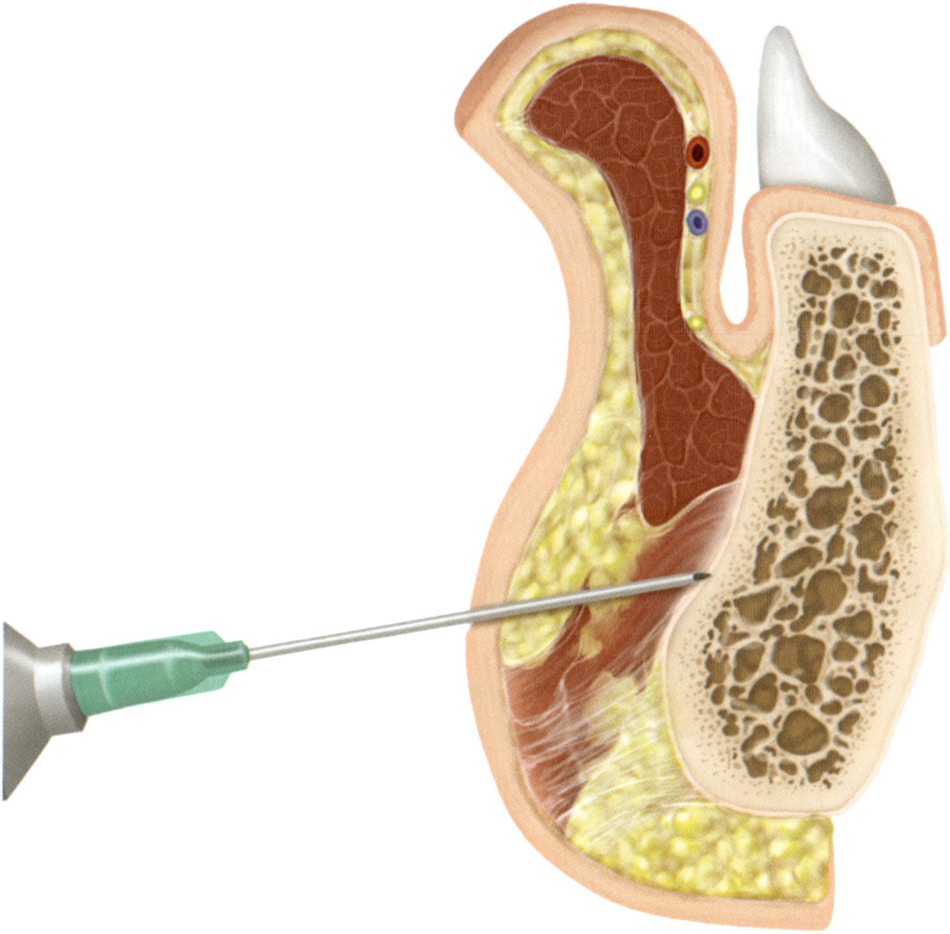

Figure 8 Correction of the chin region: injection technique

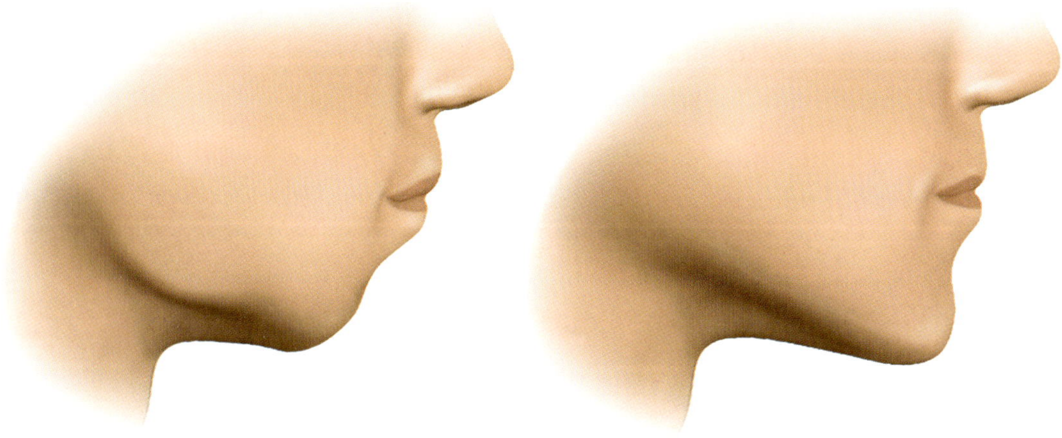

Figure 9 Secondary distension of the mandibular region

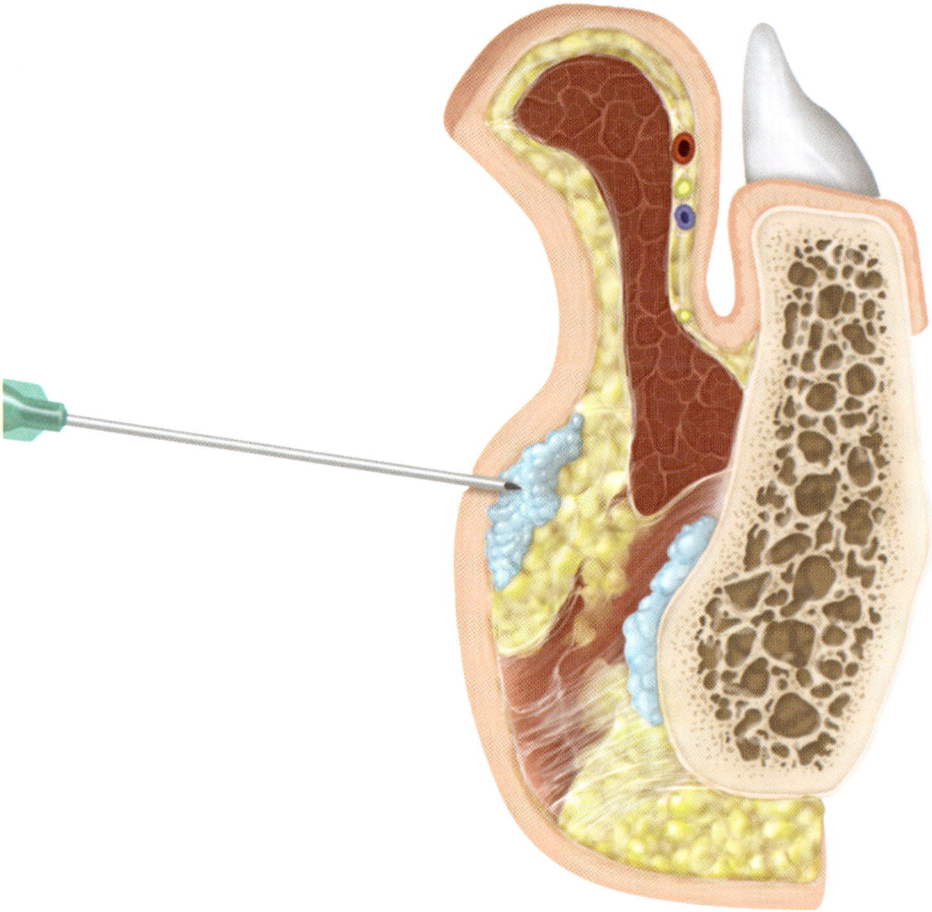

Figure 10 In cross-section: chin region correction technique

chin with hyaluronic acid-based filler, a dense and substantial product is recommended, to provide support. Alternatively, the dual plane technique can be used, deeply injecting a more consistent and superficial filler and finishing off with a more malleable (dynamic) volumetric filler, to make the effect more natural without compromising deep support (fig. 10).
Lastly, remember that the only risk area for this technique lies below the fifth tooth in the lower mandibular arch, where the mental nerve and facial artery emerge in most cases, except for the obvious anatomical deformities, which are always possible. Their plane is located deep down, however, and must never be infiltrated with fillers (fig. 11).

Bibliography

1. Torrealba R, Fariña R, Valladares S, Sáez F. Correction of chin ptosis. Int J Oral Maxillofac Surg. 2017 Aug;46(8):1026-1029.
2. Larrabee YC, Moyer JS. Reconstruc-

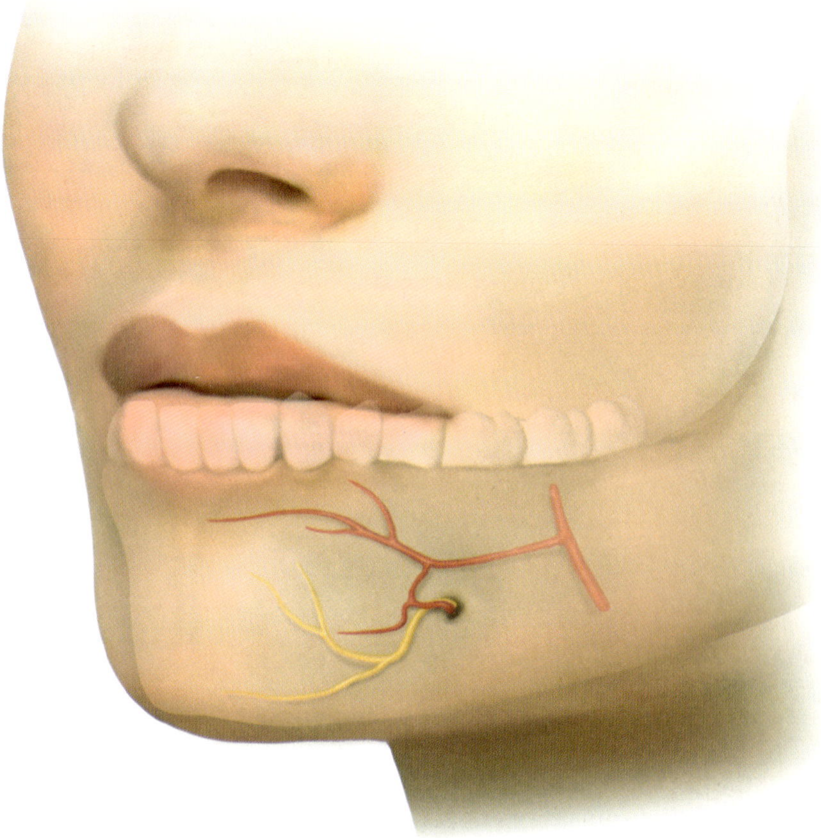

Figure 11 Innervation and vascularization of the chin region

tion of Mohs Defects of the Lips and Chin. Facial Plast Surg Clin North Am. 2017 Aug;25(3):427-442.
3. de Maio M, Wu WTL, Goodman GJ, Monheit G; Alliance for the Future of Aesthetics Consensus Committee. Facial Assessment and Injection Guide for Botulinum Toxin and Injectable Hyaluronic Acid Fillers: Focus on the Lower Face. Plast Reconstr Surg. 2017 Sep;140(3):393e-404e.
4. Sykes JM, Fitzgerald R. Choosing the Best Procedure to Augment the Chin: Is Anything Better than an Implant? Facial Plast Surg. 2016 Oct;32(5):507-12.
5. Rho NK, Chang YY, Chao YY, Furuyama N, et al. Consensus Recommendations for Optimal Augmentation of the Asian Face with Hyaluronic Acid and Calcium Hydroxylapatite Fillers. Plast Reconstr Surg. 2015 Nov;136(5):940-56.
6. Bertossi D, Galzignato PF, Albanese M, Botti C, Botti G, Nocini PF. Chin Microgenia: A Clinical Comparative

Study. Aesthetic Plast Surg. 2015 Oct;39(5):651-8.
7. Braz AV, Louvain D, Mukamal LV. Combined treatment with botulinum toxin and hyaluronic acid to correct unsightly lateral-chin depression. An Bras Dermatol. 2013 Jan-Feb;88(1):138-40.
8. Vanaman Wilson MJ, Jones IT, Butterwick K, Fabi SG. Role of Nonsurgical Chin Augmentation in Full Face Rejuvenation: A Review and Our Experience. Dermatol Surg. 2018 Jul;44(7):985-993.
9. Lorenc ZP, Bass LM, Fitzgerald R, Goldberg DJ, Graivier MH. Physiochemical Characteristics of Calcium Hydroxylapatite (CaHA). Aesthet Surg J. 2018 Apr 6;38(suppl1):S8-S12.

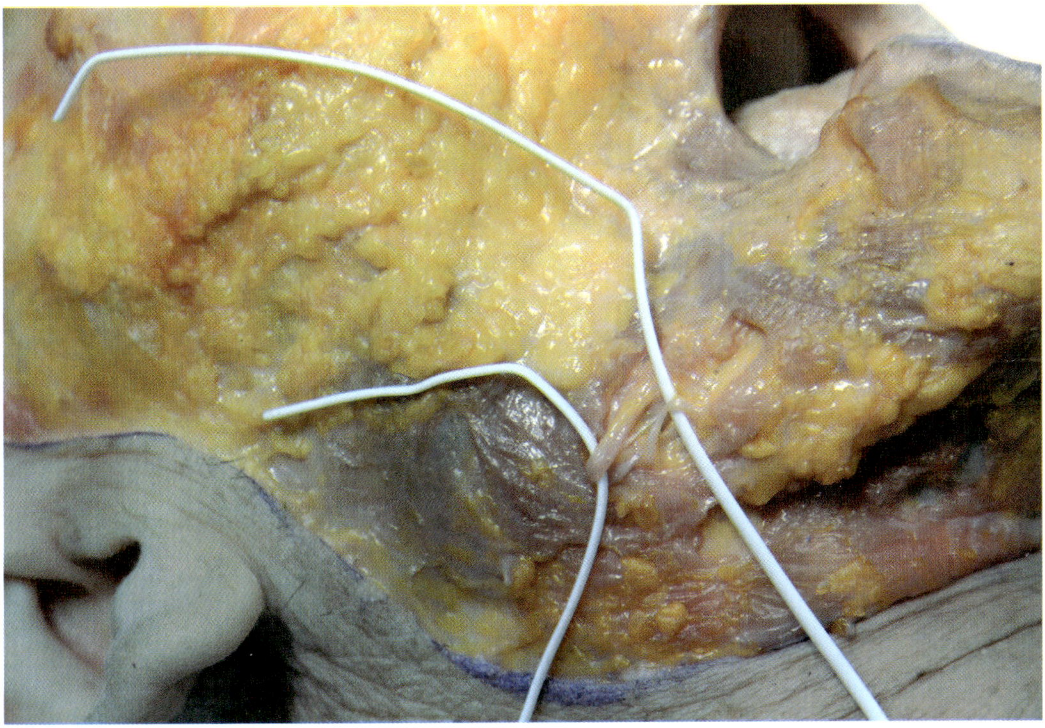

Division of the facial artery in an anatomical preparation

CLINICAL CASES

CLINICAL CASE 1

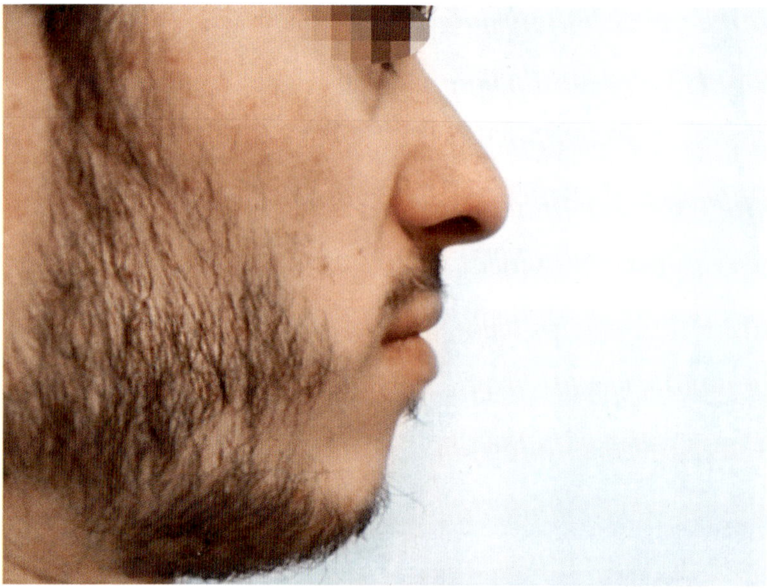

BEFORE

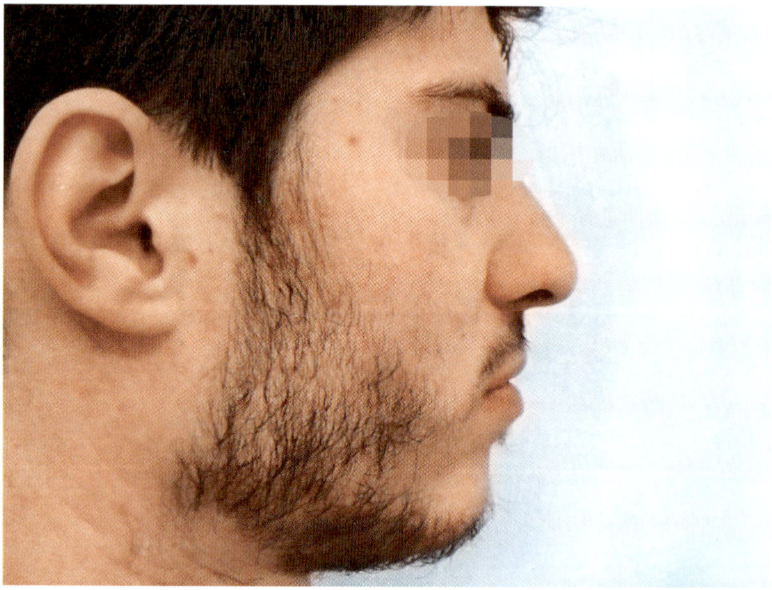

AFTER

38-year-old man with average hypoplasia of the chin for which he says he is forced to have a beard. Correction with double bolus linear technique and high density biodynamic hyaluronic acid injected with a needle, subperiosteal, using 1.8 ml of HA.

CLINICAL CASES

CLINICAL CASE 1

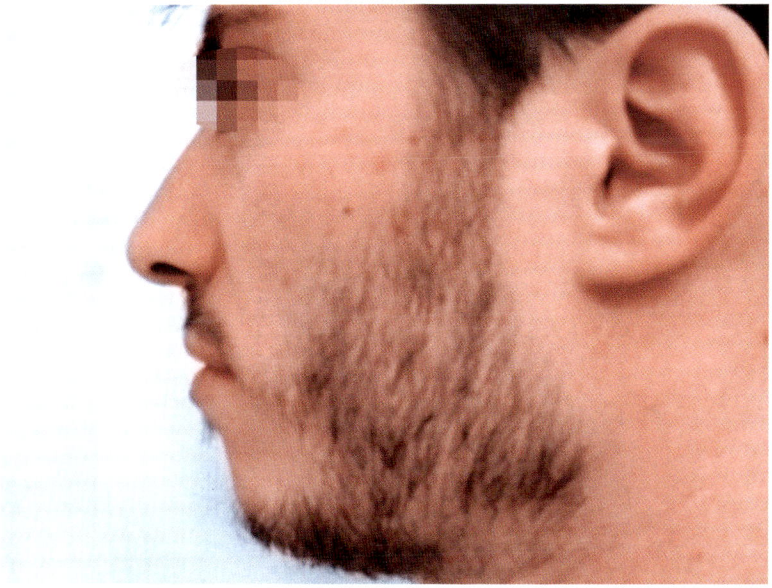

BEFORE
<

AFTER
>

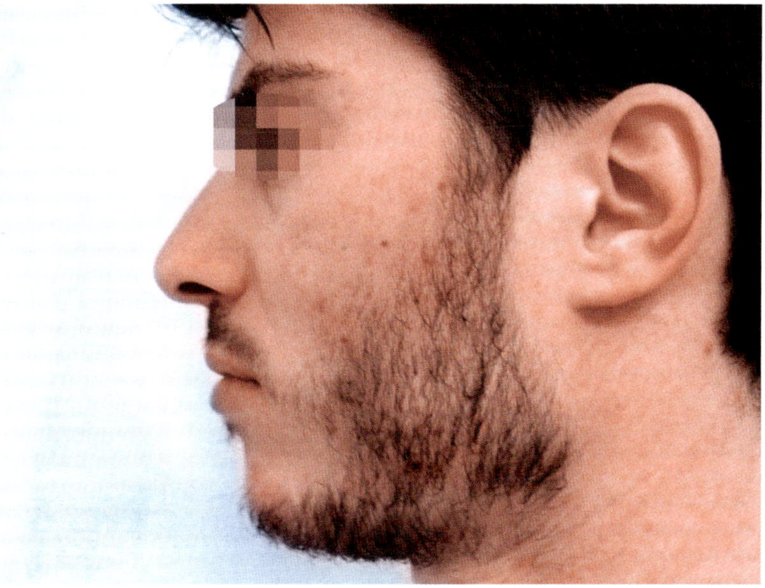

Same patient, left profile.

CLINICAL CASES

CLINICAL CASE 2

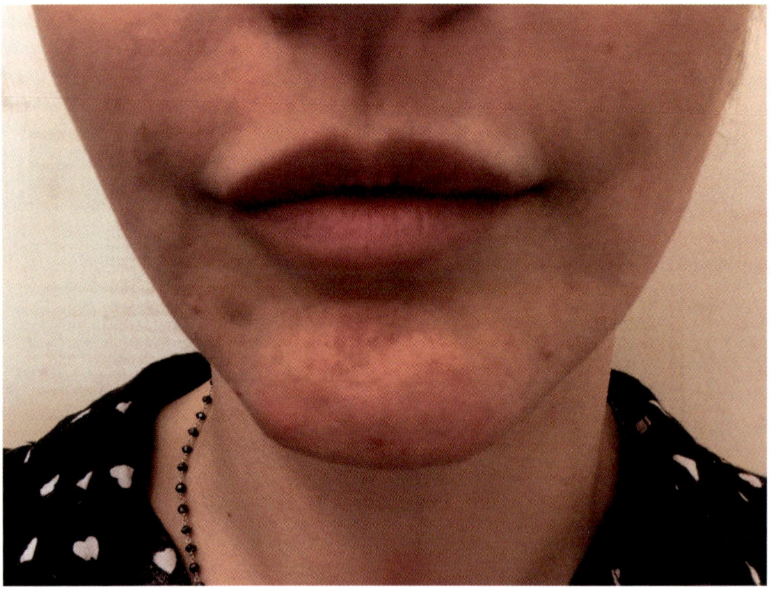

BEFORE

<

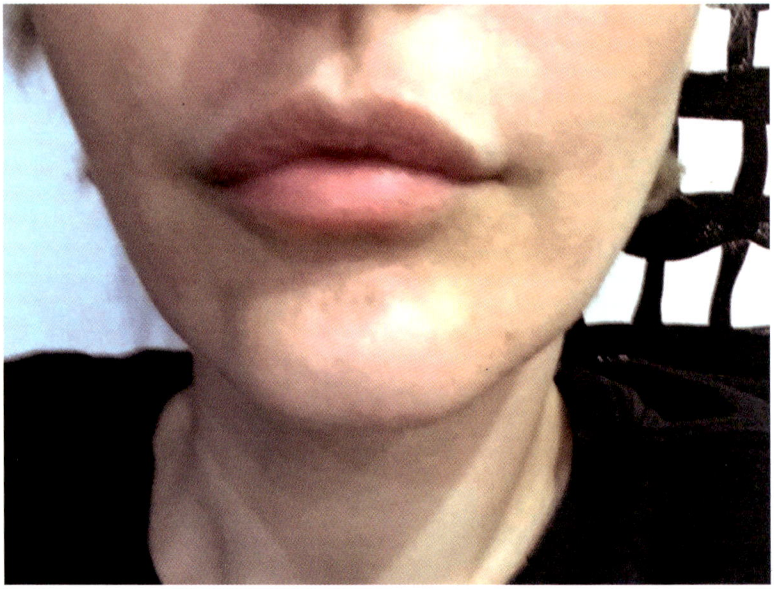

AFTER

>

29-year-old woman with hypoplasia of the chin and lips, corrected elsewhere. Correction of chin and lip hypoplasia with hydroxyapatite: 1.5 ml in double bolus and without analgesia. Post injection shaping massage.

CLINICAL CASES

CLINICAL CASE 3

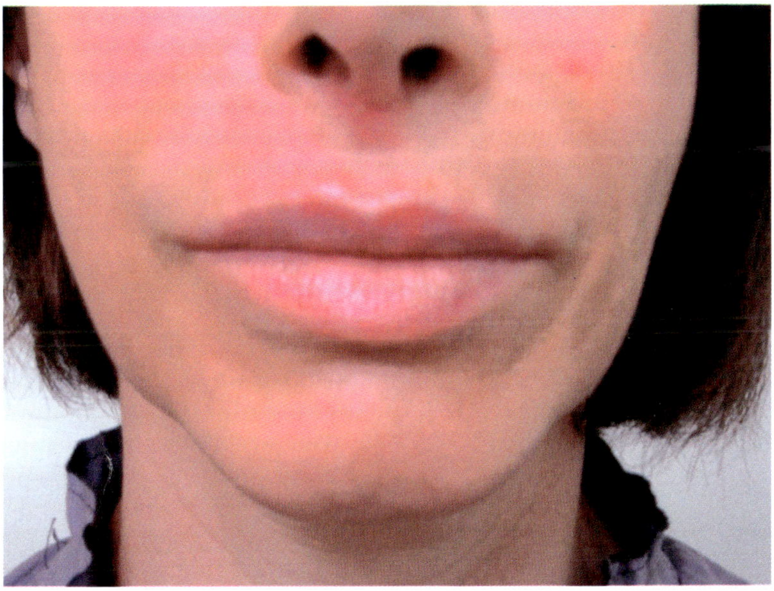

BEFORE

<

AFTER

>

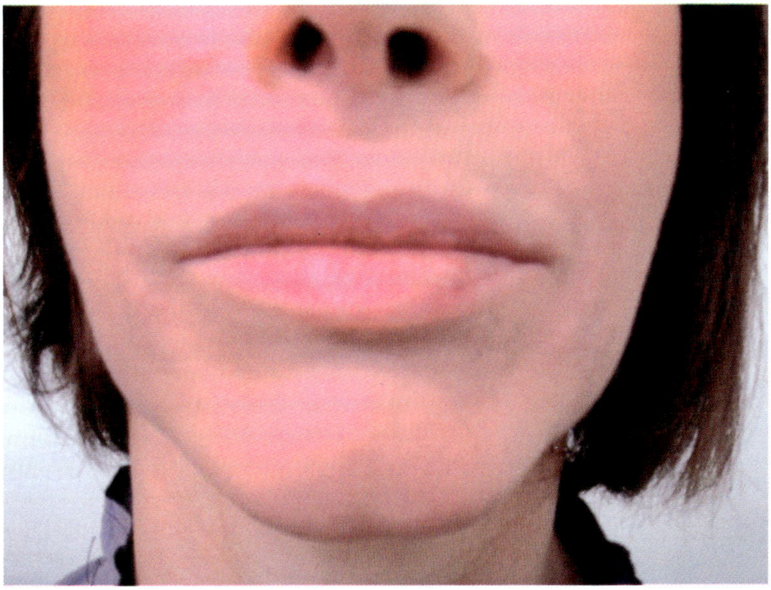

53-year-old woman, very tall (1.85 m), with marked hypoplasia of the chin. Correction with needle, subperiosteal, using approx. 1.8 ml of high G' hyaluronic acid.

CLINICAL CASES

CLINICAL CASE 3

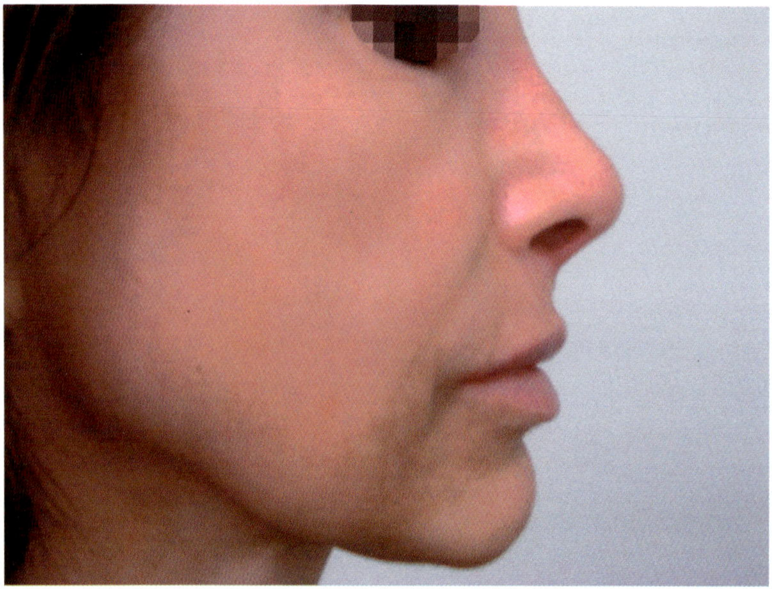

BEFORE

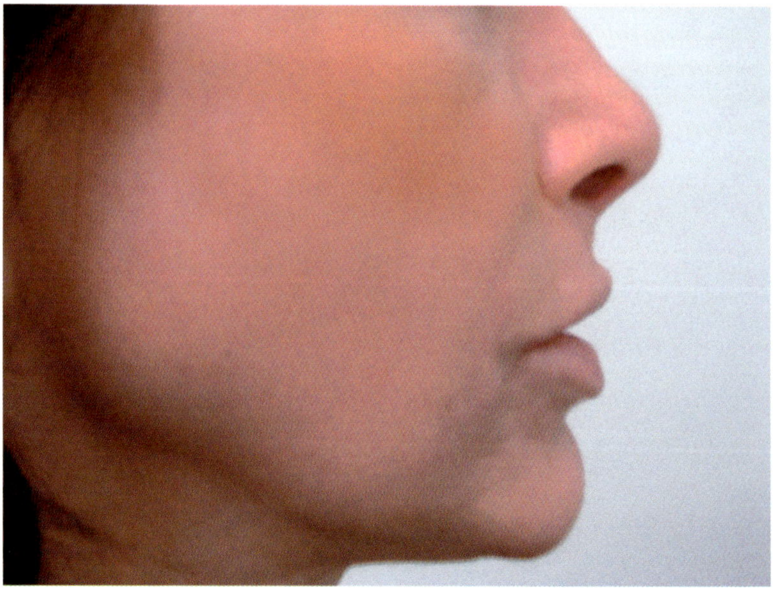

AFTER

Same patient, right profile.

CLINICAL CASES

CLINICAL CASE 3

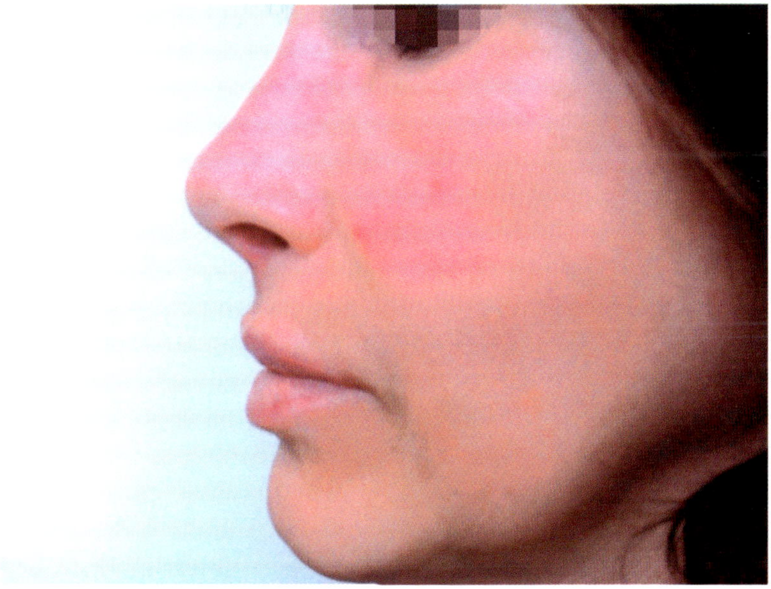

BEFORE

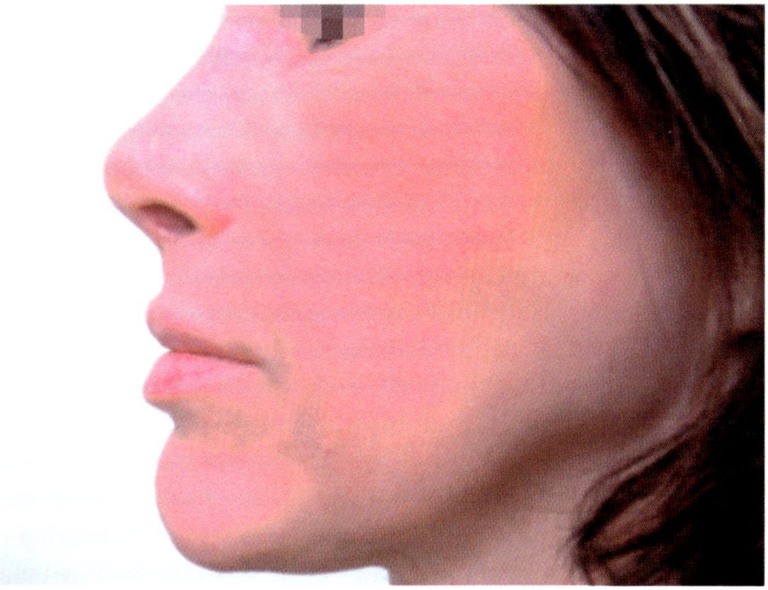

AFTER

Same patient, left profile.

10

PERIORAL REGION

Anatomy of the perioral region

Doctor Takahiko Masuda of the University of Alberta recently demonstrated, using images of real faces and digital emoticons, that the Japanese pay more attention to the eyes when interpreting other people's facial expressions, while North Americans (and Westerners in general) focus particularly on the mouth. This can only mean that, in our geographical area, the lips and perioral region takes on specific value in terms of beauty. And we do quite frequently hear talks on the small but significant details of beauty, which always include the perioral region.

Even Ovid, many and many years ago, is known to have said: "If you do not have a beautiful mouth, you will do yourself untold harm".

From an anatomical point of view, the perioral region belongs to the lower third of the face, where it is common to subdivide this already well-defined region into three further sub-regions: the upper lip region, the lower lip region and the chin region. The perioral area (fig. 1) can be subdivided into

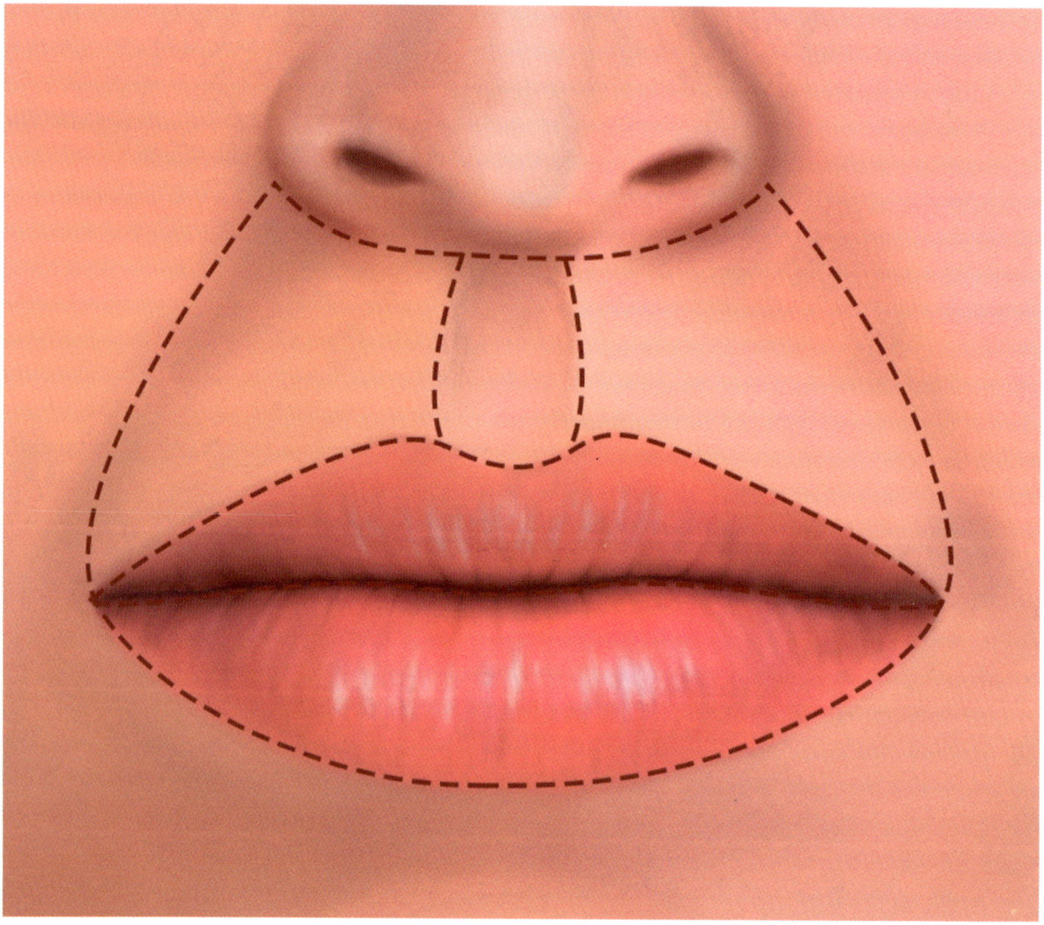

Figure 1 The subunits of the lip region

five smaller regions, all of which are of great importance, known as lateral and medial subunits.
But what is the etiopathogenesis of supralabial wrinkle formation? Undoubtedly there are several contributing factors. Intrinsic ageing, of course, which, due to the incessant movement of the orbicularis muscle, a sphincter muscle that has the sole function of opening and closing the lips, causes the formation of wrinkles due to the failed repositioning of the skin that envelops it and is no longer able to follow its continuous movements; and also extrinsic ageing and lifestyle habits. We know for certain that female smokers develop supralabial wrinkles much earlier and more deeply than non-smokers. Exposure to the sun plays an important role, as the nasal pyramid does not afford the area sufficient protection, and people rarely use adequate sunscreen. The skin also develops wrinkles due to dehydration and much more.
All this falls clearly within the anatomy of the so-called senile lip, where we see a loss of turgidity, the inversion, lengthening and flattening of the philtrum, with or without thinning of the upper lip, and excess skin tissue, found in both lips but definitely more visible in the upper lip.

Correction of the perioral region

What are the remedies and what can we reasonably do?
Besides the obvious prevention, which we must never forget to recommend, based on very rich creams with intense photoprotection properties, when supralabial wrinkles are present, there are very few options available. A good start is represented by biorevitalization or bioredensification, microinjections with a 32 G needle and possibly an electronic pen. This is a device capable of reducing algic stimuli and offering greater precision during injection, using hyaluronic acid, increasingly often with the skilful addition of minerals, amino acids and mostly antioxidants. These should be "utopistically" administered into the dermis but are more realistically injected just below, in an average of four sessions repeatable twice a year. This offers a good preparation for the skin, which must then be injected with filler to correct the defect, but we will look at that in greater detail in another chapter. Wherever there is a minus, it is always a good idea to think about how to correct it, and this can be achieved largely with dedicated fillers. So which characteristics and techniques should we use?
When we approach this correction, we must ask ourselves whether it is healthy, effective, lasting and free of side effects. The choice of filler must fall, as always but especially here where the injection space is extremely limited, to a dynamic filler that adapts to the movements of the lips. A filler that is very fluid and does not cause oedemas and undesirable swelling, which would take a long time to disappear.
The technique must also observe the rules of absolute delicacy; injection following the morphology of the wrinkle upwards, prolabium, towards the nose, using the retrograde injection technique, releasing the filler while withdrawing the needle; it must be extremely

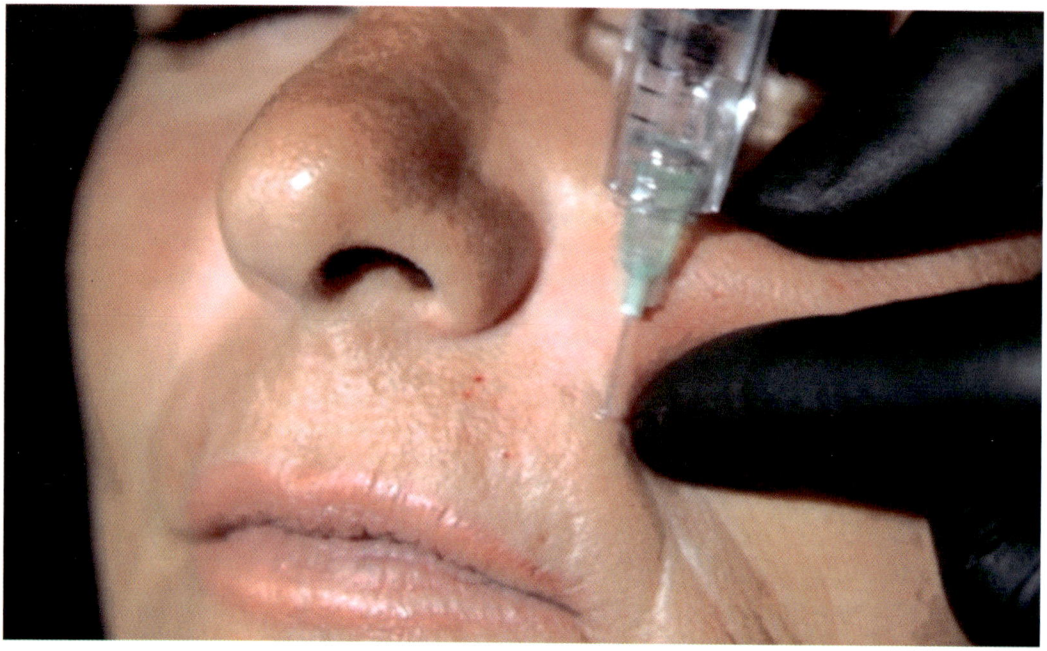

Figure 2 Correction of the perioral region: injection technique

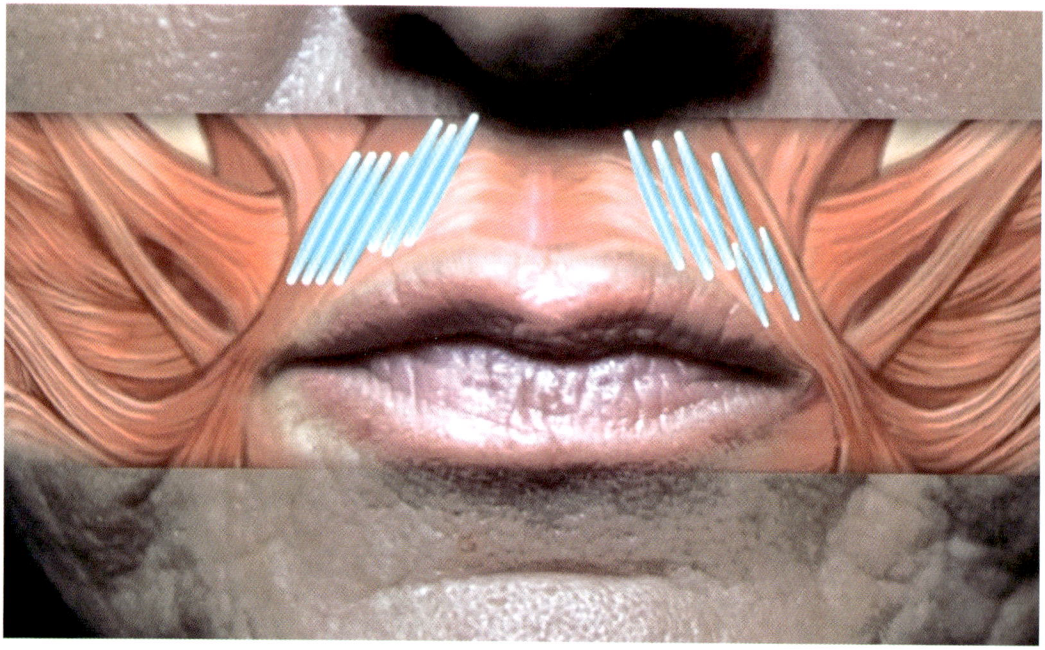

Figure 3 Correction of the perioral region: positioning the filler

gentle and leave no accumulations that could form unsightly papules, which could easily become an unpleasant and long-lasting result.
Another much more complex method is the so-called vertical linear technique, involving a series of injections that follow the perioral wrinkles in a linear way, but starting from the top, downwards to the contour of the vermilion. This enables us to simultaneously correct the supralabial wrinkles and the vermilion contour. However, we must be very careful not to go beyond the vermilion contour with the needle, because this would be very painful and would result in an unnecessary waste of filler.
Pain can be successfully overcome by applying a 32% lidocaine officinal ointment, never to be used over large areas, ten minutes beforehand, and using an electronic pen. This device, as mentioned earlier, improves the precision of the injection while reducing the imperceptible movements of the hand which cause damage and pain.
Shaping massage immediately after the injection is always helpful.

Bibliography

1. Pascali M, Quarato D, Carinci F. Filling Procedures for Lip and Perioral Rejuvenation: A Systematic Review. Rejuvenation Res. 2018 Dec;21(6):553-559.
2. Wollina U. Facial rejuvenation starts in the midface: three-dimensional volumetric facial rejuvenation has beneficial effects on nontreated neighboring esthetic units. J Cosmet Dermatol. 2016 Mar;15(1):82-8.
3. Moradi A, Shirazi A, Moradi-Poehler J, Turner J, Howell DJ. A blinded, randomized, split-face pilot study of bruising and pain with hyaluronic acid for correction of perioral lines using no lidocaine, lidocaine alone, and lidocaine and epinephrine. Aesthet Surg J. 2015 May;35(4):443-55.
4. Wollina U. Perioral rejuvenation: restoration of attractiveness in aging females by minimally invasive procedures. Clin Interv Aging. 2013;8:1149-55.

CLINICAL CASES

CLINICAL CASE 1

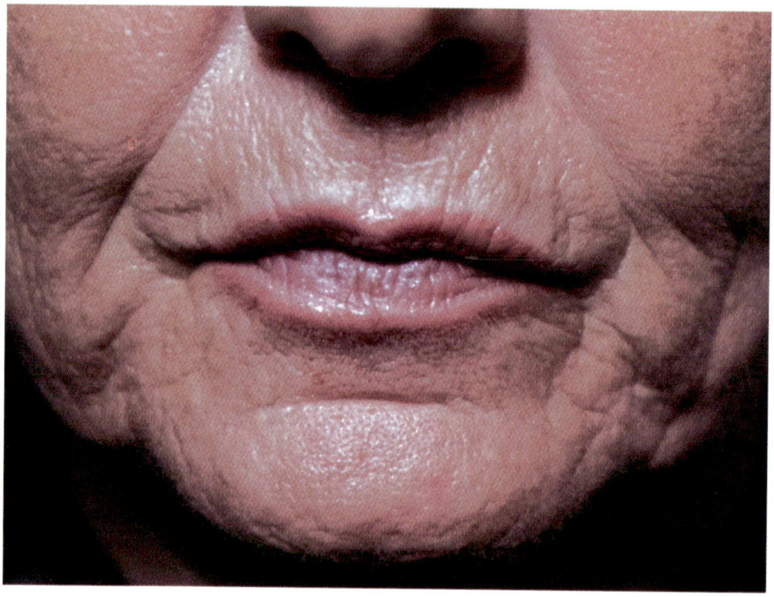

VIDEO 1

Correction of perioral wrinkles with anatomical details and graphic representation of the correction

BEFORE

VIDEO 2

Correction of perioral wrinkles comparing the linear technique with the vertical technique

AFTER

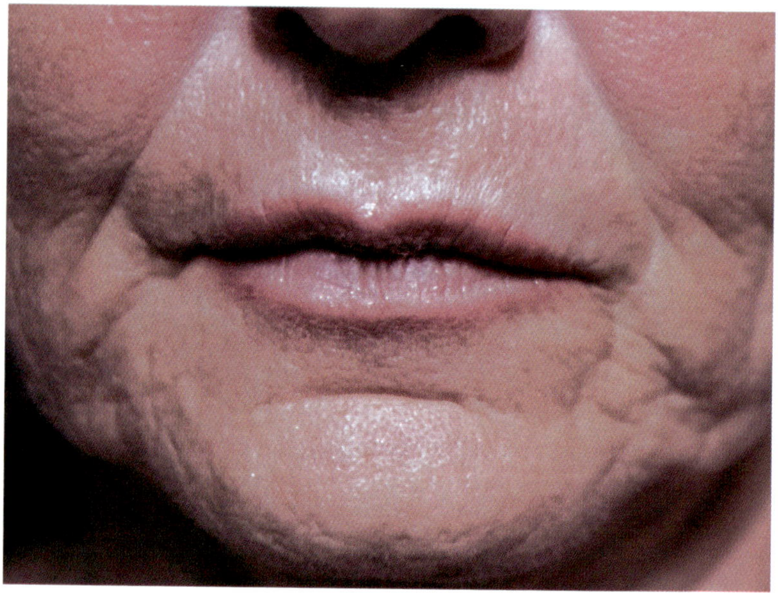

60-year-old patient, smoker, with marked photoaging. Correction of supralabial linear wrinkles, with biodynamic HA to promote adaptability to the region, injecting about 1 ml with the linear technique. Post injection shaping massage.

11

LIPS

Luana Consolini and Giuseppe Sito

Anatomy of the lips

A recent British study claims that a man's attention is drawn to the lips, especially those wearing lipstick. His eyes remain focused on them for about nine seconds, with this time falling to less than two for bare lips, dedicating less than a second to eyes and hair. But why?

It is clear that the lips, which are an important organ for more than one function, are also considered a certain sign of beauty and sensuality. This is why aesthetic doctors spin the tale that a talent for lips is tantamount to building a pension, because once a woman regains the perfect lip tone she will be hooked forever. It is no mere coincidence that, in recent years (1), lip rejuvenation and lip augmentation treatments have become some of the most sought-after aesthetic interventions. If we think of female lips, those of famous actresses such as Angelina Jolie and Scarlett Johansson immediately spring to mind. We instinctively associate the concept of fleshy lips with youth and beauty. And this is perhaps also the reason why we are inclined to exaggerate, building lips that are increasingly unrealistic, with dimensions that have completely lost touch with anatomy and physiology.

We are well aware that the beauty of the lips is a matter of just a few millimetres. Tiny corrections can make two previously anonymous lips beautiful (2). But what do we mean when we talk about "beautiful" lips? Full lips (3), proportioned and defined, set in a perioral context with no evident wrinkles (4). Aesthetic treatments should therefore focus not

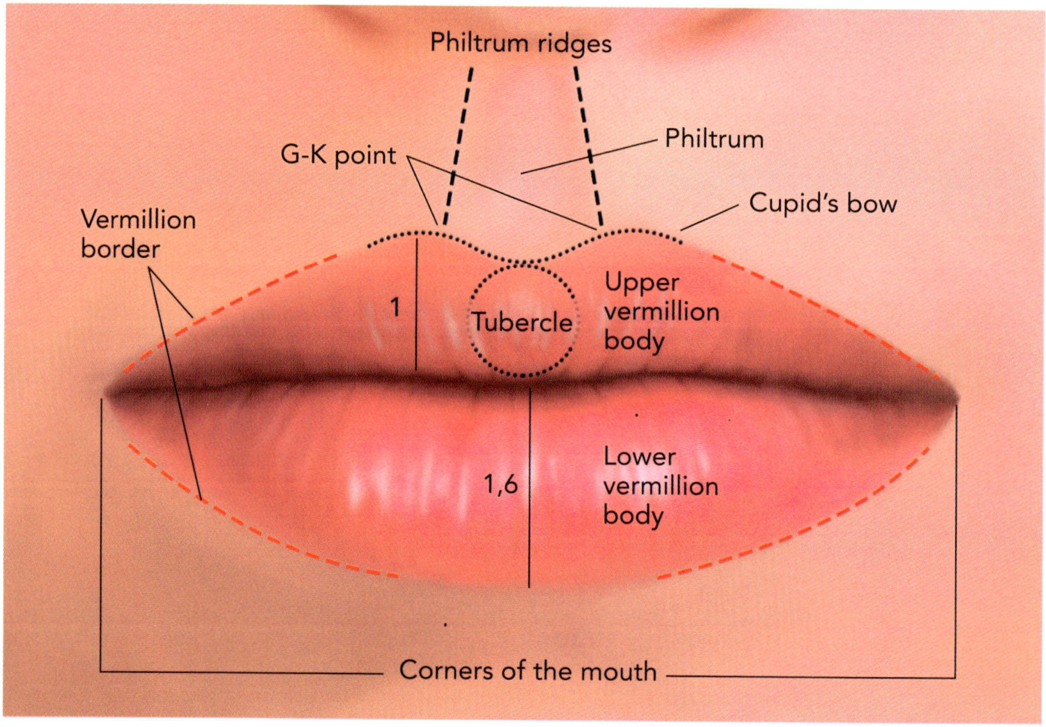

Figure 1 Macroanatomy of the mouth

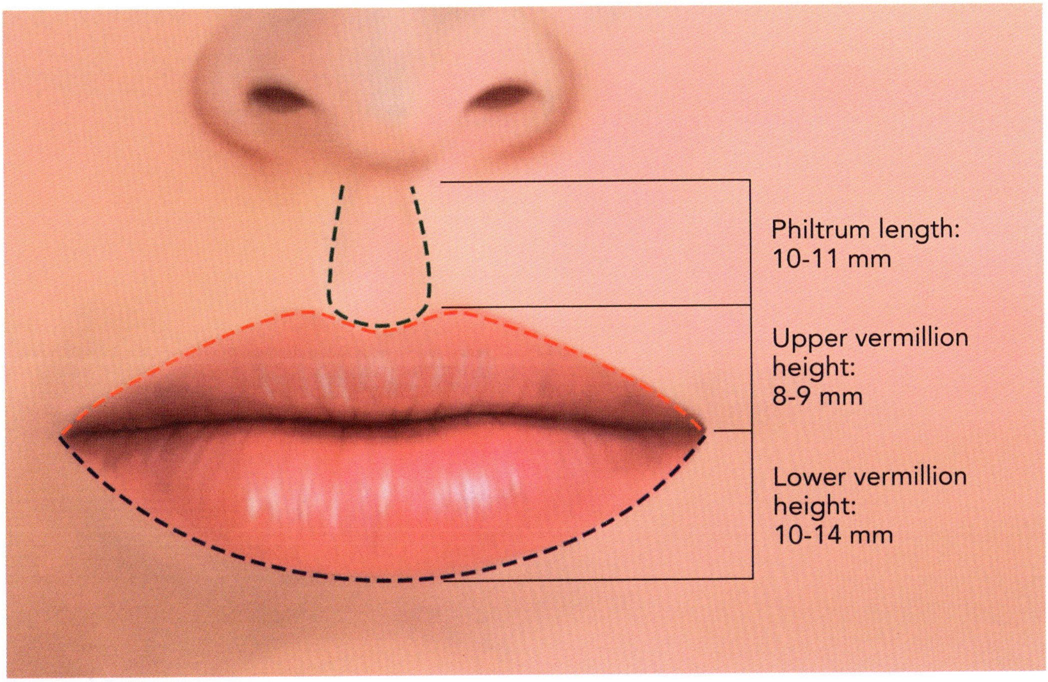

Figure 2 Microareas of the perilabial region

only on the vermilion, but on the entire area surrounding the lips (5), which includes two macro-regions (fig. 1):

> the upper lip, consisting of the upper vermilion and the white lip. The latter represents the skin area furrowed centrally by the philtrum and bordered above by the nasal base, below by the border of the upper vermilion and laterally by the nasolabial folds;;

> the lower lip, which extends from the lower vermilion to the lateral commissure and the mandible (below).

The macro-regions then include three different microareas, each characterised by a defined ideal height, which changes over time.

Lips that capture our attention, which we unconsciously find attractive, have specific measurements. There seems to be a perfect combination of characteristics that allows us to classify certain types of lips as objectively beautiful. According to Hoefflin (2), lips should have an upper vermilion height of 8-9 mm and a lower vermilion height of 10-14 mm (fig. 2). Similarly, when proportioned, the lips have a Cupid's bow and a defined lip contour, as well as a golden ratio of 1:2 between the volume of the upper and lower lips (6) (fig. 1). This specific proportion has been the key factor for the harmony of a face since ancient times. Suffice to say that the same ratio also governs the length and width of the face, for example, the position of the mouth in relation to the chin and eyes or the lip contour.

Literature also indicates the ideal dimensions of the philtrum, which would seem to correspond to a length of 10-11 mm (2) and a width of 12-15 mm (7) (fig. 2). Like every other area of the face,

VIDEO 1

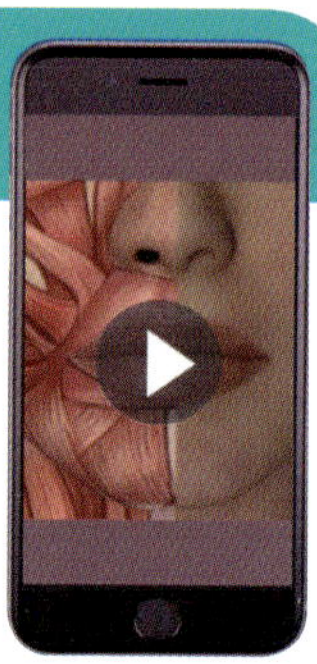

Graphic representation of the anatomy of the lips

this too is subject to an incessant ageing process that involves its progressive lengthening and flattening to values of over 20 mm (7,8,9).

Young lips share some common characteristics. In the upper lip we find a typical, centrally positioned protrusion (median tubercle), which complements a depression in a specular position on the lower lip. This is flanked by two lateral tubercles responsible for the typical lower lip protrusion. In addition to this we have the Cupid's bow, with its characteristic M shape, which perfectly outlines the ridges of the philtrum (10) (fig. 3).

The overall ageing of the perioral region is highly subjective and depends on different processes (photoaging, genetics, maxillo-mandibular bone resorption, smoking, etc.) which often occur simultaneously. These factors can affect the volume and length of the lips, their shape, the degree of vermilion inversion and the length of the

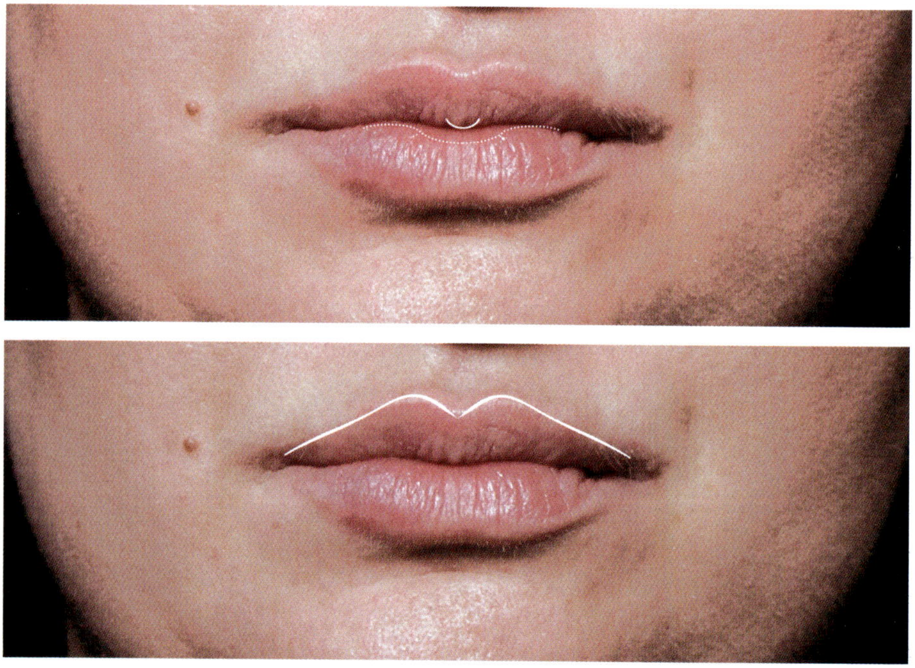

Figure 3 Above, upper vermilion (highlighting the central tubercle) and lower vermilion (highlighting the median depression and two lateral tubercles). Below, the detail shows the typical youthful shape of the Cupid's bow

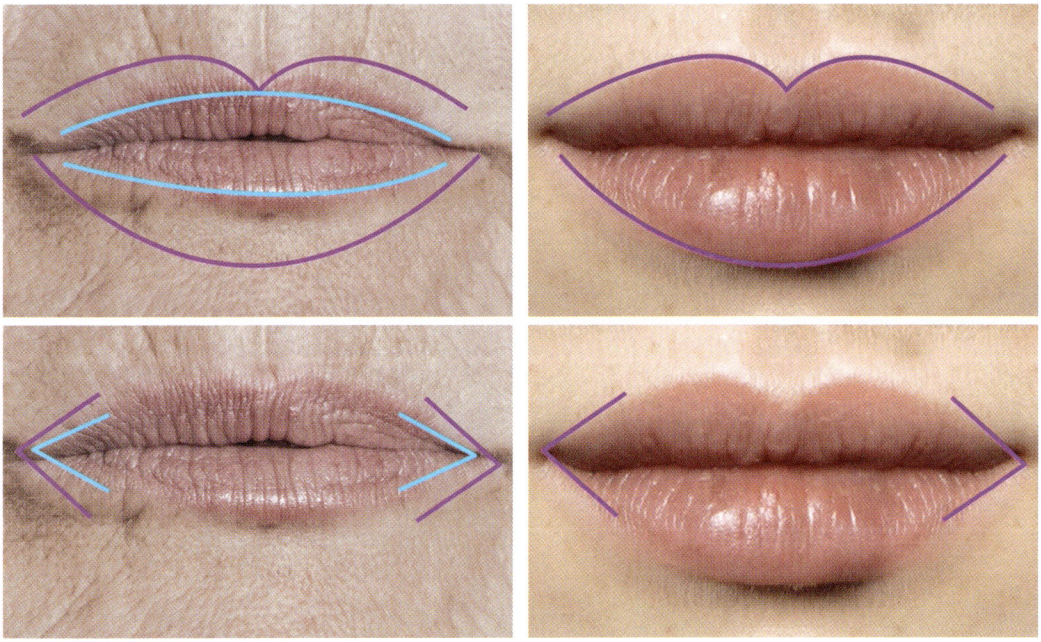

Figure 4 Comparison of lip shape, length and volume. Left: a 68-year-old woman. Right: a 25-year-old woman

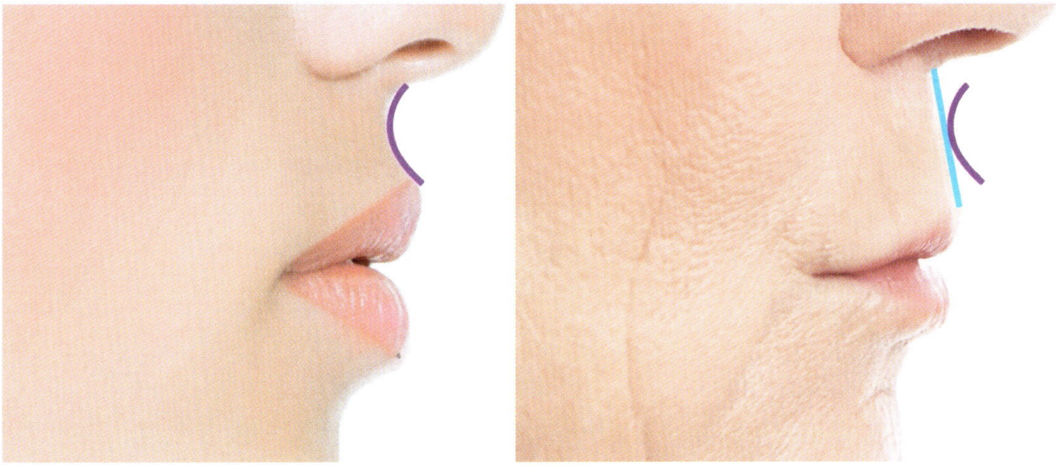

Figure 5 How the lips change as we age: comparison of lip profile. Left: concave profile (25 years old). Right: flat and convex profile (68 years old)

philtrum. Contrary to popular belief in the past, recent studies have shown that, in most cases, lip thinning is due to a redistribution of the muscular volume of the lip rather than a real loss of volume (11) (fig. 4).

In other words, the length of the lips increases while the height of the vermilion decreases, with thinning of the skin, degeneration of collagen and elastin

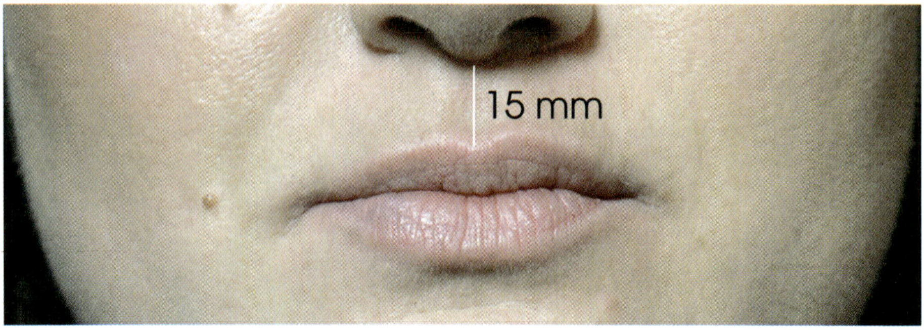

Figure 6 Slight-moderate elongation of the philtrum (15 mm)

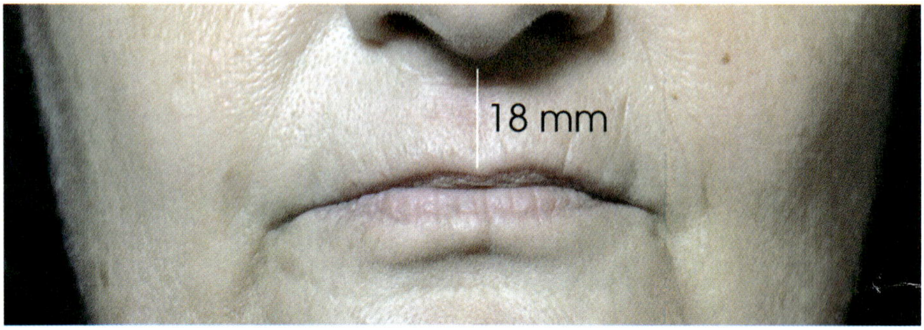

Figure 7 Advanced elongation of the philtrum (18 mm)

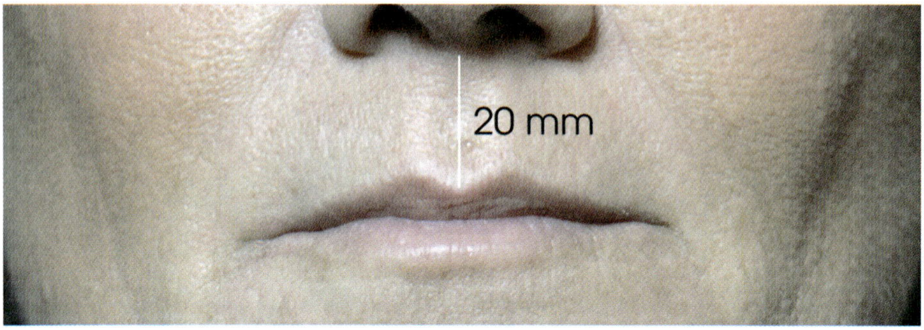

Figure 8 Severe elongation of the philtrum (20 mm)

fibres and an overall reduction in the curvature of the orbicularis oris muscle, which reduces lip projection and results in an unsightly inversion of the upper vermilion (labial ptosis) (10). The Cupid's bow, previously defined by marked G-K points (Glogau-Klein points) (fig. 1), becomes flat (12).
Seen from the side, the lips lose their characteristic concavity, the philtrum becomes flat and long. The lips droop towards the chin area (fig. 5).
As demonstrated by numerous studies, the lengthening of the philtrum seems to be proportional to age (7,13,14). Three different age classes can be identified (7). The first, between the ages of 25 and 45, undergoes light-moderate

philtrum elongation to between 15 and 17 mm (fig. 6). The second, between the ages of 45 and 65, presents advanced elongation to between 17 and 19 mm (fig. 7). And the last, over the age of 65, presents severe philtrum elongation to more than 19 mm (fig. 8). The upper vermilion becomes thinner and more introflected as a result of the lengthening of the philtrum and the resorption of fatty tissue and alveolar bone. The narrow, concave Cupid's bow (fig. 9) takes on a convex profile with a flattened, elongated vermilion (fig. 10).

In addition to the elongation of the philtrum and the thinning of the vermilion, many patients also complain of the formation of perioral wrinkles. The ptosis of the perioral skin tissue, combined with the loss of tone in the angular depressive muscle of the mouth, changes the characteristic angle of the labial commissure. From being concave with a slight upward bend (fig. 11a), the lateral commissures first become horizontal (fig. 11b), before rotating and taking

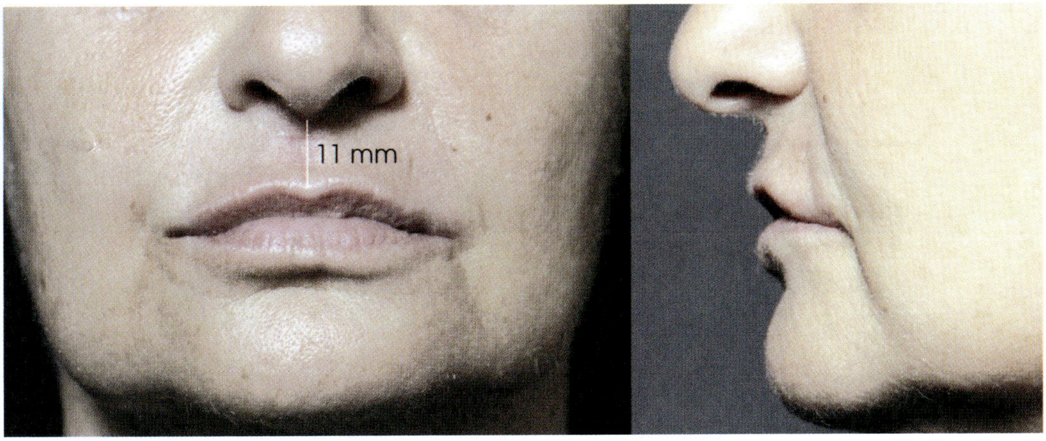

Figure 9 Youthful lips: defined Cupid's bow and lip contour, philtrum with ideal length

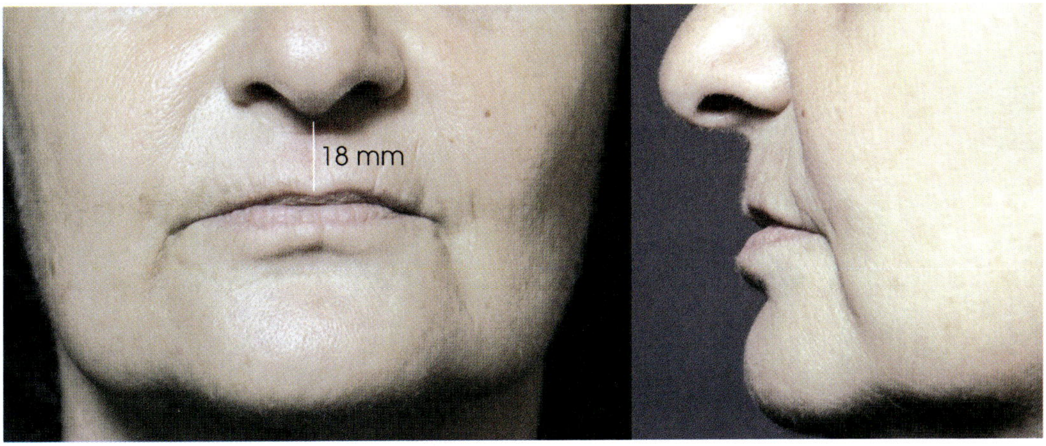

Figure 10 Aged lips: thinning and elongation of the upper vermillion, reduction of the labial projection (inversion of the upper vermillion)

on a characteristic downward curve (10) (fig. 11c). Overall, the nasolabial folds and labiomental creases become accentuated, forming what are known as marionette lines (10) (fig. 12).
The impact of all these parameters on the beauty and harmony of the lips is broadly acknowledged. Just think about the lip characteristics that our mind associates with youth and those it associates with being old. Almost all observers will think of thin lips that have lost their characteristic heart shape and elongated philtrum as being aged lips (15,16).

Lip treatment technique

Thanks to the results obtainable and the excellent safety profile, hyaluronic acid is now the most widely used substance for the treatment of ageing lips and perioral area (6). There is no fatty tissue plane in the lips, so hyaluronic acid can be injected superficially (dermis) or deeply (submucosa, above the orbicularis oris muscle), depending on the specific rheology of the gel (fig. 13).

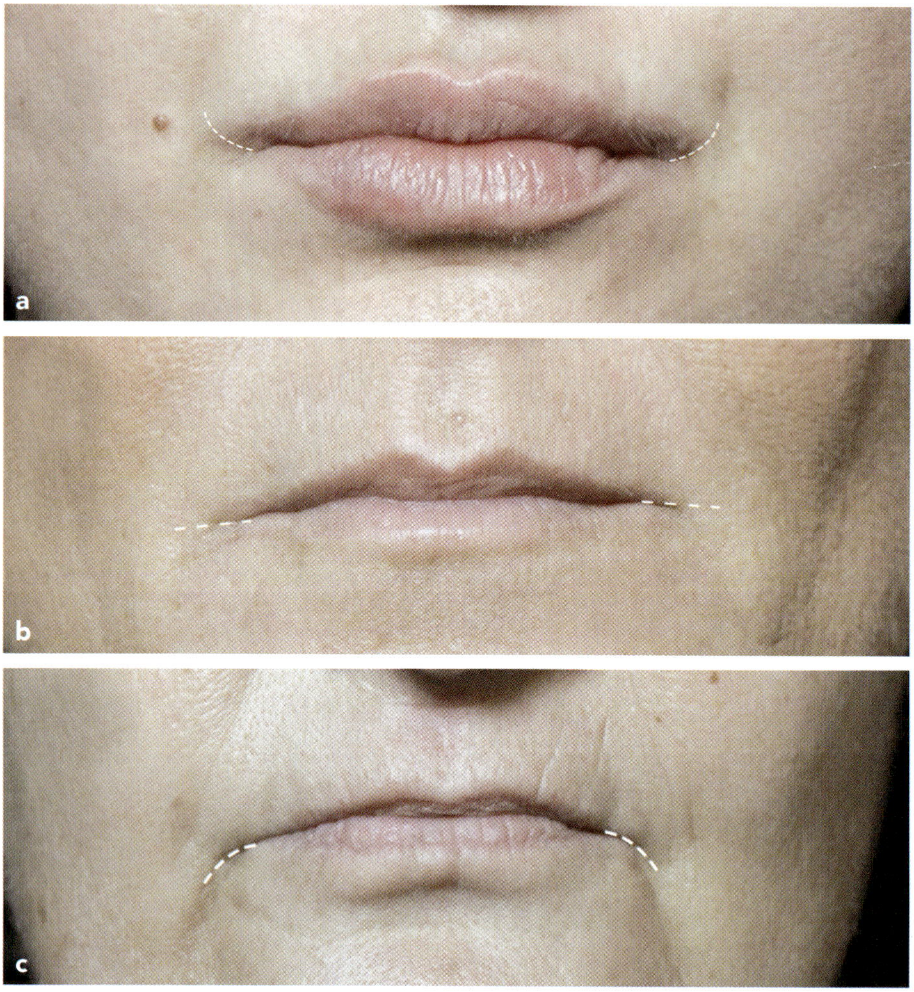

Figure 11 Ageing of the mouth: alteration of the lip commissures with age

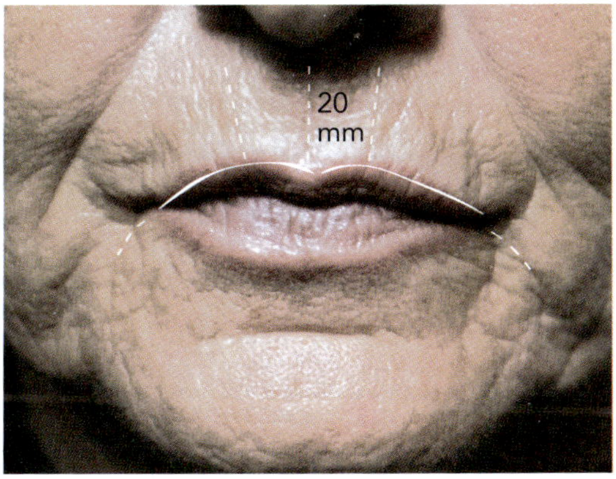

Figure 12 Ageing of the mouth: alteration of the lower third with age

VIDEO 2

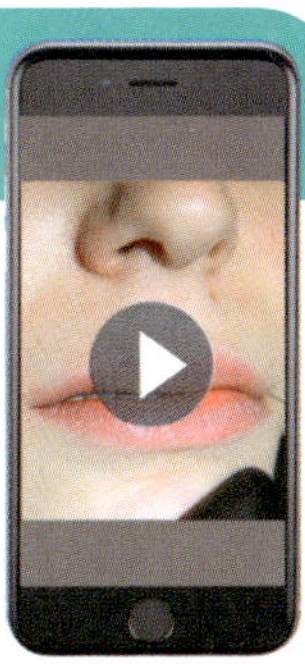

Lip correction with electronic syringe

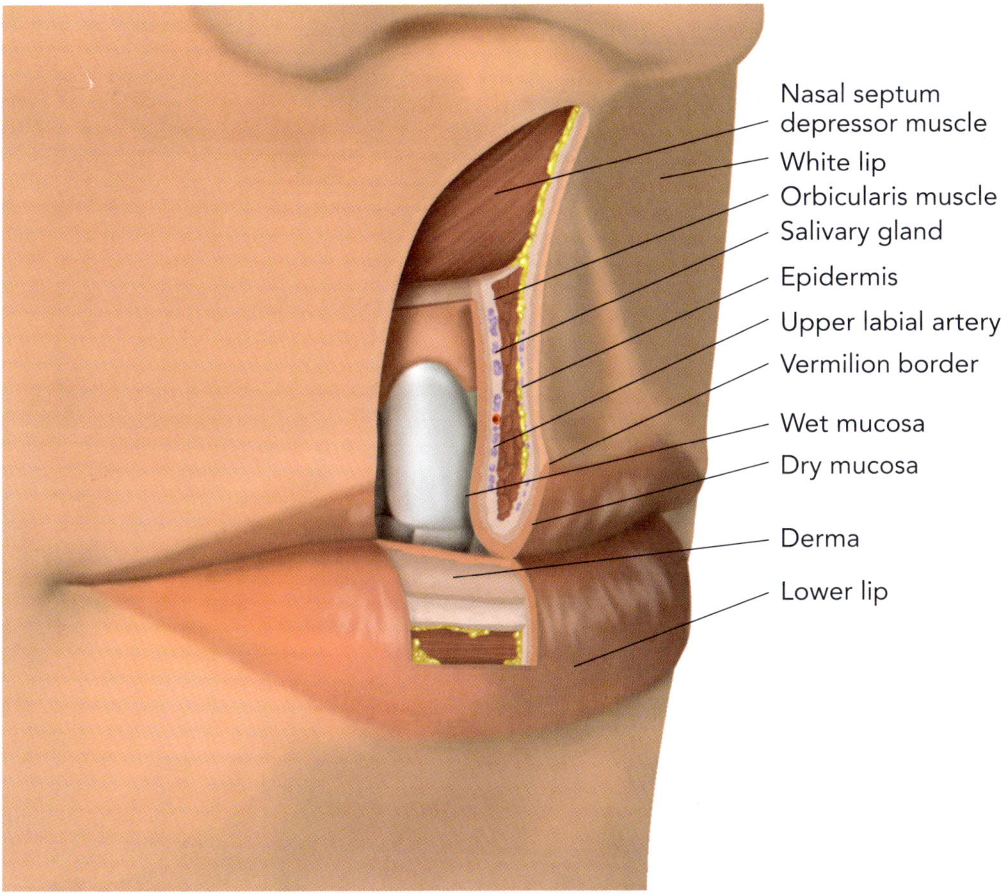

Figure 13 Cross-section of the graphic anatomy of the lip

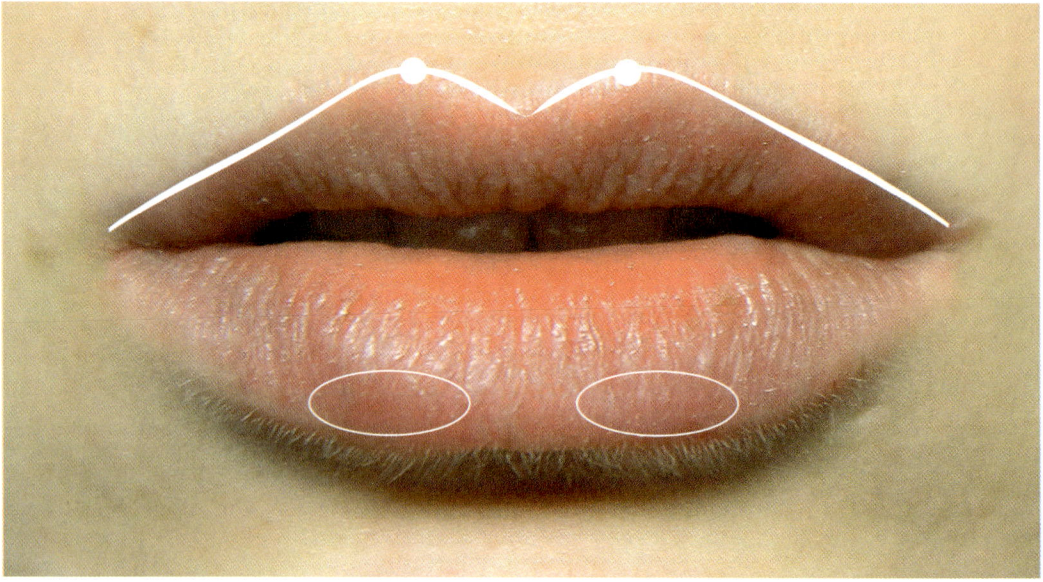

Figure 14 Treatment of the lip contour: upper and lower vermillion border, G-K points

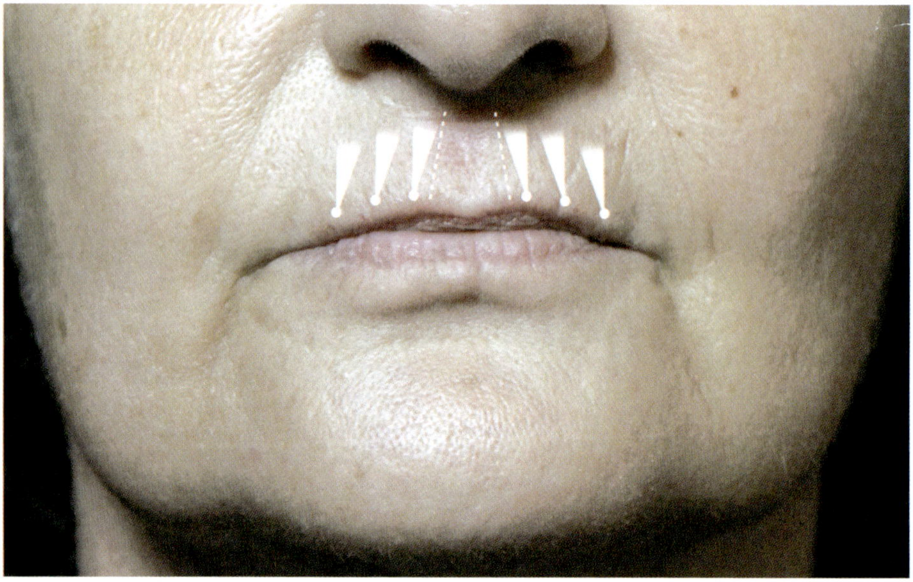

Figure 15 Treatment of the white lip

It should never be injected in intramuscular positions, due to the short duration of the deposit (and consequently the correction), and to the real risk of intravascular injections.

The procedure usually begins with the correction of the shape of the lips, with injection at the border of the vermilion (fig. 14). This is followed by the treatment of the white lip and a redefinition, if necessary, of the philtrum ridges (fig. 15). Lastly, when you want to increase the

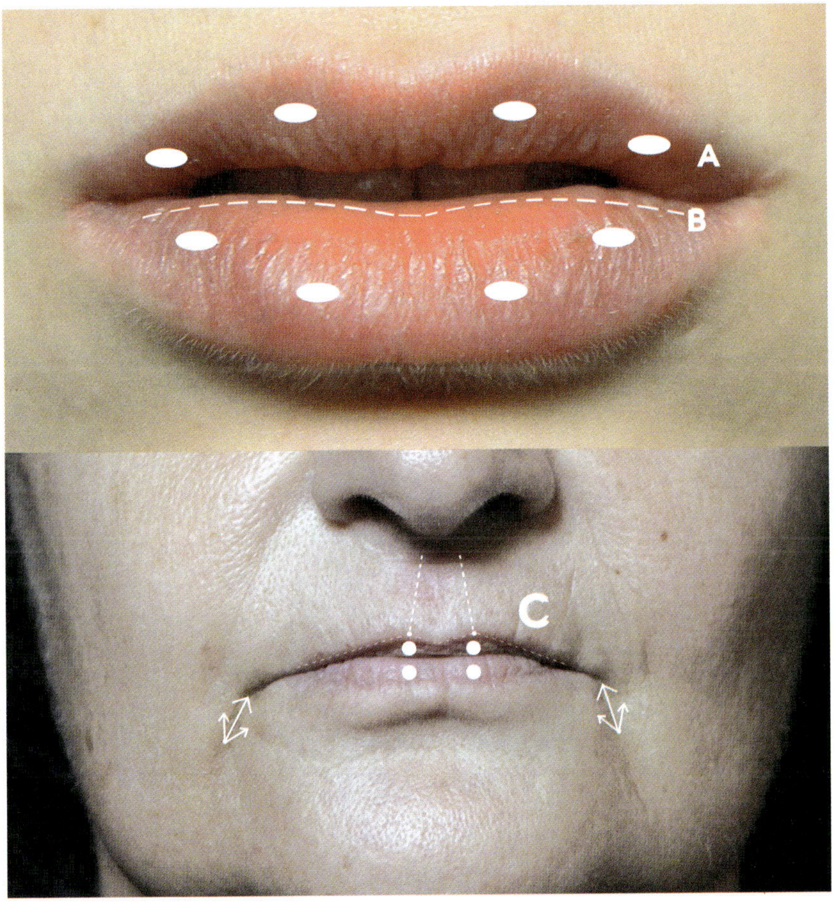

Figure 16 Lip augmentation. A) Positioning of the filler just below the vermilion border; B) positioning of the filler immediately between the dry mucosa and the orbicularis muscle; C) positioning of the filler in the vermilion body (submucosal)

volume of the lips or improve the proportion between the upper and lower lips, inject deep into the body of the upper and/or lower vermilion (10,17,18) (fig. 16).

Vermillion line treatment

We start with a slow injection along the border of the upper vermilion, from the sides to the Glogau-Klein points of the Cupid's bow (fig. 14).

> Product quantity: 0.6-0.7 ml.
> Position: between the red lip and the white lip (at about 1/3 of the height of the white lip), to redefine the lip contour.
> Technique used for the vermilion border: linear retrograde.
> Technique used to define the Cupid's bow: Paris lip or injection from the centre towards the G-K points.

Aesthetic result: demarcation of the lip contour and Cupid's bow, overall lifting of the upper lip, increase in vermilion projection, reduction in perioral wrinkles (10).

Perioral wrinkles on the upper and lower lips

Inject into the white lip, along the perilabial wrinkles, from the border towards the centre of the upper lip (fig. 15). If necessary, the lower white lip can also be treated.

> Product quantity: 0.3-0.4 ml, occasionally 0.5-0.6 ml.
> Position: deep subcutaneous, to avoid the formation of lumps.
> Technique used: layering also in microboluses using the electronic device and a 32 G-0.4 mm needle.

Aesthetic result: restoration of the typical concavity of a young lip, delicate redefinition of the philtrum ridges, reduction of the philtrum length, reduction of perioral wrinkles around the upper and lower lips (10).

Lip augmentation

Inject into the upper and lower vermilion bodies and into the lateral commissures.

> Product quantity: 1 ml.
> Position A: just below the border of the vermilion, at a height of 1.5-2 mm and 2 mm from the lip contour (10). Suggested for slight correction of the lip volume (fig. 16A).
> Position B: in the border of the dry mucosa (10). Recommended for increasing the height and volume of the upper lip (fig. 16B).
> Position C: deep injection (submucosal) into the body of the vermilion, level with the incisors. Should be followed by massage to reduce the perception or visibility of the filler. In particularly thin lips, follow up with slight correction of the lip contour and near the philtrum (fig. 16C). Recommended to increase the volume of the upper and/or lower lip and for the correction of flat and thin lips.

Aesthetic result: increase in volume, correct proportion between upper and lower lips, restoration of convexity and correct projection of the lips (upper lip inversion).

Lastly, when it comes to the treatment of thin lips, we must consider that:

> often the lack of fullness of the lips depends on the flattening and lengthening of the philtrum rather than on the lips themselves. In these cases, inject superficially into the border of the vermilion and/or the white lip, in particular to redefine the philtrum ridges. The linear retrograde technique is used. This treatment improves the inversion of the upper lip and reduces the perceived length of the philtrum;
> in young patients, the increase in volume is concentrated mainly in the central third of the vermilion body, but it is sufficient to correct the lip contour to obtain fuller lips, avoiding exaggerated correction;
> in elderly patients, injection deep into the entire body of the vermilion is recommended, also to encourage a reduction in frequently associated vertical lip wrinkles. However, it is necessary to consider the progressive atrophy endured by the lips over time (11). We know that the greater the atrophy, the greater the risk of an unnatural aesthetic result. In senescent lips, it can be helpful to reduce the amount of hyaluronic acid injected into the vermillion body, associating the treatment with a

more superficial redefinition of the lip contour and philtrum ridges (19). Naturally, a more fluid, less viscous and strongly elastic hyaluronic acid should be preferred;

> injection can be carried out using different techniques, including linear retrograde, preferably, or multibolus injection. The linear technique is highly recommended too, starting from the anti-oral margin and descending with the needle. It must always be extremely superficial without ever crossing the prolabium, but the utmost attention must be paid to avoid perforating the border of the vermilion, which would be extremely painful and imprecise. The correct plane is deep, never intramuscular, but more submucosal.

Materials: filler characteristics

When considering which is the most appropriate treatment for the patient, in addition to the technique and the right injection plane, it is essential to consider the rheological characteristics of the filler. The ideal rejuvenation of the lips is based on two factors: an increase in the volume of the vermilion, the definition of its contour and of the structure of the philtrum.

Filler for lip augmentation

From a rheological point of view, the filler must have a G′ elastic modulus and intermediate cohesion, allowing it to maintain its shape and conferred projection, as well as to resist decomposition and the forces of compression generated by the contraction of the underlying labial muscles (6,20). To avoid the perception of the implant, the correct position is on a deep plane, and always submucosal, particularly in elderly patients or patients with thin lips.

Filler for lip contour enhancement

Frequently requested by young patients with normal to fleshy lips or by older patients as a complement to augmentation (6,19). From a rheological point of view, the gel should be soft, with low G′ and cohesion, high stretching capacity and minimal hygroscopic activity. This is a highly dynamic area, subject to repeated mechanical stress due to contraction and stretching. We advise against the use of rigid fillers or fillers with high viscoelasticity, which could cause unevenness and unsightly accumulations of the product. Lower viscoelasticity combined with high stretching capacity increases the dermal integration of the gel, stabilising its position and favouring a natural correction.

Lastly, we must remember that the continuous stress placed on the lips increases the risk of gel fragmentation and oedema. This is why it is important to use a filler with a high and proven resistance to decomposition. The availability of new dynamic rheology fillers (medium-high stretch and strength values, lower G′, high tissue integration) could represent an interesting opportunity for this type of correction.

The specific rheology of dynamic fillers depends on the preservation of the natural bonds of the hyaluronic acid molecule, impossible until now with traditional methods (21,22). Dynamic

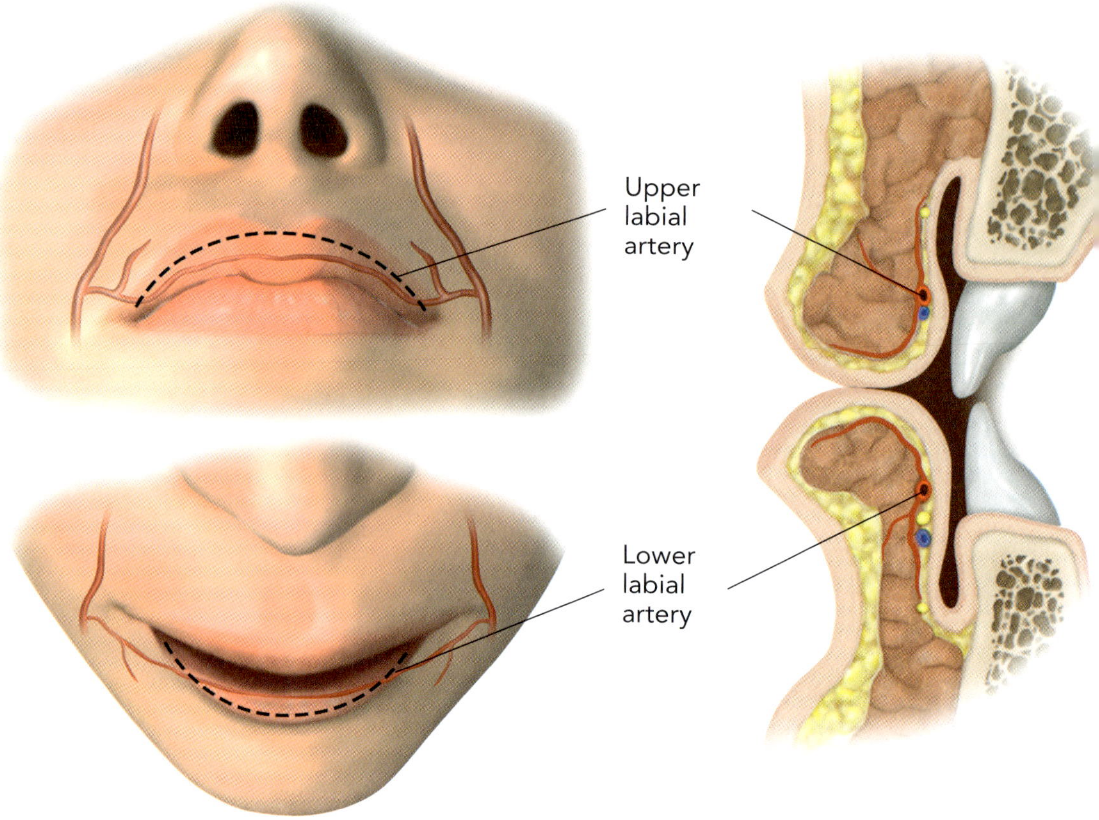

Figure 17 Vascularization of the lips

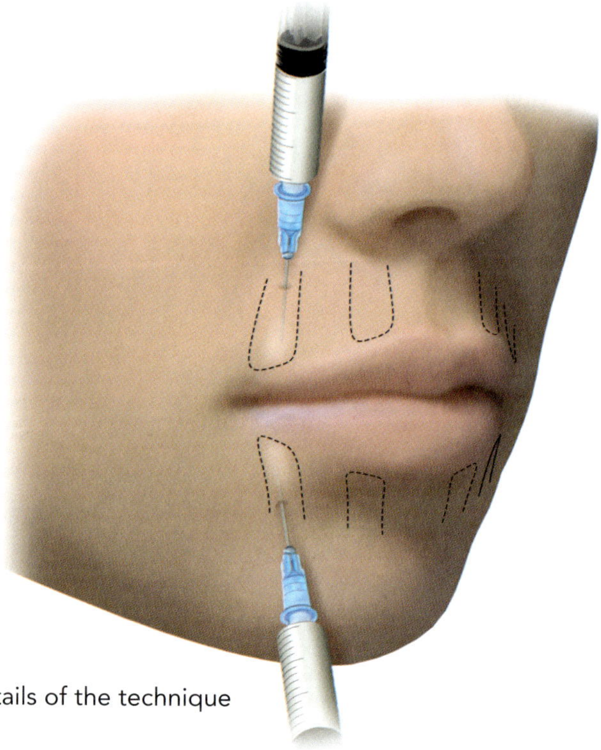

Figure 18 French Kiss: details of the technique

VIDEO 3

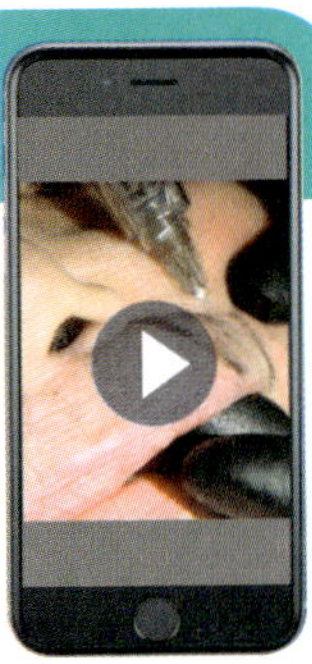

Lip correction using the French Kiss technique and electronic syringe

rheology studies (23,24) have shown that it is precisely the preservation of these bonds that preserves the length of the hyaluronic acid chains, allowing reduced fragmentation of the gel in hydrophilic and hydrophobic environments. All this translates into a higher safety profile (less risk of oedema) and a lower risk of asymmetry.

As far as positioning is concerned, the filler is injected into the superficial dermis using very thin needles. In conclusion, the technique is standardised and very simple. Retrograde injection of modest amounts of product along the entire border of the vermilion and into the philtrum ridges, if required and if necessary.

The French Kiss technique

One last technique has recently appeared in the already vast panorama of aesthetic techniques for the lips: French Kiss. This is a method dedicated to the inversion of the vermilion, both in the upper and lower lips, which is not free from risks and, most importantly, must be practised with the necessary experience and by very expert hands.

From cadaveric observation we know that the distance of the superior and inferior lip arteries, both of which are direct branches of the facial artery, varies between 0.4 mm and 0.7 mm: minimal distances that must place us at a sufficient distance from the risk of embolization (fig. 17).

The first phase is represented by using a pen to draw the division of each upper hemilabrum into three equal parts; this will give us a starting point that coincides with the apex of the commissure, an intermediate point at 1/3 and another point, after another 1/3. The same goes for the other upper hemilabrum.

On the lower lip, starting from the midline, we will draw just two points, 1/3 from the midline.

Keeping a gloved finger in the prolabium, we will cross the distance from the dry to the wet lip with the needle, remembering the average distances of the labial arteries and avoiding them, injecting about 0.2 of dedicated lip filler, obtaining from four to six accumulations that will be palpable inside the prolabium. We will then vigorously massage them, so that the patient goes home with no noticeable swelling and after scrupulously observing that there are no blanched areas, which could indicate initial ischemia.

The clinical effect will noticeably lift the area concerned, enhancing the projection (fig. 18).

It is important to observe the lips in the immediate vicinity of the implant, to identify the need for partial and not total correction, because beauty is made up of details, not size.

Bibliography

1. Byrne PJ, Hilger PA. Lip Augmentation. Facial Plast Surg. 2004. Feb; 20(1): 31-8.
2. Hoefflin SM. The Definition of Facial Beauty. In Aesthetic Surgery of the Facial Mosaic 43-51. Springer, Berlin, Heidelberg, 2006.
3. Segal L, Ellis DA. Therapeutic options for lip augmentation. Facial Plast Surg Clin North Am. 2007 Nov; 15(4): 485-90.
4. Dickinson BP, Roy I, Lesavoy MA. Temporalis fascia for lip augmentation. Ann Plast Surg. 2007 Feb; 23(1):21-6.
5. Cartier H, Trevidic P, Rzany B, Sattler G, Kestemont P, Kerrouche N, Dhuin JC. Perioral rejuvenation with a range of customized hyaluronic acid filler: efficacy and safety over six months with a specific focus on the lips. J Drugs Dermatol. 2012 Jan; 11(1 Suppl): s17-26.
6. Sarnoff DS, Gotkin RH. Six steps to the "perfect" lip. J Drugs Dermatol. 2012;11(9):1081-1088.
7. Zankl A, Eberle L, Molinari L, Schinzel A. Growth charts for nose length, nasal protrusion, and philtrum length from birth to 97 years. Am J Med Genet. 2002;111(4):388-391.
8. Ramirez OM, Khan AS, Robertson KM. The upper lip lift using the 'bull's horn' approach. J Drugs Dermatol. 2003;2(3):303-306.
9. Perenack J. Treatment options to optimize display of anterior dental esthetics in the patient with the aged lip. J Oral Maxillofac Surg. 2005;63(11):1634-1641.
10. Azib N, Charrier J-B, Cornette de Saint Cyr B, Criollo-Lamilla G, Dmitrieva I, Garcia P, Gout U, Iblher N, Lemaire T, Noël X, Padey H, Pavicic T, Penna V, Surlemont Y, Stark G.B, Trévidic P, Verner I; Clinical Analysis of the ageing lip. In: Patrick Trèvidic, Stèphanie Heavey, eds. Anatomy & Lip Enhancement. Vitry-sur-Seine France: E2e Medical Publishing Expert; 2013: 54-55.
11. Iblher N, Kloepper J, Penna V, Bartholomae JP, Stark GB. Changes in the aging upper lip--a photomorphometric and MRI-based study (on a quest to find the right rejuvenation approach). J Plast Reconstr Aesthet Surg. 2008;61(10):1170-1176.
12. Klein AW. In search of the perfect lip: 2005. Dermatol Surg. 2005;31(11 Pt 2):1599-1603.
13. Feingold M, Bossert WH. Normal values for selected physical parameters: an aid to syndrome delineation. Birth Defects Orig Artic Ser. 1974;10(13):1-16.
14. Farkas LG. Anthropometry of the head and face. Raven Press, 1994.
15. Aiache AE. Rejuvenation of the perioral area. Dermatol Clin. 1997;15(4):665-672.
16. Guerrissi JO. Surgical treatment of the senile upper lip. Plast Reconstr Surg. 2000;106(4):938-940.
17. Chiu A, Fabi S, Dayan S, Nogueira A. Lip Injection Techniques Using Small-Particle Hyaluronic Acid Dermal Filler. J Drugs Dermatol. 2016;15(9):1076-1082.
18. Lemperle G, Anderson R, Knapp TR. An index for quantitative assessment of lip augmentation. Aesthet Surg J. 2010;30(3):301-310.

19. Penna V, Stark GB, Voigt M, Mehlhorn A, Iblher N. Classification of the Aging Lips: A Foundation for an Integrated Approach to Perioral Rejuvenation. Aesthetic Plast Surg. 2015;39(1):1-7.
20. Pierre S, Liew S, Bernardin A. Basics of dermal filler rheology. Dermatol Surg. 2015;41 Suppl 1:S120-S126.
21. Pomarède N. Injection d'acide hyaluronique [Hyaluronic acid injection]. Ann Dermatol Venereol. 2009;136 Suppl 6:S287-S289.
22. Practical Aspects of Hyaluronan Based Medical Products. CRC Press (2005). Available at: https://www.crcpress.com/Practical-Aspects-of-Hyaluronan-Based-Medical-Products/Kuo/p/book/9781420037647. (Accessed: 12th March 2018)
23. Converset-Viethel S, et al. Safety and effectiveness of three new dynamic fillers for the treatment of moderate to severe nasolabial folds: An 18-month randomized controlled trial versus competitors. AMWC 2016 Monaco Available at: https://teoxanetrainingcenter.com/sites/default/images/downloads/studi_clinici/RHA_Studio_clinico_18_mesi.pdf. (Accessed: 12th March 2018)
24. Sundaram H, Rohrich RJ, Liew S, et al. Cohesivity of Hyaluronic Acid Fillers: Development and Clinical Implications of a Novel Assay, Pilot Validation with a Five-Point Grading Scale, and Evaluation of Six U.S. Food and Drug Administration-Approved Fillers. Plast Reconstr Surg. 2015;136(4):678-686.

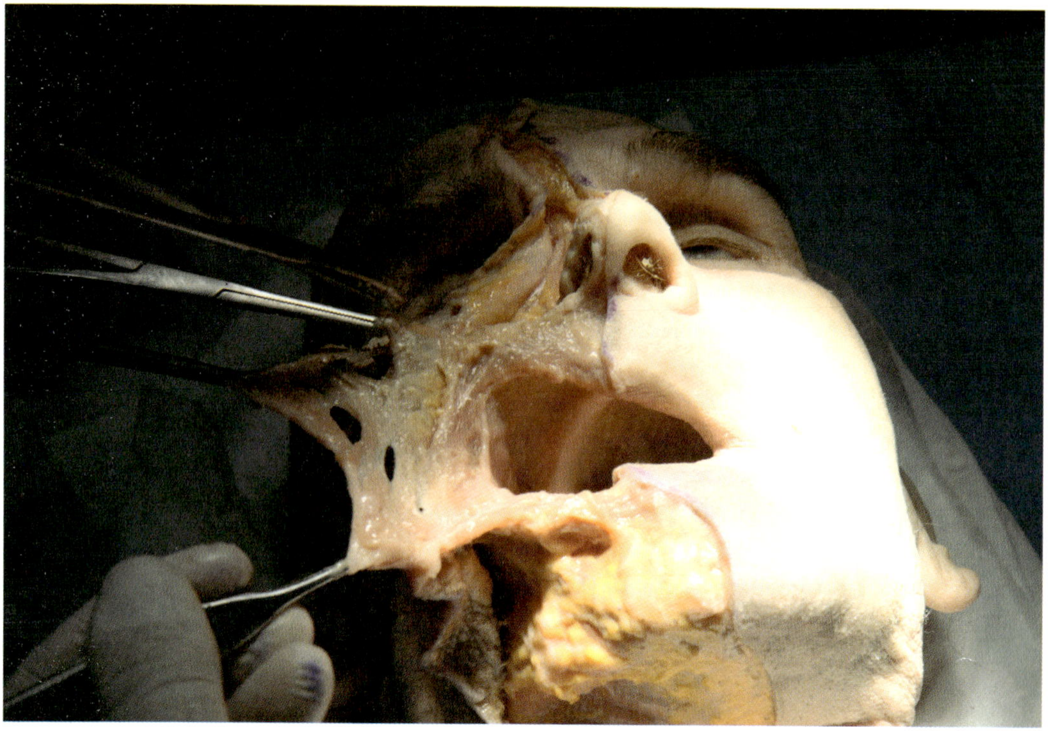
Facial artery in an anatomical preparation

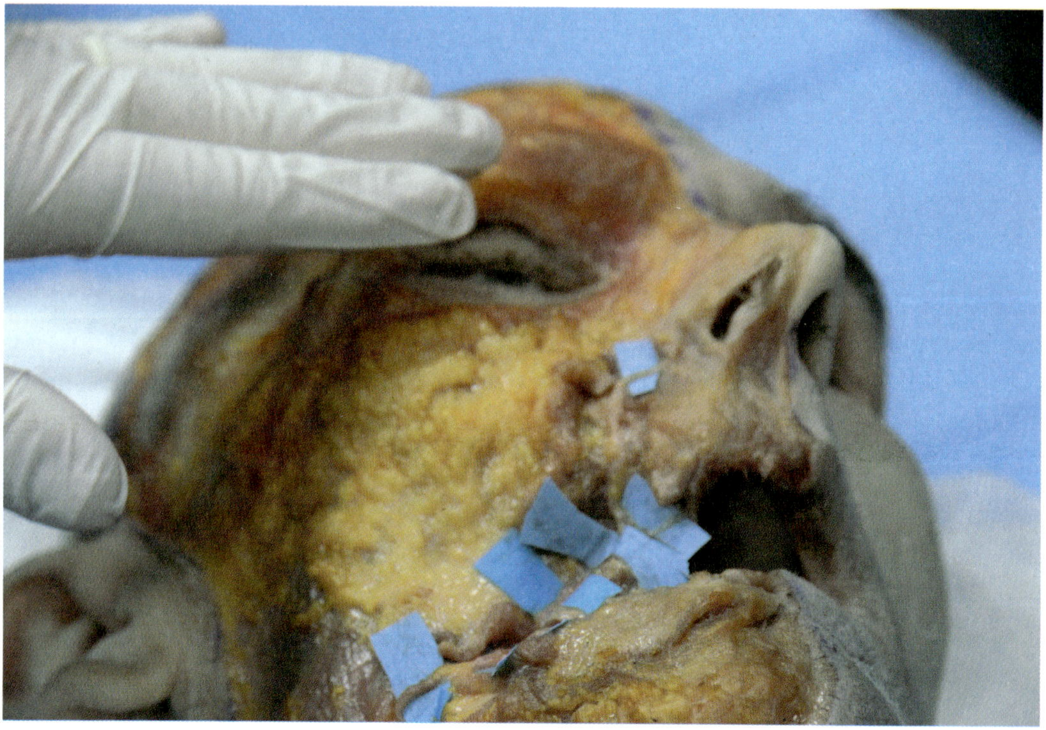
The progress of the facial artery in an anatomical preparation

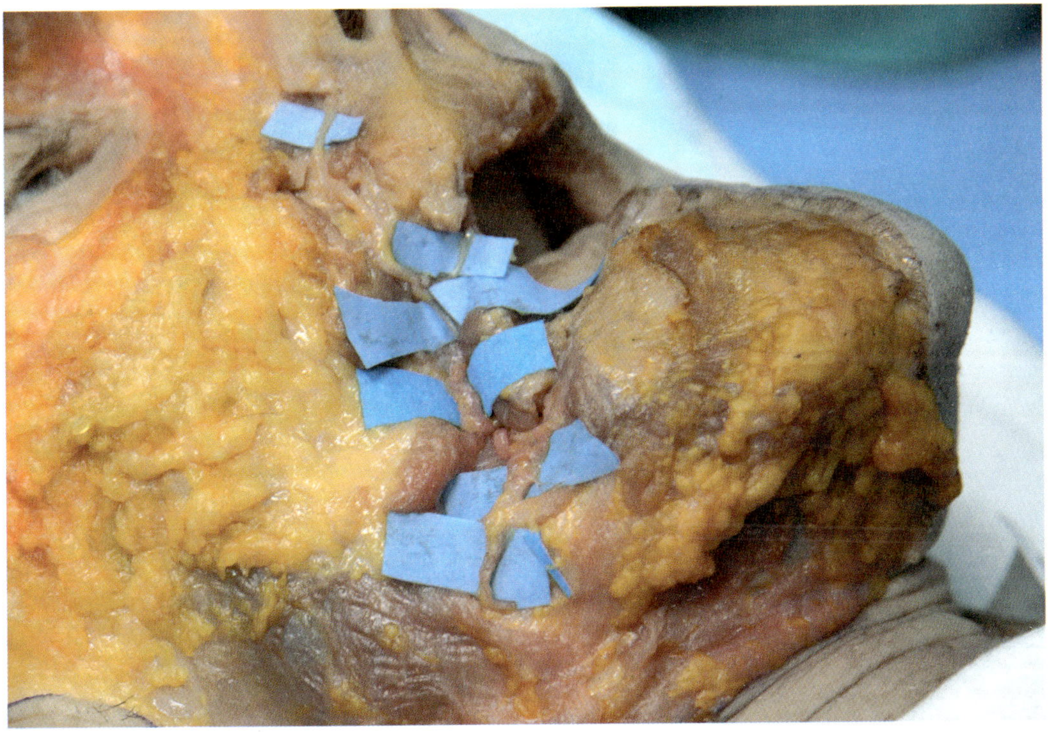

Origin of the labial arteries in an anatomical preparation

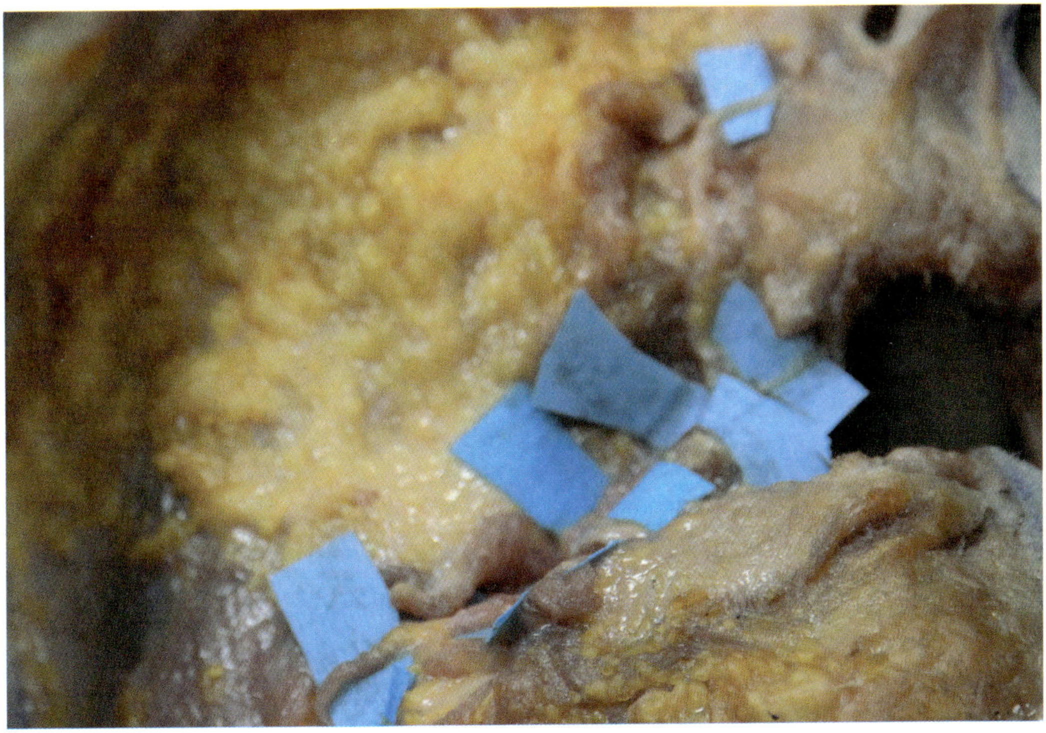

Detail of the progress of the facial artery

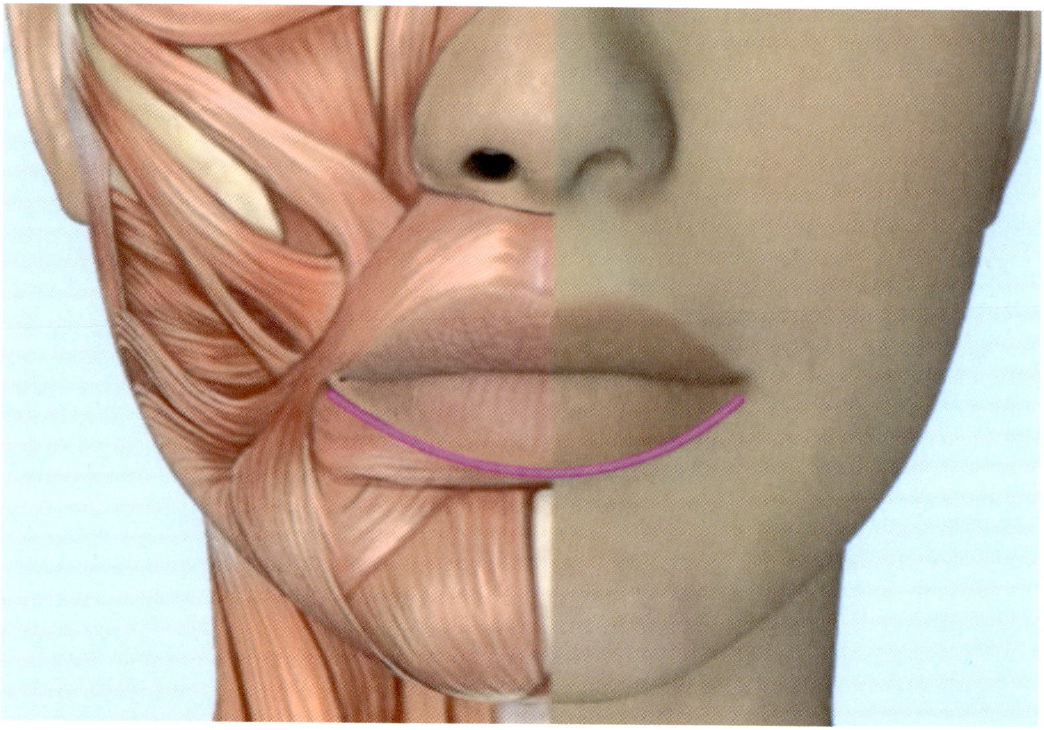

Graphic representation of the anatomy of the lips

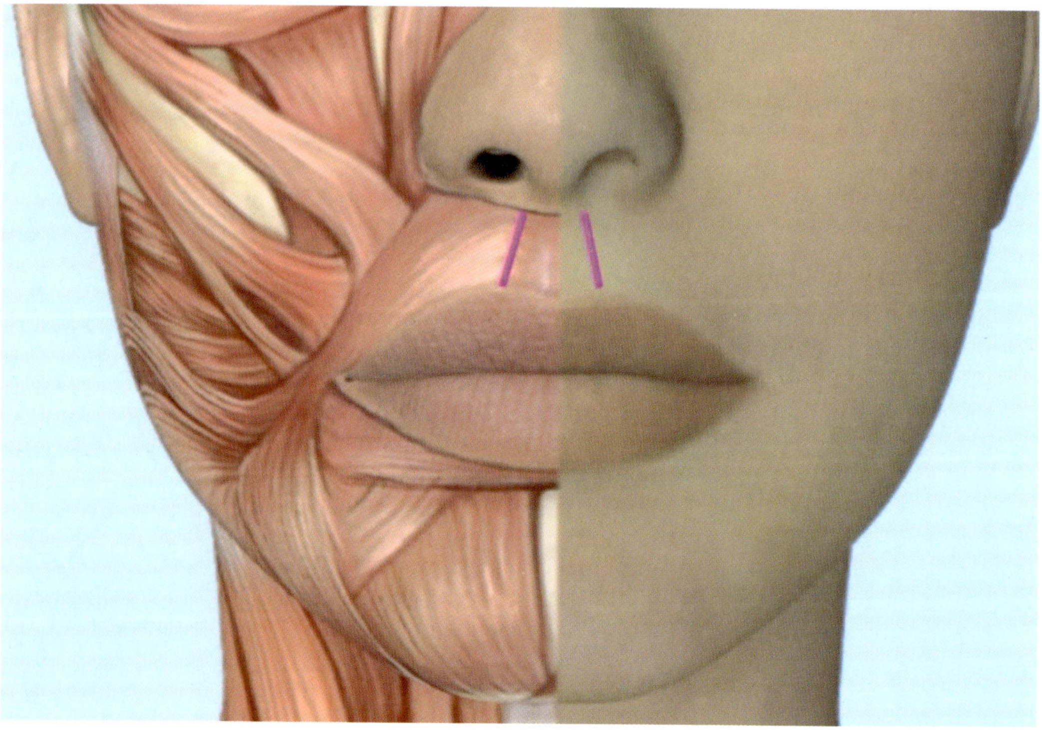

Graphic representation of the anatomy of the lips

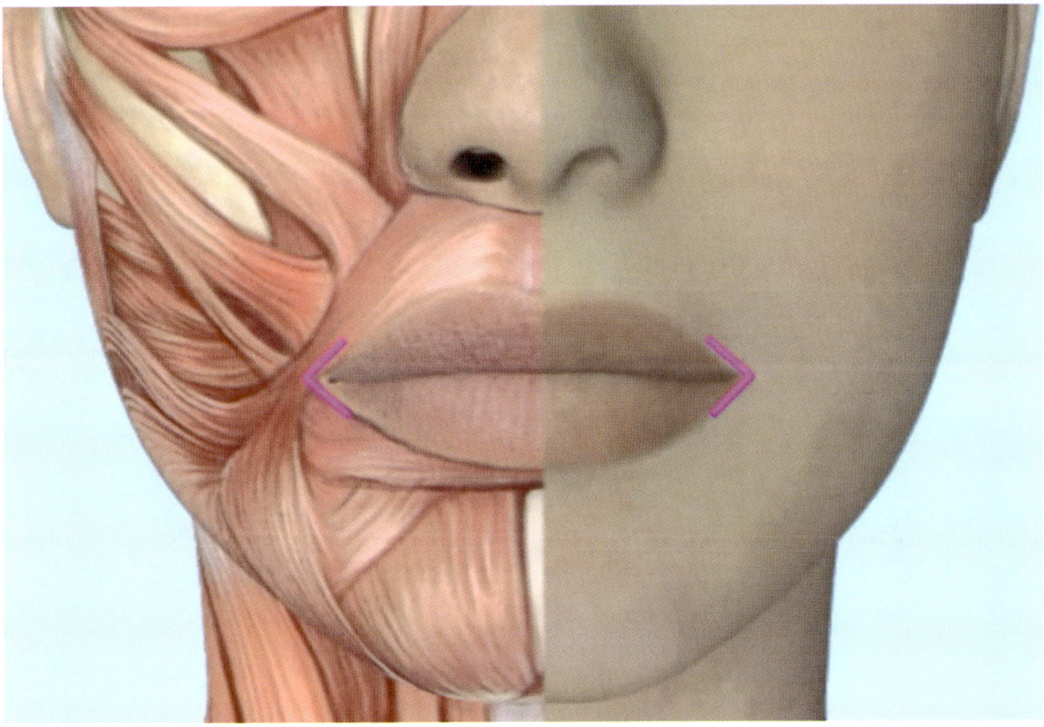

Graphic representation of the anatomy of the lips

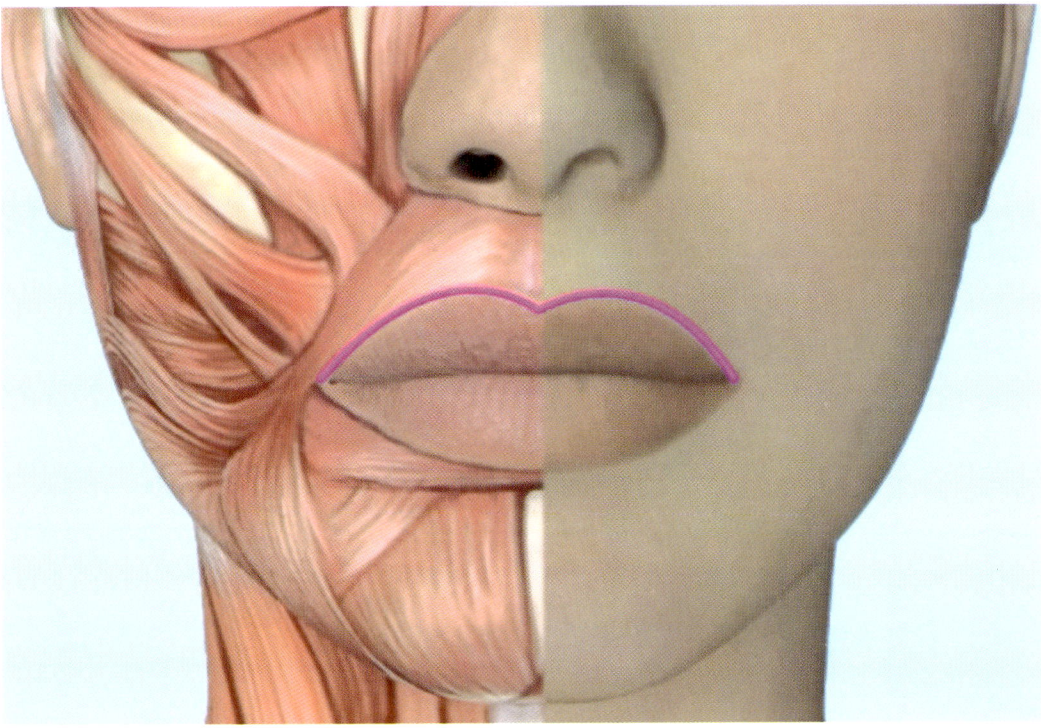

Graphic representation of the anatomy of the lips

CLINICAL CASES

CLINICAL CASE 1

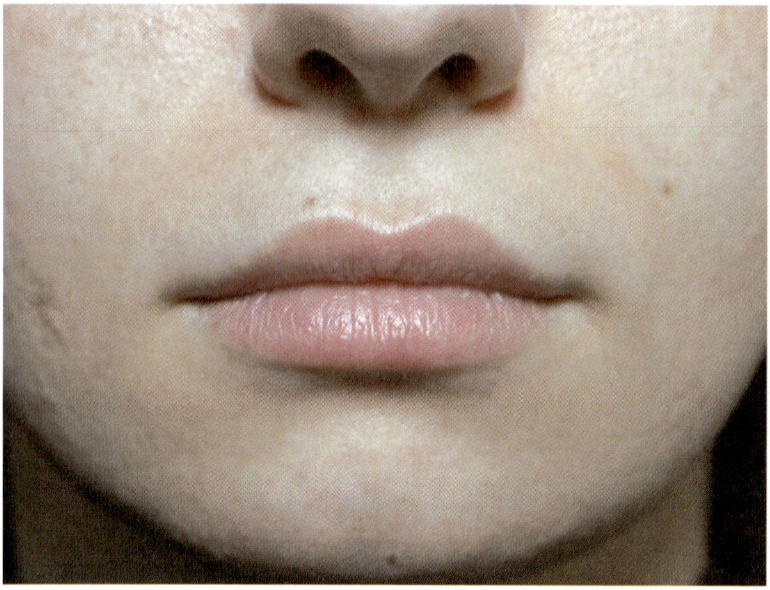

BEFORE

<

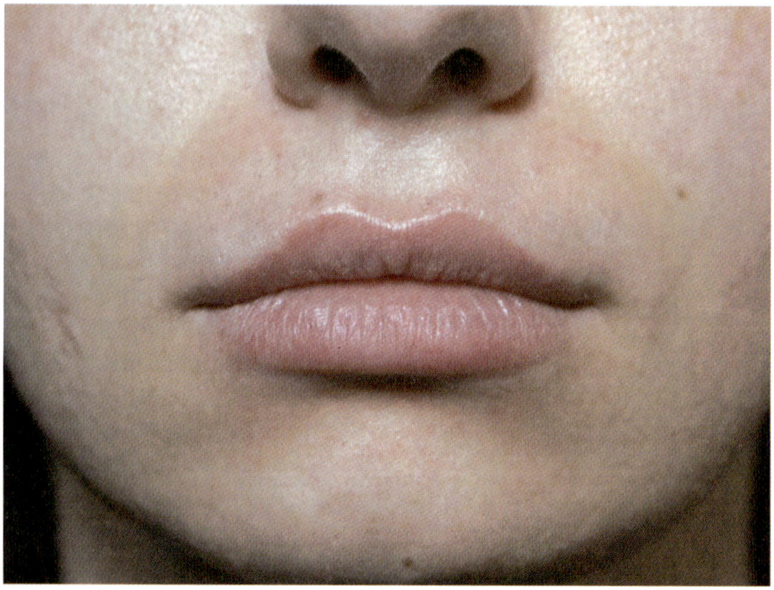

AFTER

>

30-year-old patient requiring emphasis of the lips. Injection of 1 ml of medium G′ HA in order to emphasise the contour. Injection into the vermilion line.

CLINICAL CASES

CLINICAL CASE 2

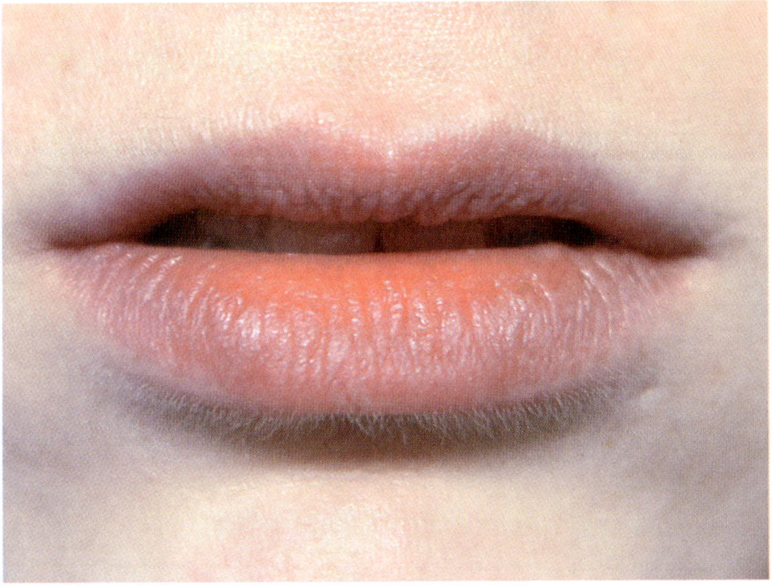

BEFORE

AFTER

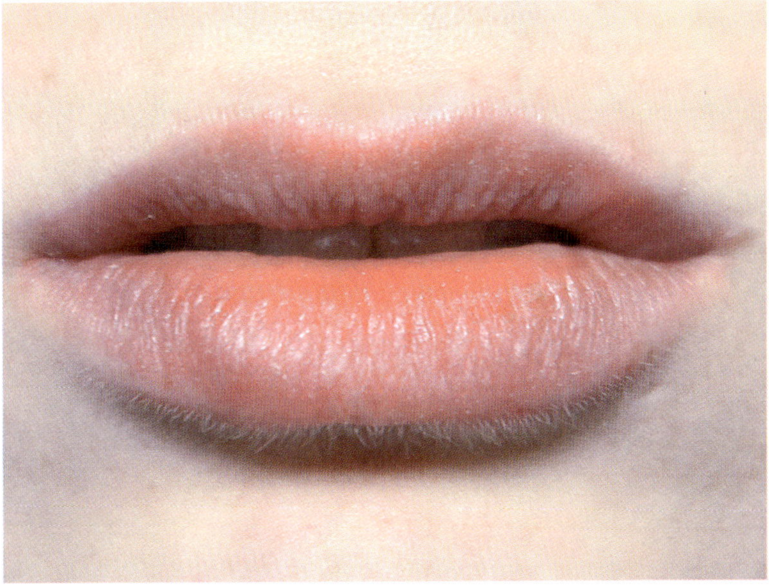

Young patient with good existing lip representation. Desire for enhanced significance. Injection of 0.7 ml of HA, with 0.4 ml in the lower lip and 0.3 ml in the upper lip, using the linear technique in the vermilion. Resilient hyaluronic acid in order to provide volume and duration.

CLINICAL CASES

CLINICAL CASE 3

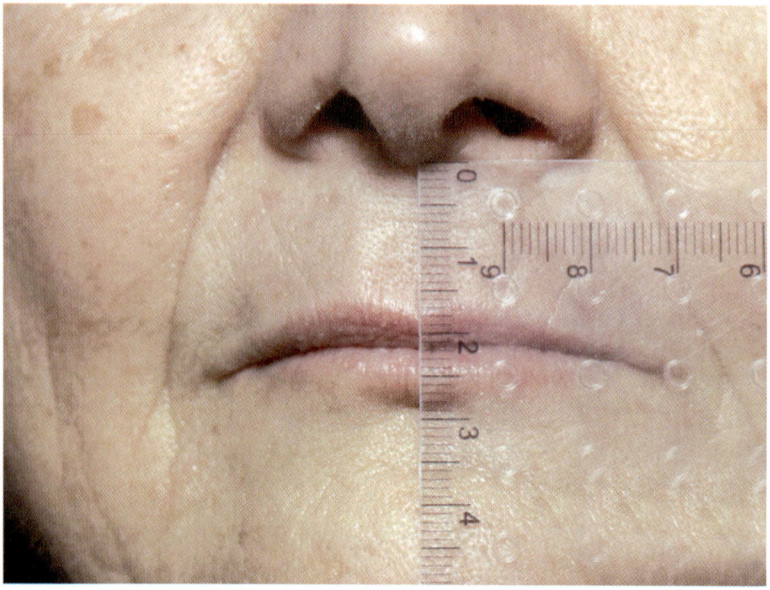

BEFORE

<

AFTER

>

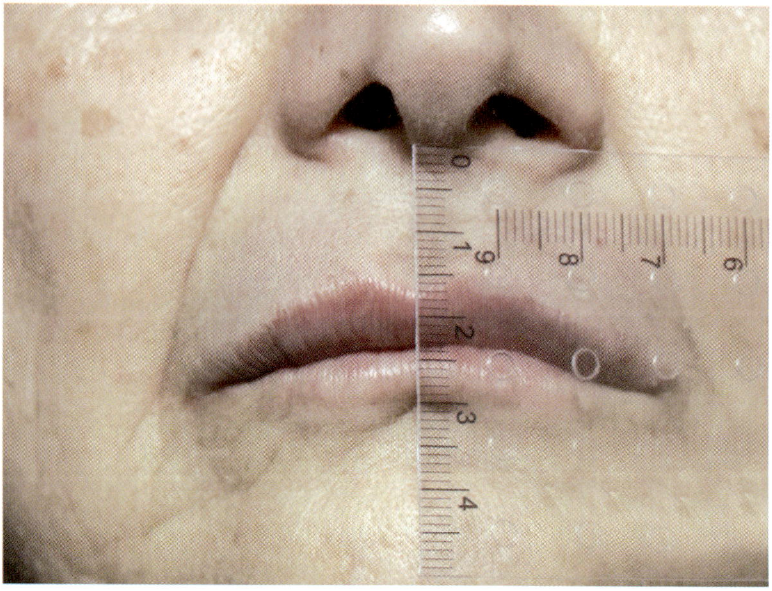

Senescent patient with elongated philtrum (1.8 cm) and almost complete disappearance of the philtrum ridges. Correction with 1.5 ml of medium density, biodynamic HA, with reconstruction of the philtrum and its ridges, and augmentation of the upper and lower lips. Note the considerable shortening of the philtrum ridges.

CLINICAL CASES

CLINICAL CASE 3

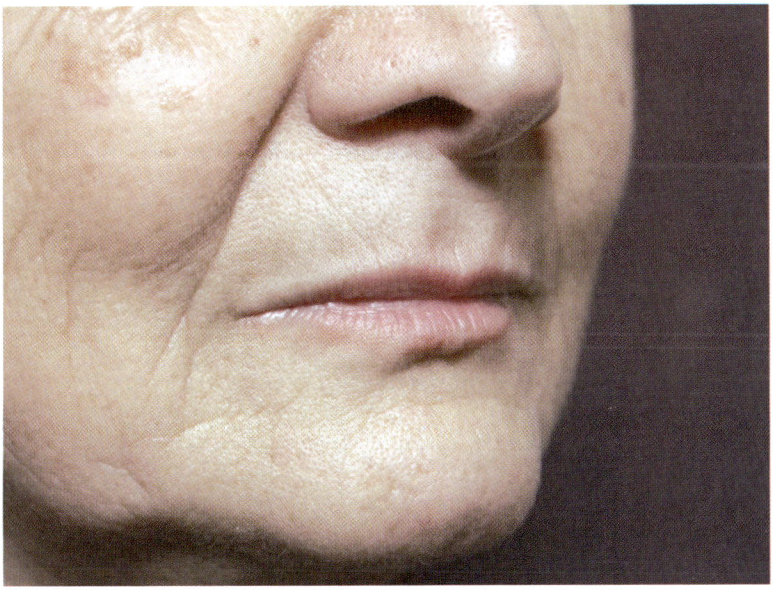

BEFORE

<

AFTER

>

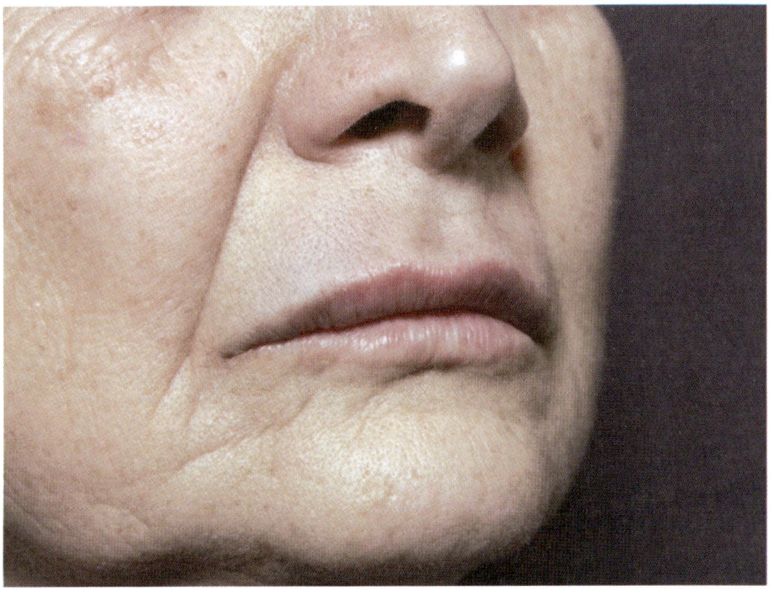

Same patient seen from the side.

12

EYEBROWS, TEMPLES AND EARLOBES

Anatomy of the eyebrow

Beauty doesn't have to be blinding. It isn't all about aggression, fleshy lips, miniskirts and big breasts. Beauty is also about harmony and details, little touches that make us appreciate the true symphony of forms.

This is why, when we look at a face, we are struck not only by the overpowering presence of heavy make-up, but also, and above all, by the sense of classic balance that characterises it.

Let's start with the eyebrows, from the Latin *supracilium*. Eyebrows are short piliferous formations surrounding the orbit, above the upper eyelids, and they protect the eyeball from atmospheric agents, particularly dust and

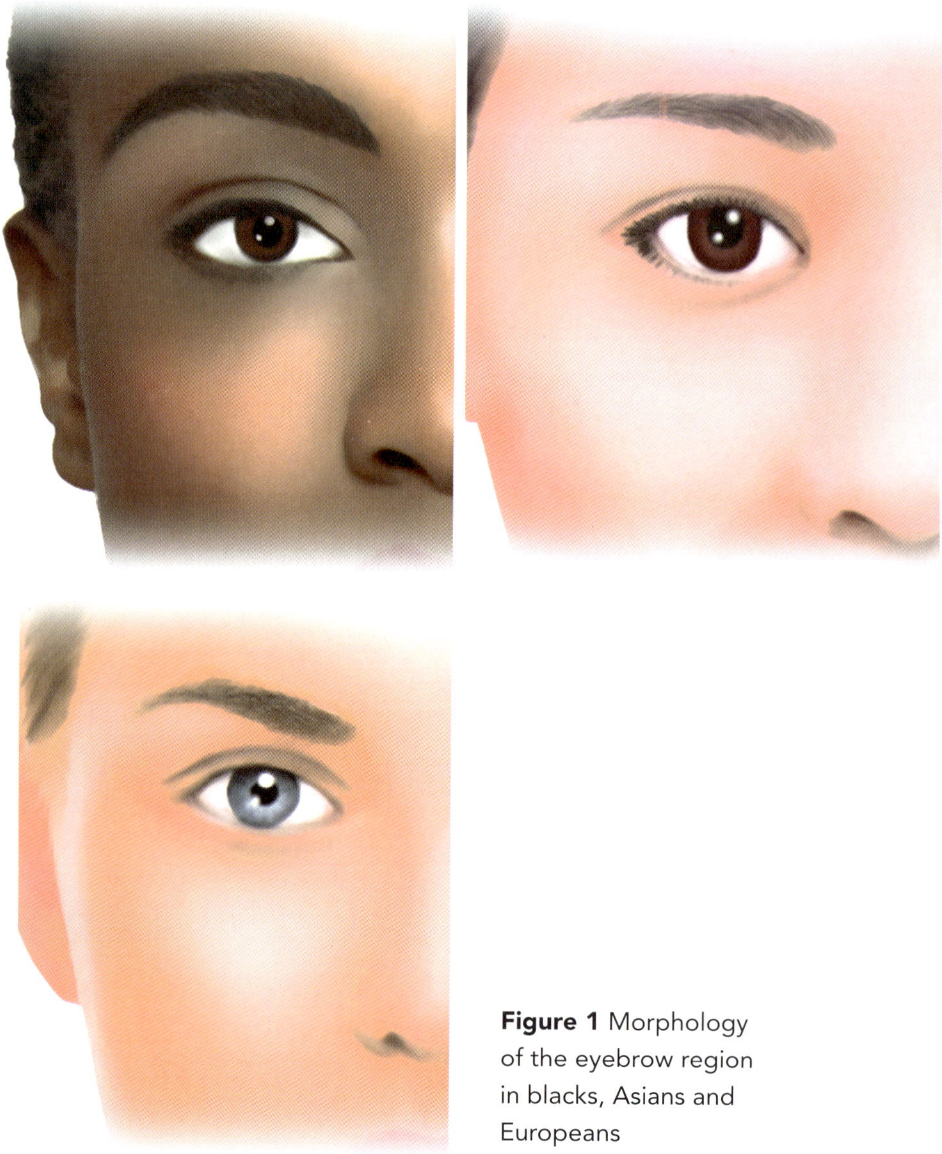

Figure 1 Morphology of the eyebrow region in blacks, Asians and Europeans

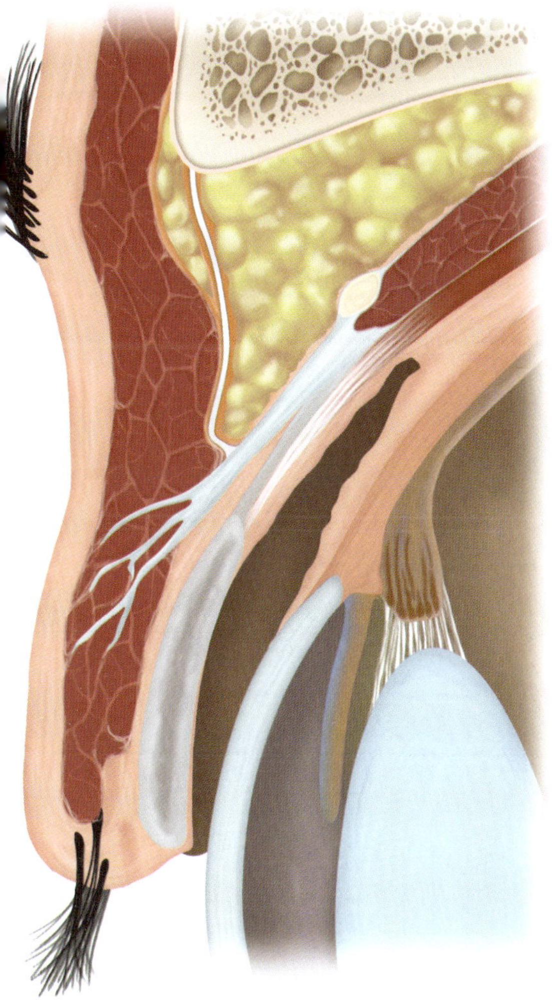

Figure 2 Graphic anatomy of the eyebrow region, in cross-section

rain. Shaving them off completely is not only anti-aesthetic, it can also damage our eye function over time.

Eyebrows differ considerably according to sex, age and race (fig. 1), and people have always had a desire to alter them. Many women shave them off altogether, committing an anatomical aberration, only to then draw them back on or have them replaced with tattoos, and both men and women often have them pierced.

Eyebrows are often used, quite artfully, as a form of expression.

In anatomy, the eyebrow is defined as an arched skin relief (fig. 2), with a concavity below it, made up of:

> skin;
> a subcutaneous layer (layer of muscle);
> periosteum of the frontal bone.

Correction of the eyebrows

Due to its anatomical complexity, which is only seemingly simple, eyebrow lifting, like many aesthetic procedures, has frequently been possible exclusively with surgery, with the application of a wide range of procedures:

> skin removal;
> suspension with threads;
> brow pexy through the upper eyelid;
> the less violent alternatives include endotine, a small device with sharp points to raise the brow, endoscopic lifting, which is also suitable in few cases and is not widely practiced, and botulinum toxin.

A lot of research into this small but aesthetically important area has been carried out in aesthetic medicine in recent years and it is now possible to obtain the lifting and physiological enhancement of the brow using fillers, sometimes combined with botulinum toxin.

The outer third of the eyebrow, the so-called tail, where the greatest number of hairs are present, is usually slightly augmented, with a retrograde injection of 0.4-0.6 ml of preferably resilient

VIDEO 1

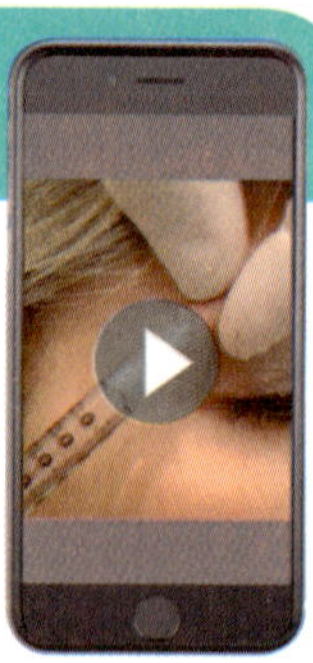

Correction of the eyebrow using the linear technique

VIDEO 2

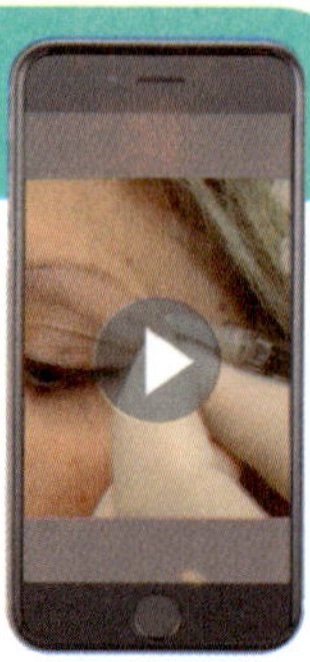

Eyebrow correction technique

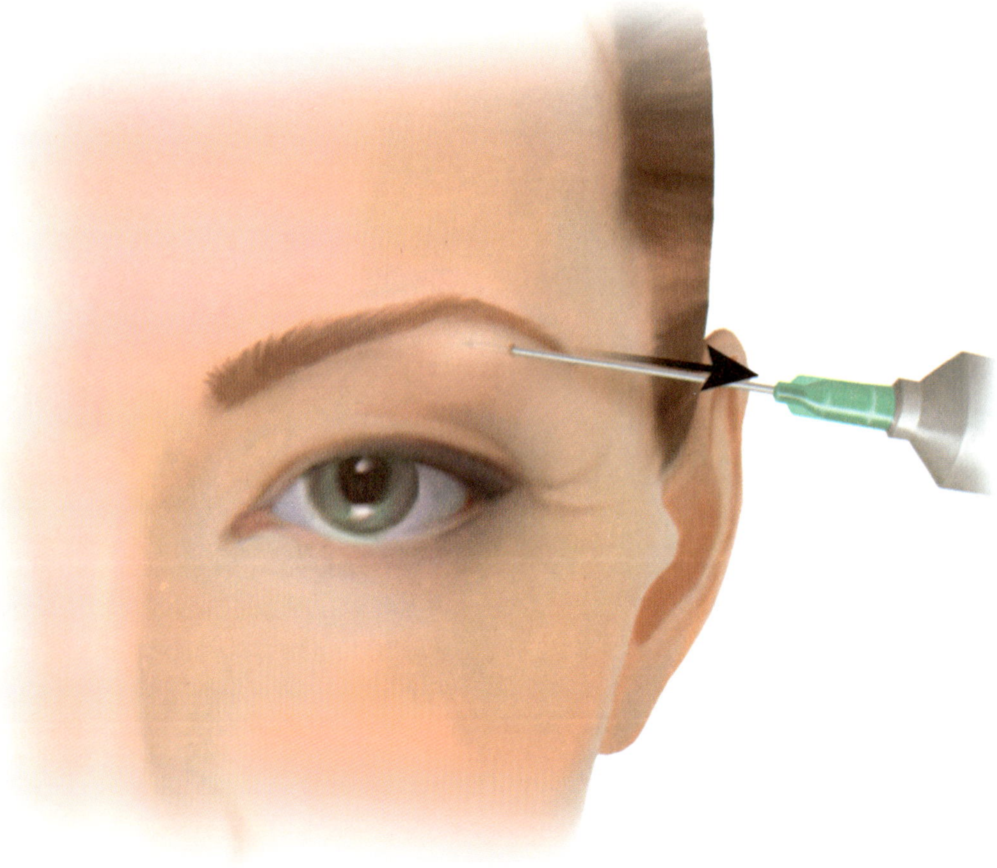

Figure 3 Eyebrow correction technique

and biodynamic hyaluronic acid (fig. 3), capable of following the movements of the face while staying in place with a corrective effect, with a medium G'. Then we perform a shaping massage, with a roll up movement that leaves the product in place.
This has no complications and has an average duration of 8-9 months, with very high levels of satisfaction.
If it is associated with botulinum toxin, it is best to carry out the conventional blockage of the orbicularis first, followed by reshaping with filler 15 days later.

Anatomy of the temples

A face without roundness is always a sign of a face that is "wasted", unhealthy, aged or somehow lacking the curves that make beauty an alternation of concavities and convexities.
Of course, there is no univocal interpretation of beauty: beauty is something that attracts, that impresses, that makes the gaze linger, without repressing wonder and even going so far as induce a state of ecstasy.
Many have tried their hand at describing beauty. Seneca said that true beauty lies in harmony and proportion: "A woman is not beautiful when her ankle or arm wins compliments, but when her total appearance diverts admiration from the individual parts of her body".
And how long does beauty last? Oscar Wilde claimed that: "Beauty is the only thing that time cannot harm. Philosophies fall away like sand, creeds follow one another, but what is beautiful is a joy for all seasons, a possession for all eternity".
Many people say that beauty lies in the body, but cannot be traced back to the body, like Mahatma Gandhi: "True beauty, after all, consists in purity of heart", or anonymous: "The beauty of a woman is not in the clothes she wears, the figure that she carries, or the way she combs her hair. The beauty of a woman is seen in her eyes, because that is the doorway to her heart, the place where love resides".
And to stress the importance of a region as neglected as the temples, all we have to do is think of Ghandi's temples.
Hippocrates, to whose rules all doctors swear an oath, was the first to describe the *facies hippocratica* which he attributed to people who were about to die, with sunken cheeks and temples and protruding eyes (fig. 4).
In the difficult art of "building" beauty, it is time to indulge the movements of the face, the emotions of the soul; beauty is in the eye of the beholder. We also need to achieve a longer duration, following what is commonly known today as morphobiodynamics.
A youthful appearance depends on the presence of a fair amount of fat in the right place, and the loss of tissue in the temporal area creates exactly the emaciated effect that we have to fight (fig. 5).
The loss, redistribution and accumulation of fat in the ageing process results in a loss of facial volume in several areas, such as the forehead and cheeks.
We are aided in our choice of the most suitable therapy by Rohrich, who has studied the facial fat compartments. After many dissections, and we will never tire of repeating that being able to see up close and touch an anatomical preparation, a human head, provides a

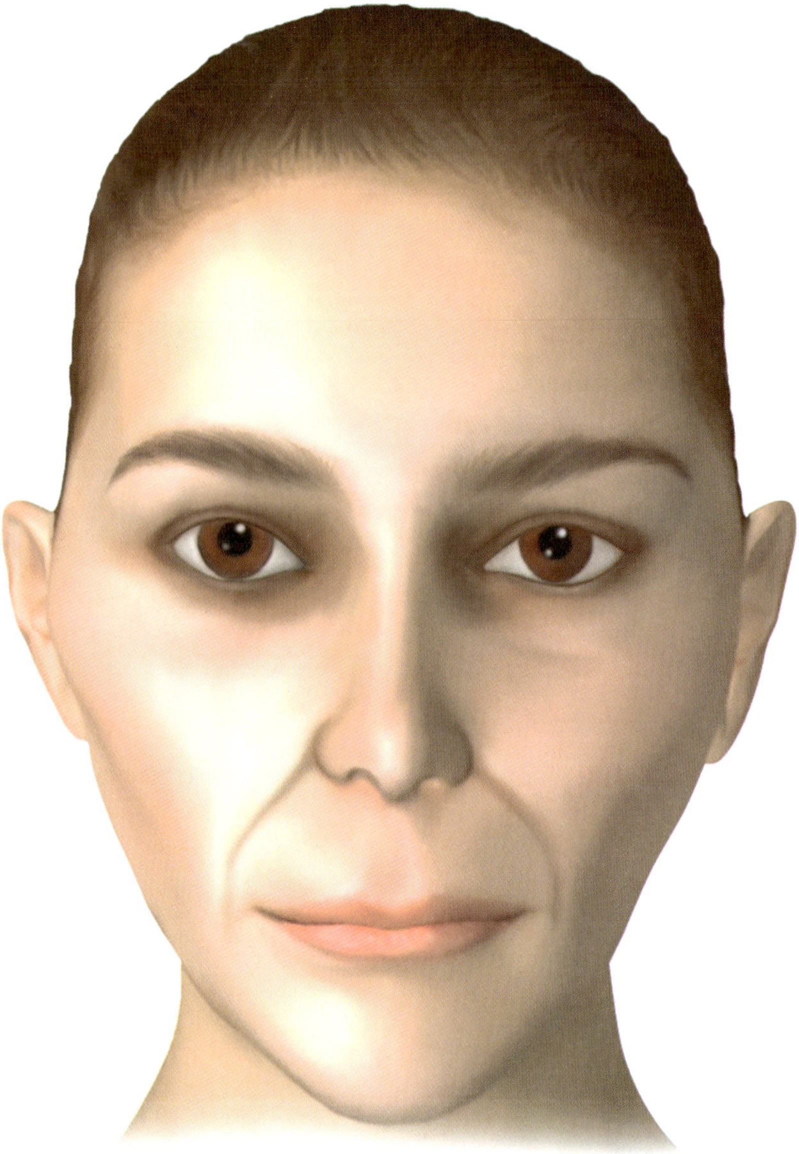

Figure 4 Facies hippocratica

very useful experience that will never be forgotten, Rohrich discovered that there are numerous fat compartments in the face, about seven to eight per hemiface. They are not connected to one another but separated by fibroelastic septa (fig. 6).

So, if we want to fill the cheekbones, for example, that is where we have to work and not on contiguous or higher areas. And if we have a temporal deficit, that is where we have to intervene, not in other areas. The ageing of the skull in particular causes a shift in the

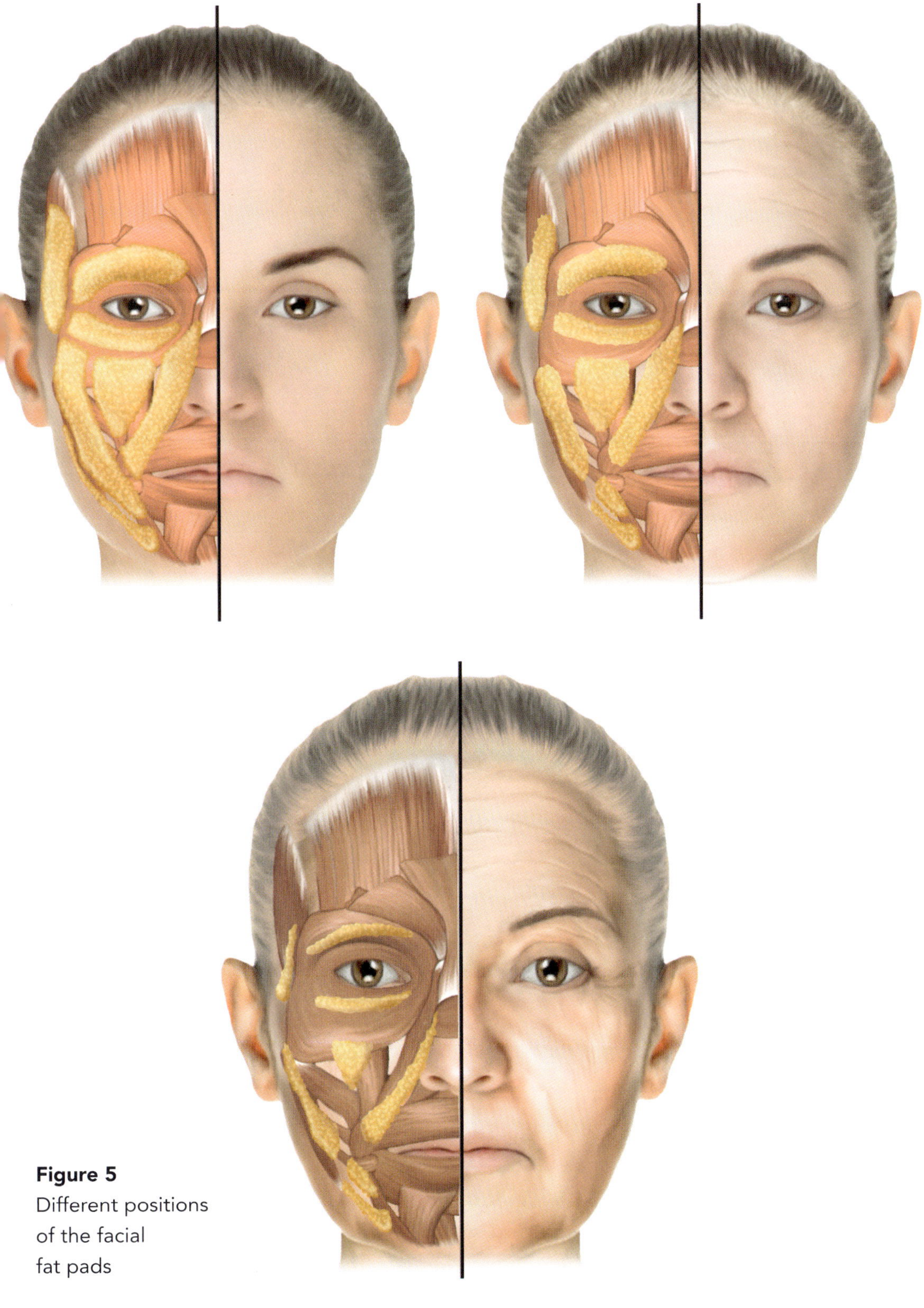

Figure 5
Different positions of the facial fat pads

natural balance between bone resorption and regeneration and consequently a loss of bone mass.
The redistribution of fat in senescence leads to the atrophy of some pads and, paradoxically, to the hypertrophy of others, as happens when we see the formation of jowls. We can never

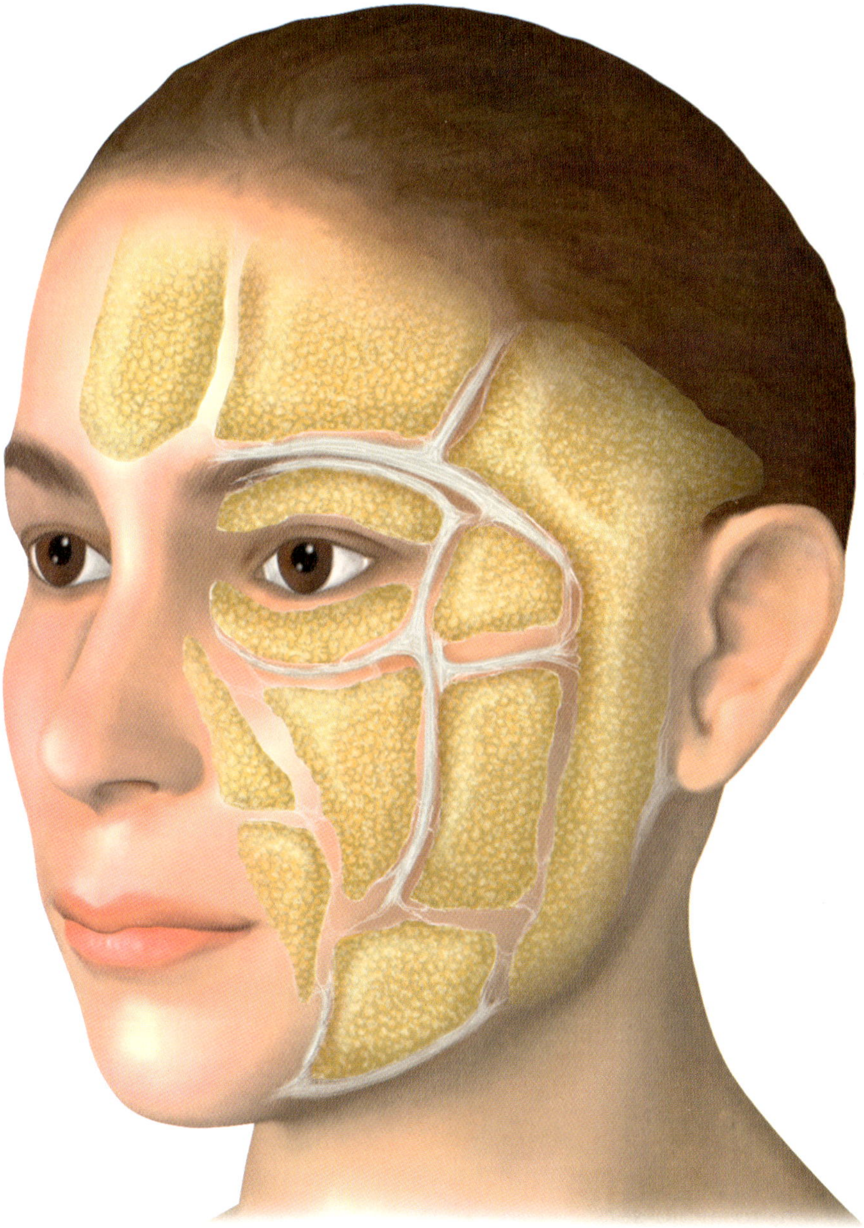

Figure 6 Fibrous septa and division of the facial fat pads into compartments

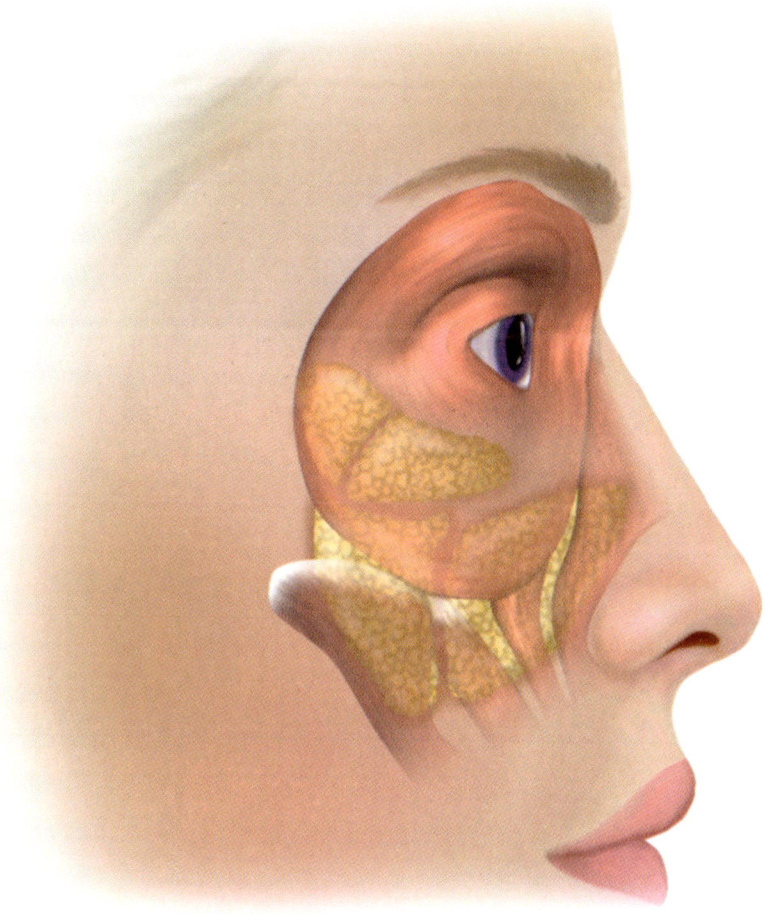

Figure 7 Fat compartments in the zygomatic and temporal region

imagine correcting one compartment by injecting into the one next to it, which would make absolutely no sense at all (fig. 7).

Correction of the temples

Very important in the evaluation and, subsequently, the execution of the technique, is the study of arterial vascularization, to avoid serious vascular risks. To this end, an easy manoeuvre can be represented by asking the patient to lower her chin onto her chest for a few minutes (fig. 8). The superficial vessels will become swollen and can be traced with a pen, eliminating the risk of injecting into the superficial temporal artery which originates from the external carotid artery and carries a fair amount of blood before its bifurcation. This is, however, located in the parotid artery and does not pose a serious risk. As far as the deep temporal artery is concerned, it branches off to

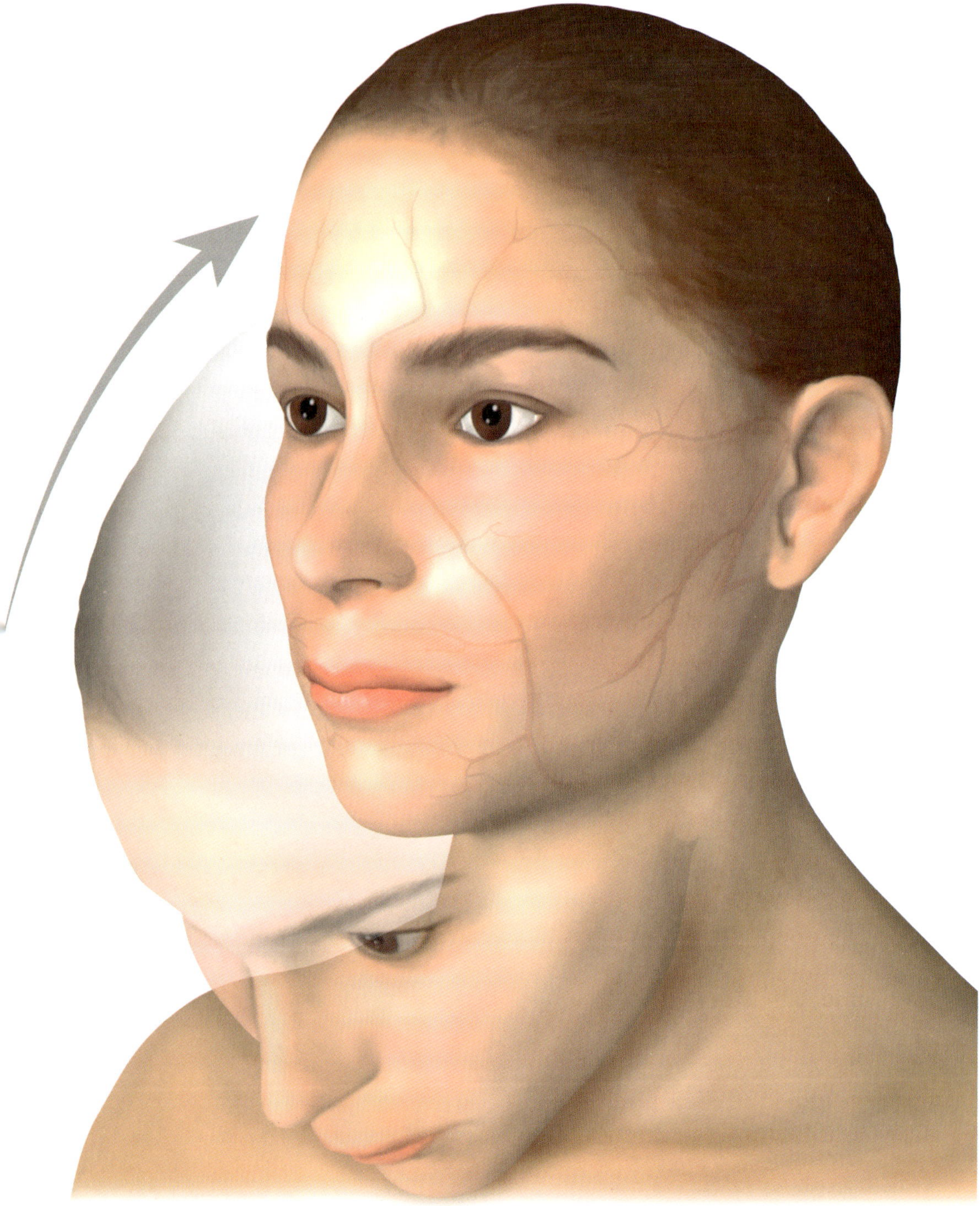

Figure 8 Semeiotic manoeuvre to highlight the veins in the temporal region

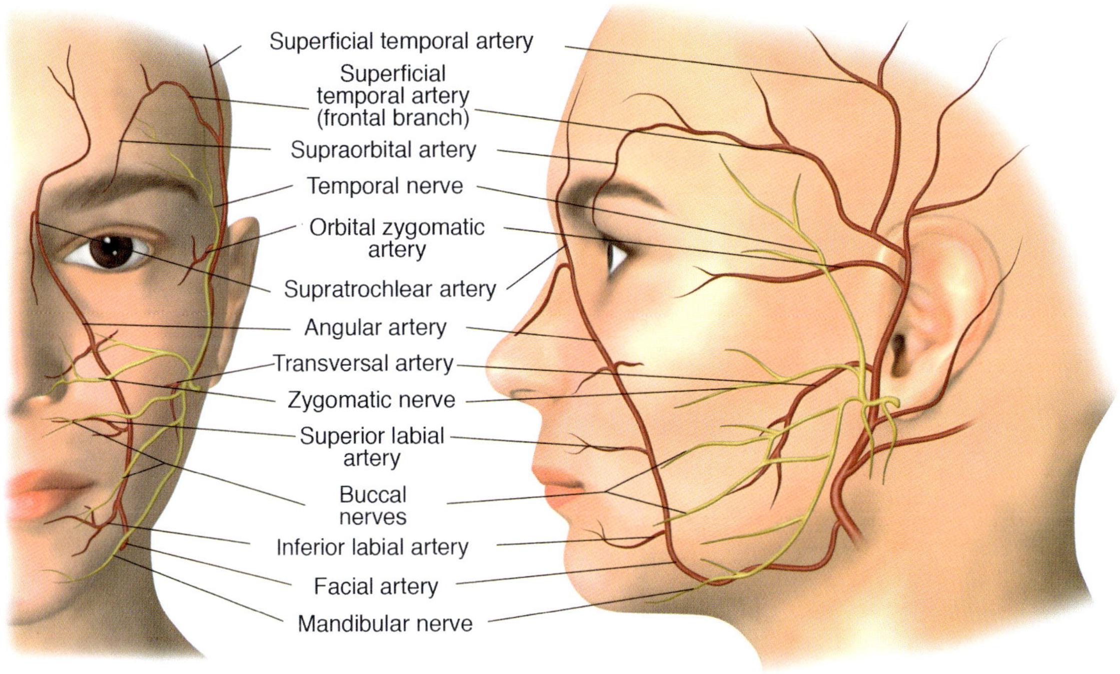

Figure 9 Facial arteries and nerves

the masseter muscle and is not a constant problem. It is therefore always advisable to avoid the superficial temporal artery, which is much more dangerous, performing a deep injection with a needle of at least 30 mm, until it reaches the deep temporal fascia or even the bone. It goes without saying that the amount of filler required for a visible and significant correction must be at least 1 ml on each side but, in the case of deeply hollow temples, even 2 ml per side. The filler must be suitable for deep corrections, with a very high G′, and capable of offering a stable result for a very long period of time, sometimes even a year.
Of course, it is also possible to use a blunt tip microcannula, preferably 25 G, with an entry point at the apex of the zygomatic process, where it becomes orbital (fig. 9).

Anatomy of the earlobe

The ear lobe is the soft, rounded part at the bottom of the outer ear. There are two types of earlobe, detached from the head and attached to it. This trait generally runs in the family and is perhaps hereditary. Then there is a third type of earlobe, one which is attached to the head as a result of a facelift, and this is what you must look for in order to tell whether or not the person in front of you has had a facelift.
Another curiosity is that the lobular artery becomes turgid during sexual arousal, making the lobe much more

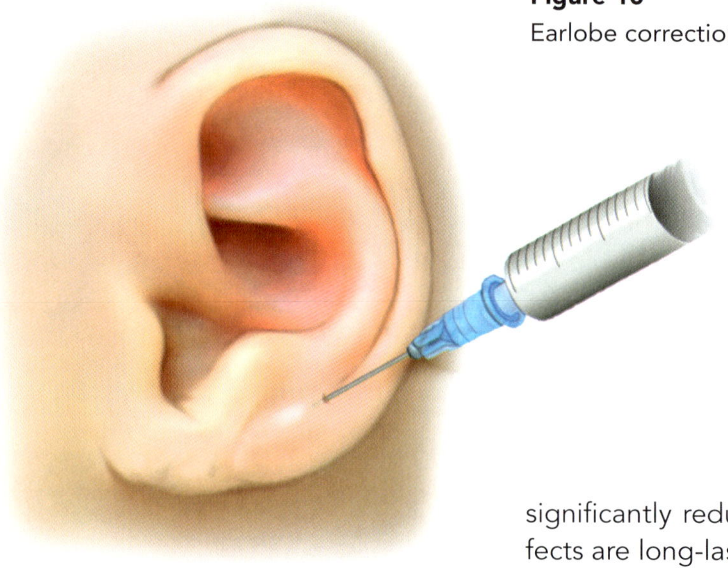

Figure 10
Earlobe correction technique

sensitive. Other clichés say that the unattached lobe indicates a free and independent spirit, while the attached lobe indicates a confident and motivated person.
In Chinese medicine, the presence of a split lobe is said to be a possible indication of heart disease.

Correction of the earlobe

During senescence, the earlobe almost always experiences lipoatrophy, resembling a prune, but this can easily be corrected with one or more infiltrations of hyaluronic acid.
After carefully disinfecting the earlobe, perform one or more injections with a 30 G needle in the most inclined point and at the apex (fig. 10), introducing a modest amount of HA (0.5 ml is usually enough), and creating a sort of grid in order to obtain an effective floor. Use a medium density, resilient filler with a low G'. There is no pain, although the use of an electronic pen is recommended to significantly reduce discomfort. The effects are long-lasting, and satisfaction is very high.
Of course, the treatment can be repeated an infinite number of times without any kind of problem.

Bibliography

1. Hanke CW, Rohrich RJ, Busso M, et al. Facial Soft-Tissue Fillers conference: Assessing the State of the Science. J Am Acad Dermatol. 2011;64(4 Suppl):S66-S85.e136.
2. Farage MA, Miller KW, Elsner P, Maibach HI. Characteristics of the Aging Skin. Adv Wound Care (New Rochelle). 2013;2(1):5-10.
3. Rohrich RJ, Pessa JE. The fat compartments of the face: anatomy and clinical implications for cosmetic surgery. Plast Reconstr Surg. 2007;119(7):2219-2231.
4. Kazemi Ashtiani A, Azarbakhsh M, Hafezi F, Naghibzadeh B. Anthropometric Analysis of the Human Skull for Developmental Left-Sided Asymmetry, New Finding. Aesthetic Plast Surg. 2020;44(1):186-190.

5. Al-Hoqail RA, Meguid EM. Anatomic dissection of the arterial supply of the lips: an anatomical and analytical approach. J Craniofac Surg. 2008;19(3):785-794.
6. Toledo Avelar LE, Cardoso MA, Santos Bordoni L, de Miranda Avelar L, de Miranda Avelar JV. Aging and Sexual Differences of the Human Skull. Plast Reconstr Surg Glob Open. 2017;5(4):e1297.
7. Badia AA. Skin aging. Clinical evaluation & treatment of aging skin. The Compounding Pharmacy of South Africa.
8. Burusapat C, Lekdaeng P. What Is the Most Beautiful Facial Proportion in the 21st Century? Comparative Study among Miss Universe, Miss Universe Thailand, Neoclassical Canons, and Facial Golden Ratios. Plast Reconstr Surg Glob Open. 2019;7(2):e2044.
9. Carey W, et al. Prime Journal. 2016. Nov/Dec: 40-3.
10. Clinical Study TEO-PEN-1403. Efficacy and safety of an injection-assisted device compared to a manual injection device in the treatment of the upper lip area. 48 Subjects injected with TEOSYAL RHA® 1 in the upper lip area including perioral rhytids.
11. Coleman SR, Grover R. The anatomy of the aging face: volume loss and changes in 3-dimensional topography. Aesthet Surg J. 2006;26(1S):S4-S9.
12. Cotofana S, Fratila AA, Schenck TL, Redka-Swoboda W, Zilinsky I, et al. The Anatomy of the Aging Face: A Review. Facial Plast Surg. 2016;32(3):253-260.
13. Cotofana S, Pretterklieber B, Lucius R, et al. Distribution Pattern of the Superior and Inferior Labial Arteries: Impact for Safe Upper and Lower Lip Augmentation Procedures. Plast Reconstr Surg. 2017;139(5):1075-1082.
14. DeLorenzi C. Complications of injectable fillers, part 2: vascular complications. Aesthet Surg J. 2014;34(4):584-600.
15. Edizer M, Ma-den O, Tayfur V, Kiray A, Ergür I, Atabey A. Arterial anatomy of the lower lip: a cadaveric study. Plast Reconstr Surg. 2003;111(7):2176-2181.
16. Fitzgerald R, Graivier MH, Kane M, et al. Update on facial aging. Aesthet Surg J. 2010;30 Suppl:11S-24S.
17. Kahn DM, Shaw RB Jr. Aging of the bony orbit: a three-dimensional computed tomographic study. Aesthet Surg J. 2008;28(3):258-264. d
18. Kar M, Muluk NB, Bafaqeeh SA, Cingi C. Is it possible to define the ideal lips?. Acta Otorhinolaryngol Ital. 2018;38(1):67-72.
19. Ma-den O, Edizer M, Atabey A, Tayfur V, Ergür I. Cadaveric study of the arterial anatomy of the upper lip. Plast Reconstr Surg. 2004;114(2):355-359.
20. Mendelson B, Wong CH. Changes in the facial skeleton with aging: implications and clinical applications in facial rejuvenation. Aesthetic Plast Surg. 2012;36(4):753-760.
21. Michaud T, Gassia V, Belhaouari L. Facial dynamics and emotional expressions in facial aging treatments. J Cosmet Dermatol. 2015;14(1):9-21.
22. Pinar YA, Bilge O, Govsa F. Ana-

tomic study of the blood supply of perioral region. Clin Anat. 2005;18(5):330-339.
23. Puizina-Ivić N. Skin aging. Acta Dermatovenerol Alp Pannonica Adriat. 2008;17(2):47-54.
24. Radlanski RJ & Wesker KH. The Face. Pictorial Atlas of Clinical Anatomy. Second edition. Quintescence Publishing. 2015.
25. Ramanadham SR, Rohrich RJ. Newer Understanding of Specific Anatomic Targets in the Aging Face as Applied to Injectables: Superficial and Deep Facial Fat Compartments--An Evolving Target for Site-Specific Facial Augmentation. Plast Reconstr Surg. 2015;136(5 Suppl):49S-55S.
26. Rinnerthaler M, Bischof J, Streubel MK, Trost A, Richter K. Oxidative stress in aging human skin. Biomolecules. 2015;5(2):545-589.
27. Rohrich RJ, Afrooz PN. Finesse in Face Lifting: The Role of Facial Fat Compartment Augmentation in Facial Rejuvenation. Plast Reconstr Surg. 2019;143(1):98-101.
28. Salti G, Rauso R. Facial Rejuvenation with Fillers: The Dual Plane Technique. J Cutan Aesthet Surg. 2015;8(3):127-133.
29. https://www.anatomynext.com/muscles-facial-muscles
30. Tansatit T, Apinuntrum P, Phetudom T. A typical pattern of the labial arteries with implication for lip augmentation with injectable fillers. Aesthetic Plast Surg. 2014;38(6):1083-1089.
31. Toledo Avelar LE, Cardoso MA, Santos Bordoni L, de Miranda Avelar L, de Miranda Avelar JV. Aging and Sexual Differences of the Human Skull. Plast Reconstr Surg Glob Open. 2017;5(4):e1297.
32. Trevidic P., Oral presentation. Upper third anatomy and filler injection: forehead and glabella, Expert-to-Expert series 2018.
33. Wan D, Amirlak B, Rohrich R, Davis K. The clinical importance of the fat compartments in midfacial aging. Plast Reconstr Surg Glob Open. 2014;1(9):e92.

CLINICAL CASES

CLINICAL CASE 1

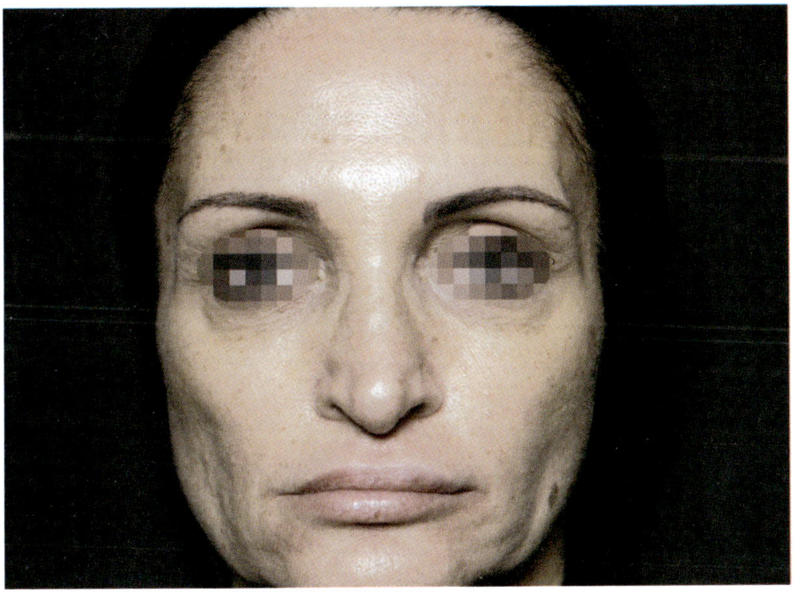

BEFORE

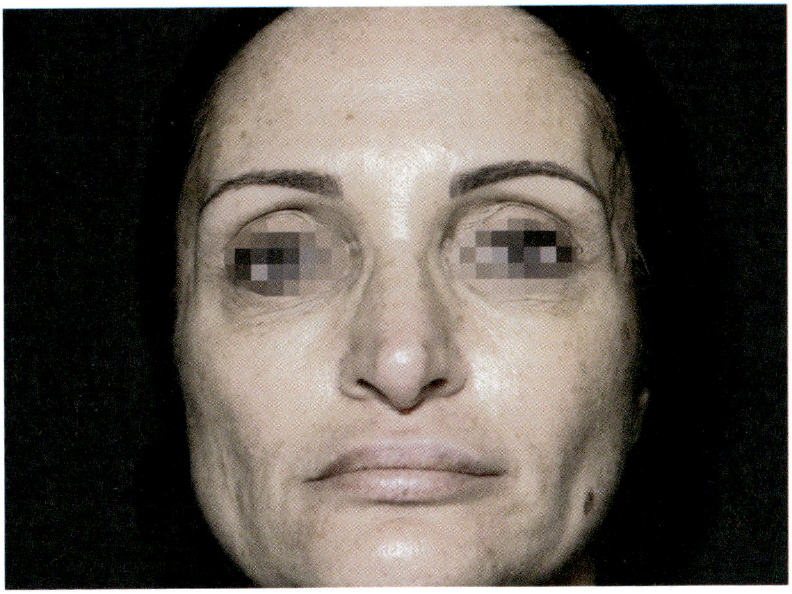

AFTER

Correction of the temporal region in a 55-year-old woman who had recently undergone severe weight loss. Correction with suprafascial injection of 1.2 cc of high G' hyaluronic acid per side.

CLINICAL CASES

CLINICAL CASE 1

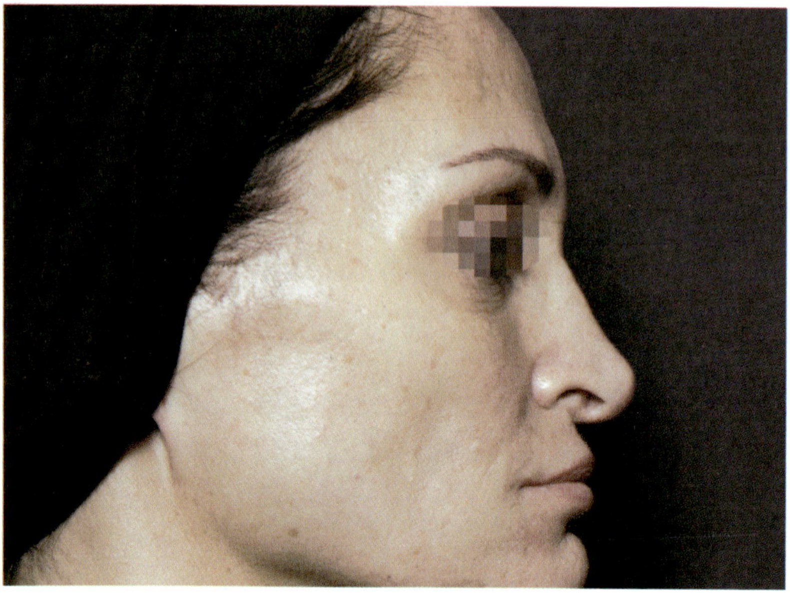

BEFORE

<

AFTER

>

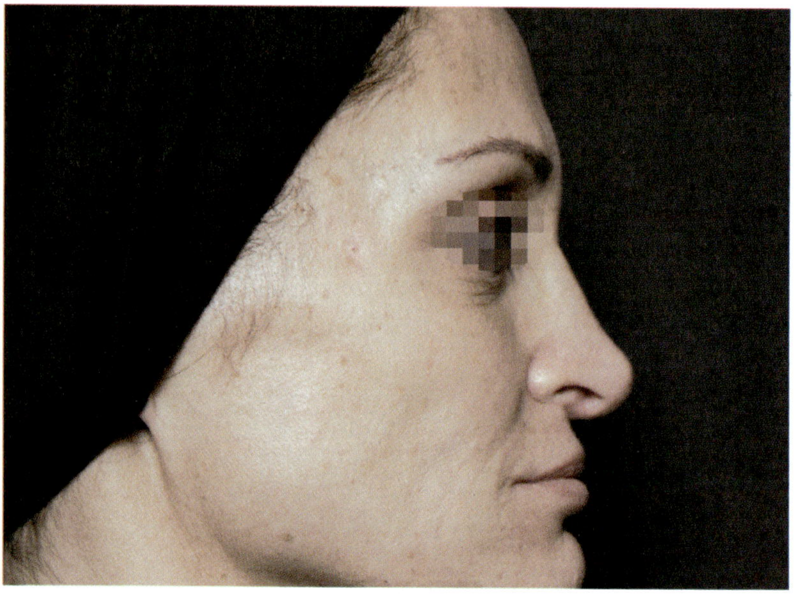

Same patient, seen from the side.

CLINICAL CASES

CLINICAL CASE 1

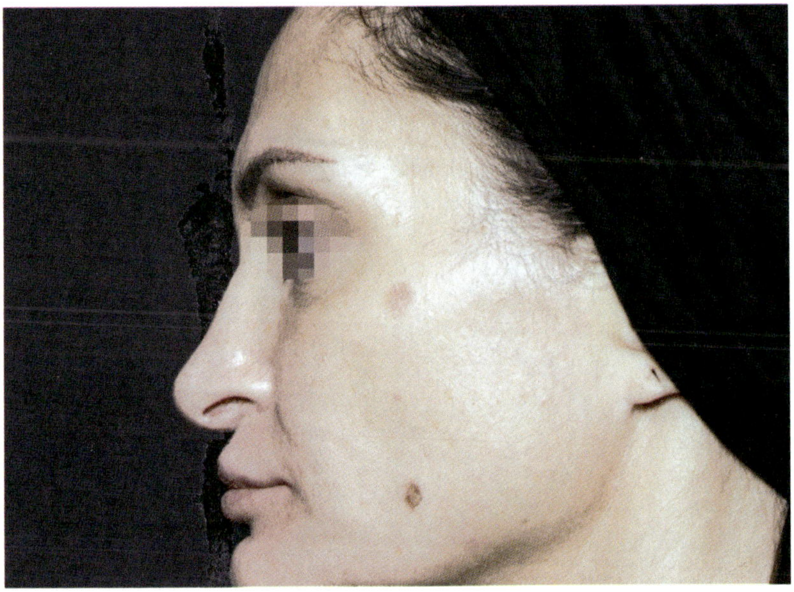

BEFORE

<

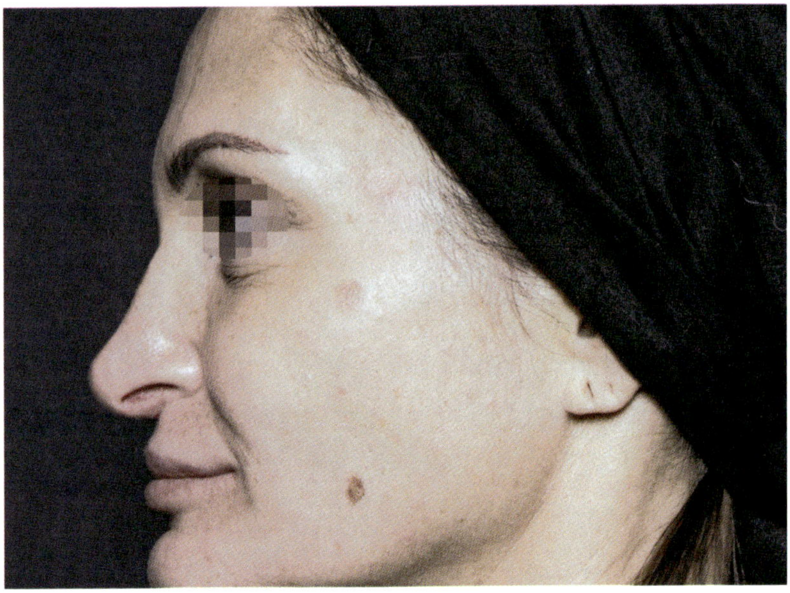

AFTER

>

Same patient, seen from the side.

CLINICAL CASES

CLINICAL CASE 2

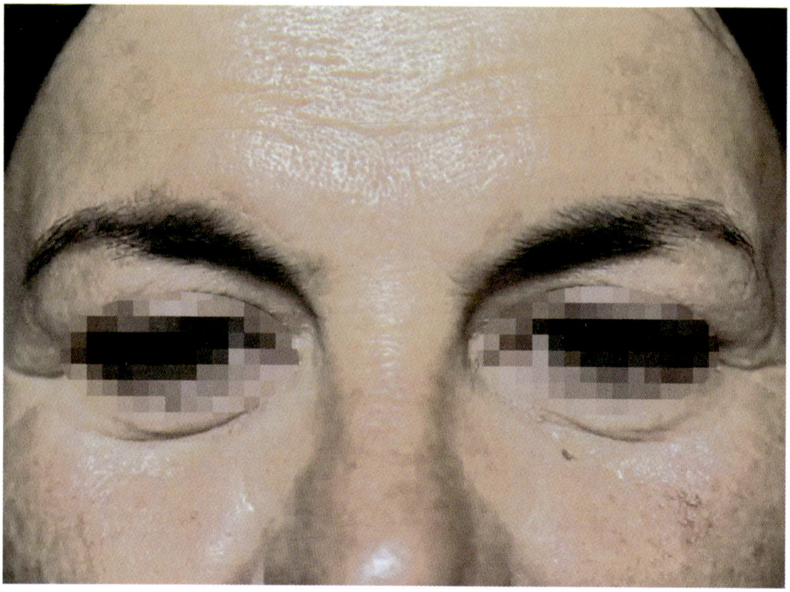

BEFORE

VIDEO 3

Temple correction technique

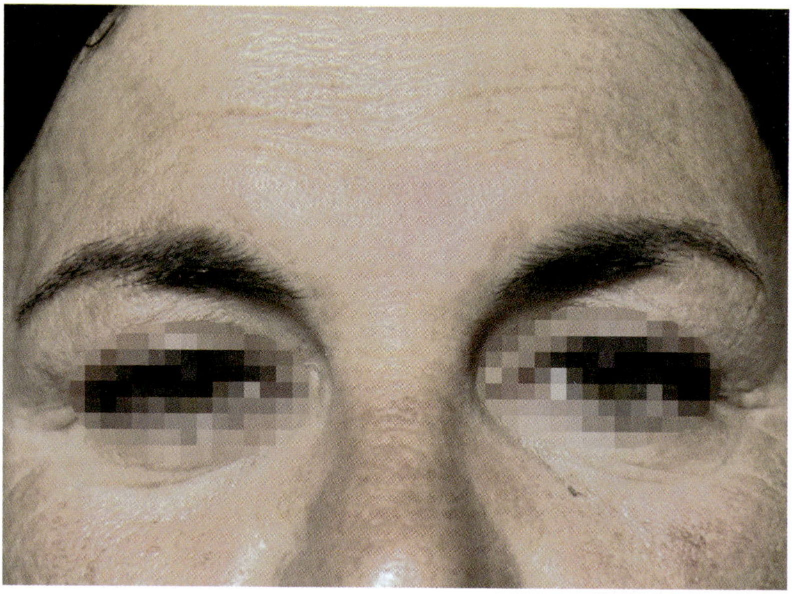

AFTER

50-year-old woman with a full, round face but with hypertrophy in the temporal region. Correction with subperiosteal injection of 1 cc of biodynamic HA per side.

13

HANDS

«When a man's hand touches
the hand of a woman, they both touch
the heart of eternity»

Kahlil Gibran

Anatomy of the hands

The hands are described in anatomy as prehensile and tactile organs situated at the end of the arms of humans and primates in general, starting from the wrist and ending with the fingers.

The skeleton of the hand is made up, in the craniocaudal direction, of the carpus, metacarpus and phalanges. It forms a division between the anterior region (or palm) and the posterior region (or wrist). Apparently it is a relatively simple anatomical formation which we use all the time, without assigning it the necessary importance.

Hands have played an increasingly crucial role in all aspects of human progress through time, especially when we consider that hands always respond to brain impulses. And hands are the second most visible part of our body, after the face, not forgetting that, in Western culture, we shake hands to greet each other, we appreciate the softness of a woman's hand or we clap our hands to acknowledge success.

In aesthetic medicine, hand rejuvenation is a relatively recent practice, but in actual fact, we have been caring for our hands since ancient times (1). The first informa-

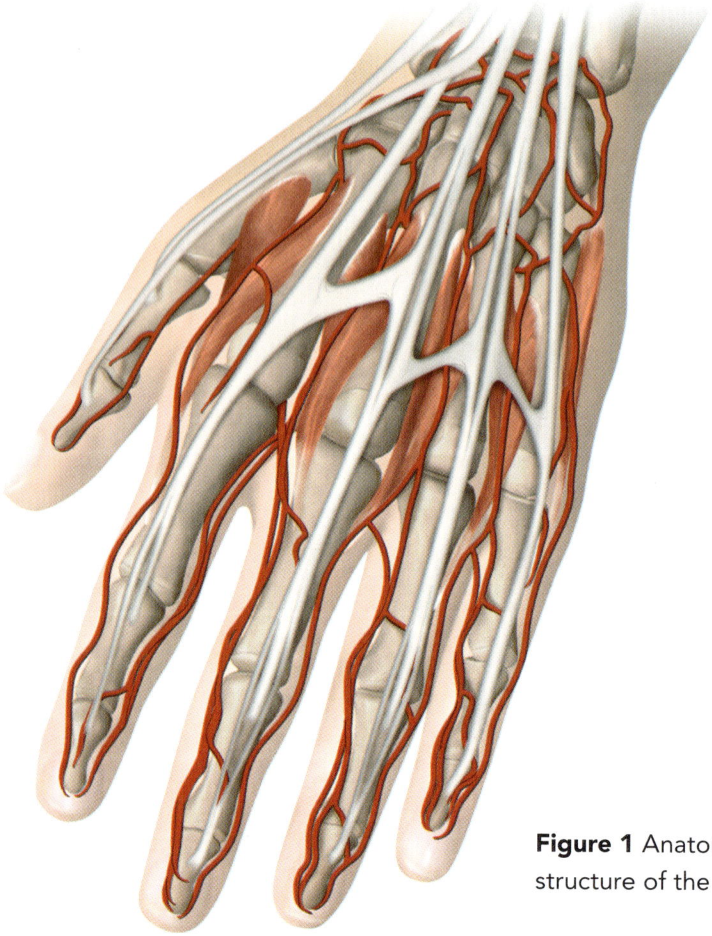

Figure 1 Anatomical structure of the hands

tion on the subject dates back to ancient Egypt and the use of limestone, mustard, sulphur and plant extracts; chemical pe-elings were also performed using lactic acid preparations made with sour milk.
The anatomy of the hands has been studied in great detail in more modern times, particularly during the Renaissance; anatomical dissections were already in use and artists such as Michelangelo and Leonardo da Vinci featured hands in many of their works. The former painted the hand of God, described as one of the greatest masterpieces in the history of art, in the Sistine Chapel.
We tend not to become involved all that frequently with hands, other than in the case of pathologies, but they undoubtedly represent a clear source of truth, as it is extremely difficult to alter their senescent appearance even in the most well-groomed and attractive women. This is one of the reasons, possibly even the most important, why, starting from the cosmetics industry, we quickly began developing hand rejuvenation techniques, which have always resulted in a high index of satisfaction among patients. In the history of hand rejuvenation, which doesn't date all that far back, the first remedies were those in use at the time, such as dermabrasion and microdermabrasion, cryotherapy, chemical peeling and, later, IPL (Intense Pulsed Light), ablative and non-ablative lasers, fractional lasers or radiofrequency (2). However, none of these remedies were able to compensate for what is a peculiar characteristic of the ageing of the hands, i.e. the loss of the fatty tissue that envelops the tendon sheaths, the absence of which highlights the presence of blood vessels and tendons, which are no longer hidden.
The anatomical structure of the hands (fig. 1) is made up of thick skin, with a highly represented horny layer that becomes increasingly present with age, to the point of frequently causing irritating hyperkeratosis, sweat glands, especially on the palm but also on the back, abundant melanocytes which, with repeated exposure to the sun, often form brown marks and hypermelanosis, a gradual decline in subcutaneous fat, blood vessels, nerves and tendons that are sometimes very evident in thin hands or become evident with age, forming real septa which are annoyingly visible. The muscles are obviously well represented both at carpal and metacarpal level, on the whole hand and in the fingers. There are at least 27 bones.
The ageing of the hands is related to intrinsic processes, associated with a decrease in the dorsal fat pads which tends to make the hand more skeletal, highlighting veins and tendons, and exacerbating tissue laxity.
The current orientation in hand ageing therapy is towards the use of fillers, mainly bioelastic hyaluronic acid, a process that some people say can be associated with the resection of excess skin tissue, but this technique is not widely practiced.
The use of calcium hydroxyapatite (6) is specifically suitable for the hands for at least two reasons: its white colour, which tends to mask the imperfections of the tissue texture for a certain length of time, and the fact that it can be injected into a deeper plane, eliminating the obvious risks.

It is important to point out that there are hundreds of fillers available today, but none of them hold specific authorisation from the FDA (Food and Drug Administration), a body to which we all refer. So, considering that there are no specifically authorised fillers, it is advisable to use substances that have been validated at least by scientific publications.
It should be remembered that the first attempt at filling a senescent hand dates back more than twenty-five years. Autologous fat was used, and this is a technique that is still practiced by some people today but which I feel unable to recommend, apart from in extremely select cases, due to the difficulty of application and delayed return to everyday life. In addition to this, it involves surgery which, while being very minor, is still surgery.
There is no doubt that, as with the correction of all facial defects, hyaluronic acid represents the treatment of choice for filling the hands, despite the fact that there are currently no specifically authorised substances of this type. Its benefits lie in its well-known biocompatibility profile (3,4,5) and its ability to offer immediate non-surgical enhancement. In addition, hyaluronic acid can be almost completely removed with the use of hyaluronidase in the event of occlusive complications, particularly vascular complications.
Among other things, the presence of volumizing subdermal fillers, which are definitely preferable in hand correction, leads us to prefer this practice over others, not forgetting the ability of hyaluronic acid to stimulate neocollagenesis.
The few existing studies on hand rejuvenation all mention considerable safety with the subcutaneous positioning of hyaluronic acid. However, there are no comparative studies between different types of filler which show that one is more suitable than another.

Materials for correcting the hands

Which materials do we need? Basically, the same as those required in other areas. Let's list them briefly:

- a sterile sheet on which to place the hands;
- sterile gloves;
- a dermographic pencil;
- sterile gauze and chlorhexidine or other similar disinfectant;
- adrenaline-free lidocaine 1%;
- 5 cc syringes for anaesthetic infiltration;
- 27 G and 30 G needles for anaesthetic infiltration;
- the chosen filler;
- 25 and 27 G cannulae;
- an 18 G needle to determine the entry point of the cannula;
- a 6 mm steri-strip to close the micro entry points.

Hand rejuvenation technique

In theory it is not very difficult to increase the volume of a hand and there are at least two possible methods.
The first is with a needle and the injection of microboluses, about 0.2 cc per bolus, following the lines determined by the tendon channels, taking care to avoid vascular formations that can easily cause significant bruising. In this case it will be necessary to press the bleeding vessel with a finger until the microhaemorrhage stops. The patient

VIDEO 1

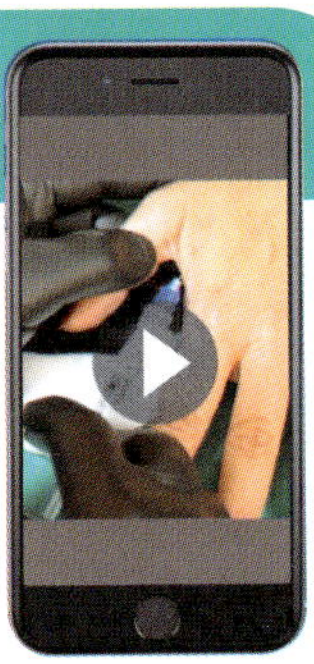

Hand correction technique with cannula

VIDEO 2

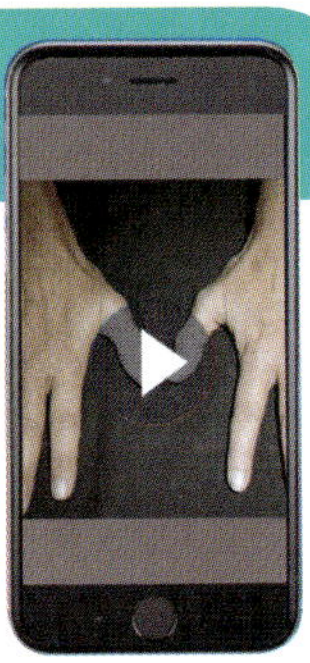

Hand correction technique with needle and electronic syringe

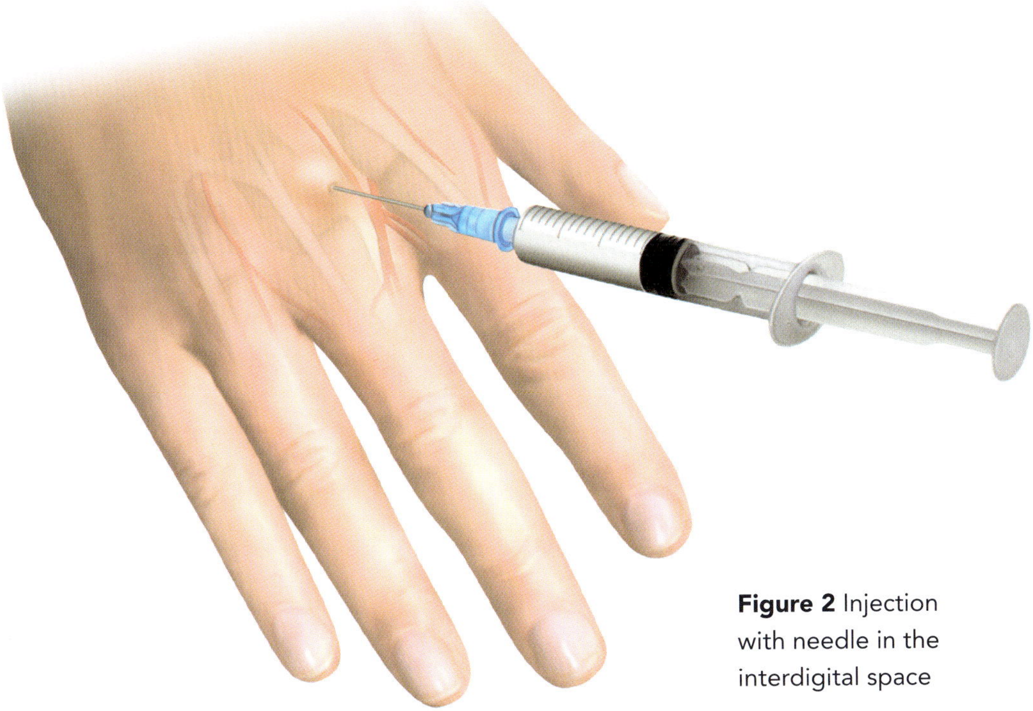

Figure 2 Injection with needle in the interdigital space

will remember it as being particularly unpleasant.
The second involves the use of a micro-cannula (9), usually 27 G or even 25 G, with the entry point in the interdigital spaces, following infiltration of 0.1 cc of lidocaine to ensure maximum patient comfort. The cannula slides into the subdermis, following the course of the tendon channels, releasing 0.2 cc of filler as it is withdrawn. It is evident, therefore, that at least 2 cc of substance will be required, 1 cc per hand.
Vigorous post-injection massage with

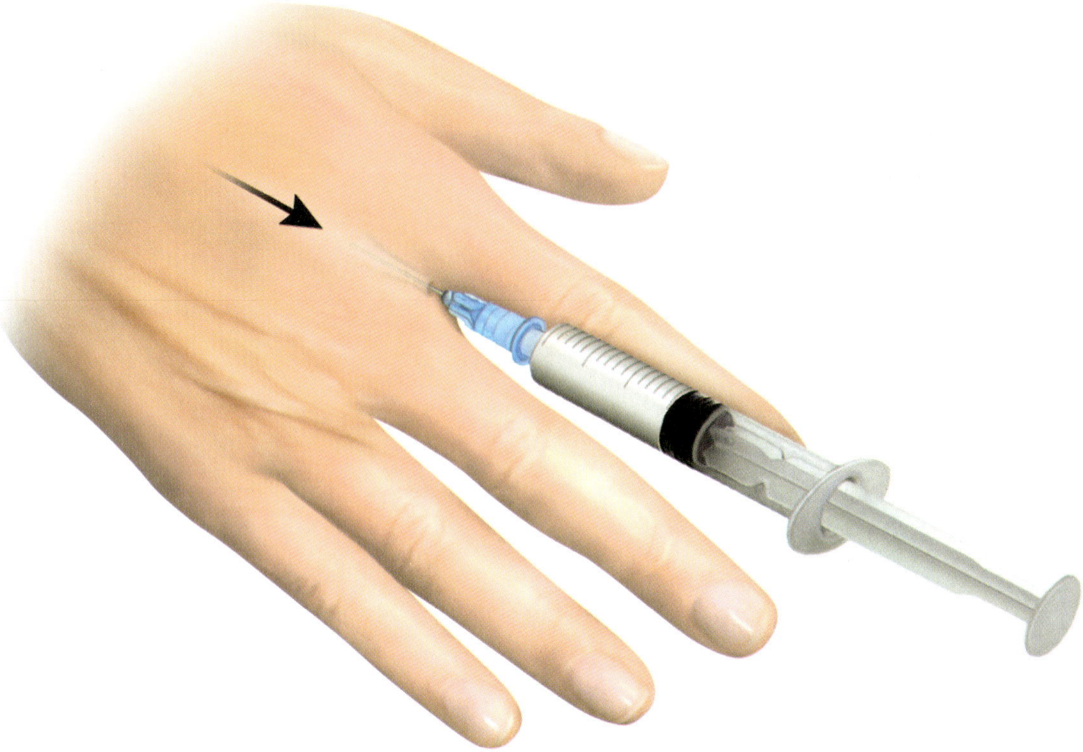

Figure 3 Injection with cannula in the interdigital space

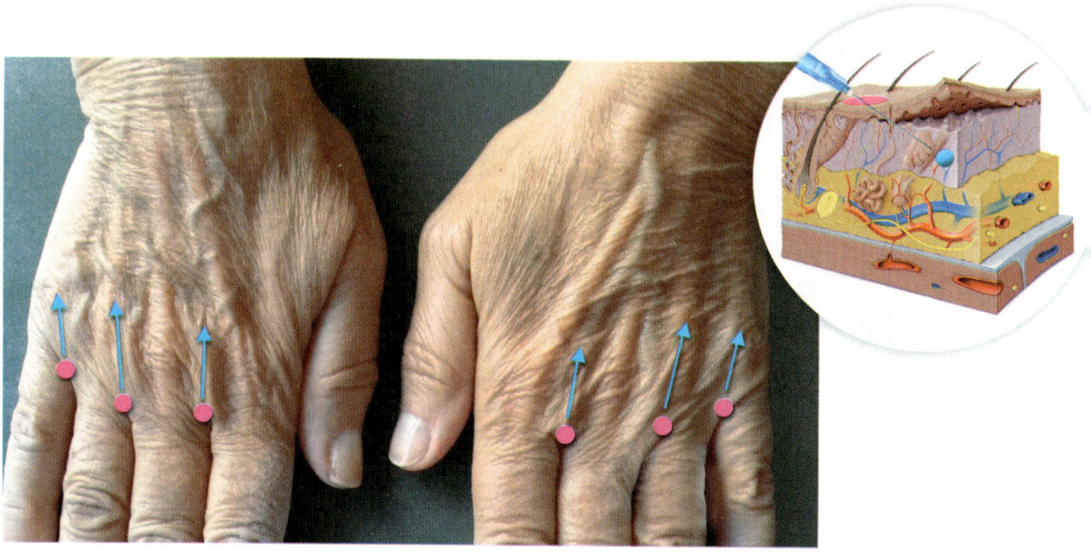

Figure 4 Layout of the injections to be practised to correct senescence

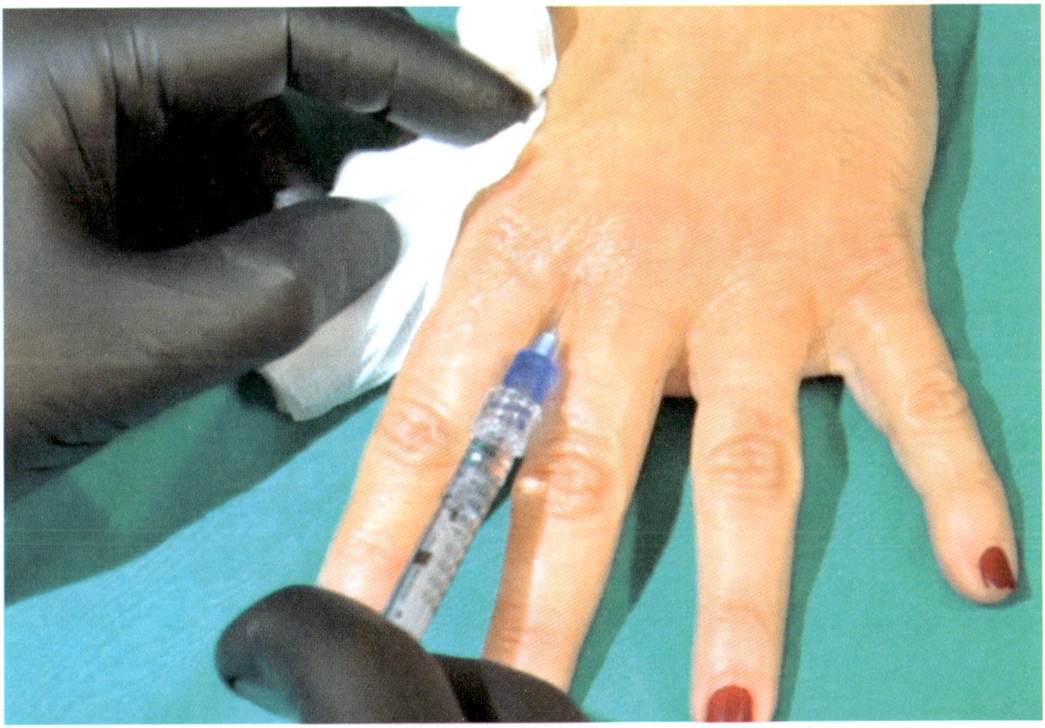

Figure 5 Correction of the hands: injection technique with cannula

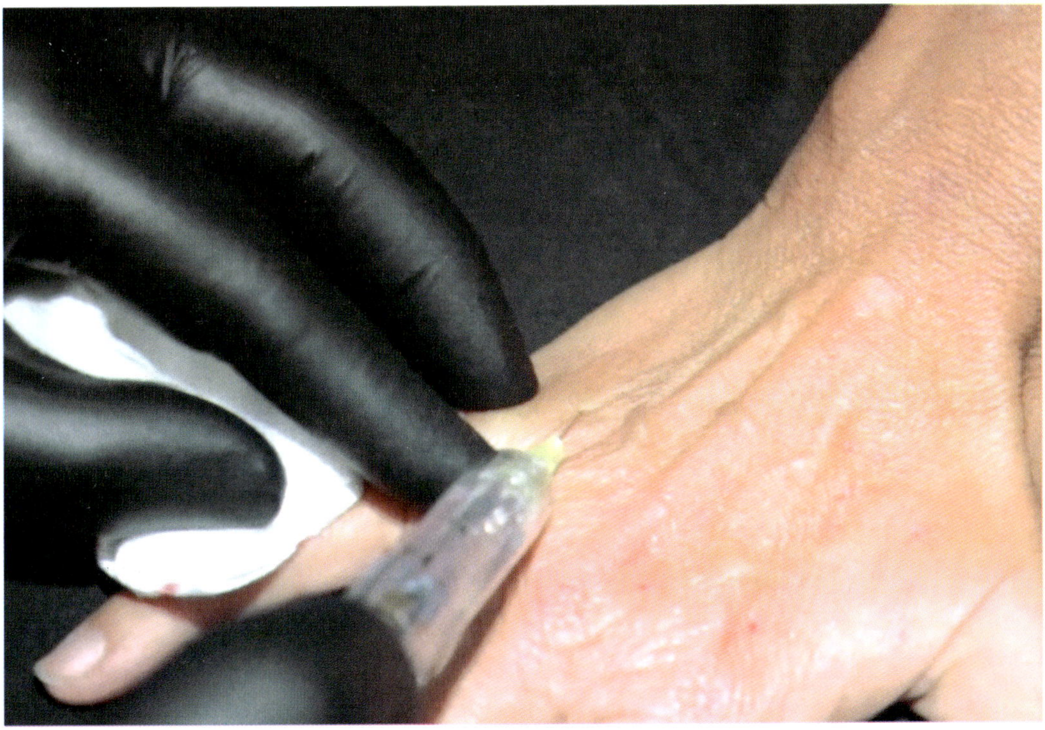

Figure 6 Correction of the hands: injection technique with needle

your open hand against the patient's hand, resting on a hard surface, is very useful, and I would even go so far as to say necessary.
Some practitioners prefer to start their injections by inserting the cannula from the wrist, but there does not seem to be any particular advantage to this (7).
Post-injection dressings are of no use and only in the case of conspicuous bruising should antibiotic treatment be prescribed.
The duration of the effects of the correction are similar whichever type of substance is used, perhaps a little longer with hydroxyapatite, lasting around a year.

Bibliography

1. Lefebvre-Vilardebo M, ed. Anatomy & Hand Medical Rejuvenation. Paris: E2e Medical 2013.
2. Riyaz FR, Ozog D. Hand rejuvenation. Semin Cutan Med Surg. 2015;34(3):147-152.
3. Gubanova EI, Starovatova PA, Rodina MY. 12-month effects of stabilized hyaluronic acid gel compared with saline for rejuvenation of aging hands. J Drugs Dermatol. 2015;14(3):288-298.
4. Fabi SG, Goldman MP. Hand rejuvenation: a review and our experience. Dermatol Surg. 2012;38(7 Pt 2):1112-1127.
5. Sterodimas A, Boriani F, Nicaretta B, Pereira LH. Hand rejuvenation by stromal enriched lipograft. J Plast Reconstr Aesthet Surg. 2018;71(10):1507-1517.
6. Graivier MH, Lorenc ZP, Bass LM, Fitzgerald R, Goldberg DJ. Calcium Hydroxyapatite (CaHA) Indication for Hand Rejuvenation. Aesthet Surg J. 2018;38(suppl_1):S24-S28.
7. Frank K, Koban K, Targosinski S, et al. The Anatomy behind Adverse Events in Hand Volumizing Procedures: Retrospective Evaluations of 11 Years of Experience. Plast Reconstr Surg. 2018;141(5):650e-662e.
8. de Melo F, Nicolau P, Piovano L, et al. Recommendations for volume augmentation and rejuvenation of the face and hands with the new generation polycaprolactone-based collagen stimulator (Ellansé®). Clin Cosmet Investig Dermatol. 2017;10:431-440.
9. Zhou J, Xie Y, Wang WJ, et al. Hand Rejuvenation by Targeted Volume Restoration of the Dorsal Fat Compartments. Aesthet Surg J. 2017;38(1):92-100.
10. Roberts WE, Colvan L, Gotz V. Topical Treatment of Aging Hands: Brief Report. J Clin Aesthet Dermatol. 2017;10(8):37-41.

CLINICAL CASES

CLINICAL CASE 1

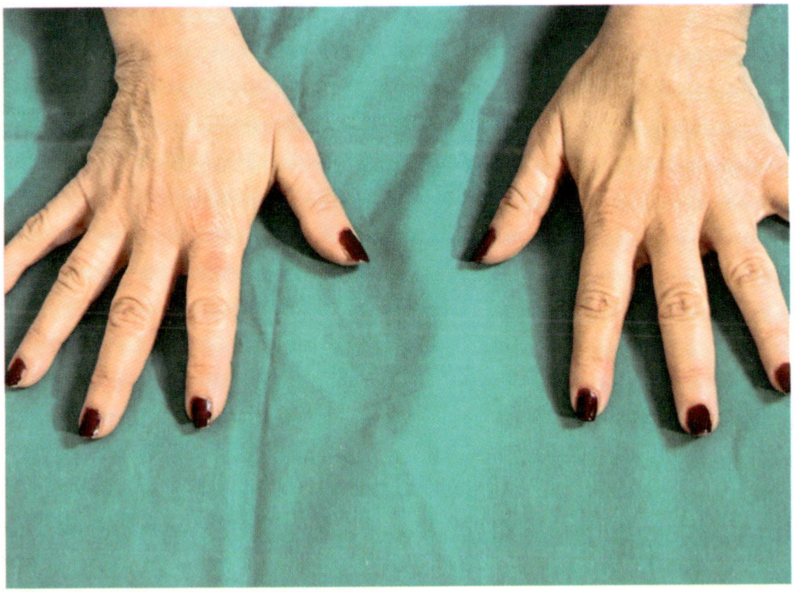

BEFORE

VIDEO 3

Correction of the hands: morphing before and after

AFTER

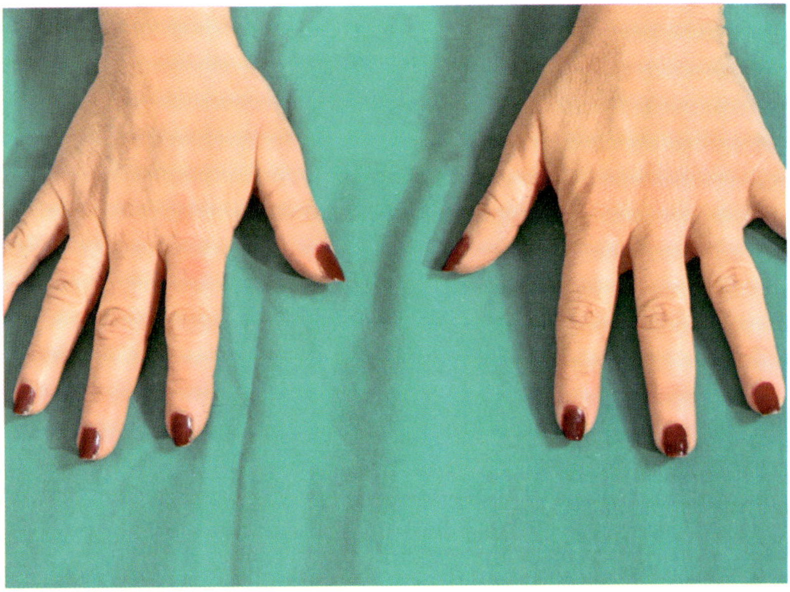

55-year-old woman. Correction with microcannula and 1.2 ml per side of medium density HA, followed by vigorous massage.

CLINICAL CASES

CLINICAL CASE 2

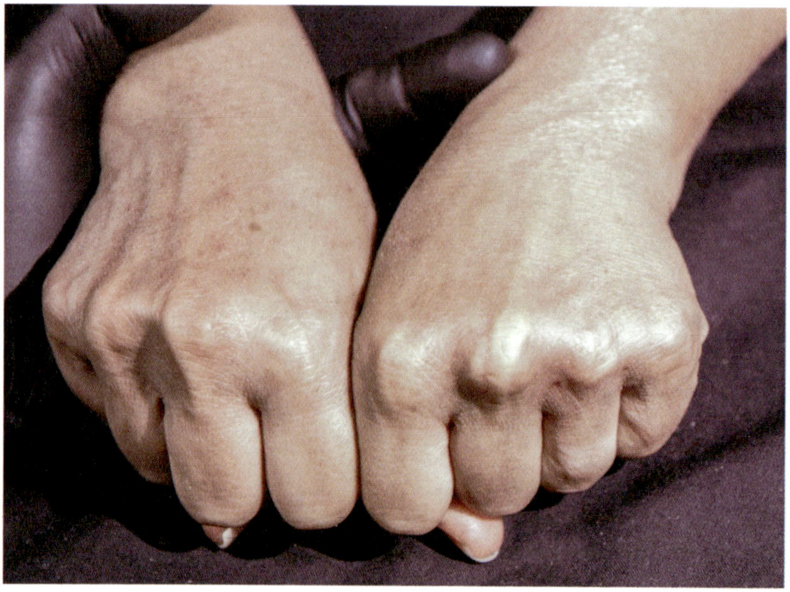

BEFORE

<

AFTER

>

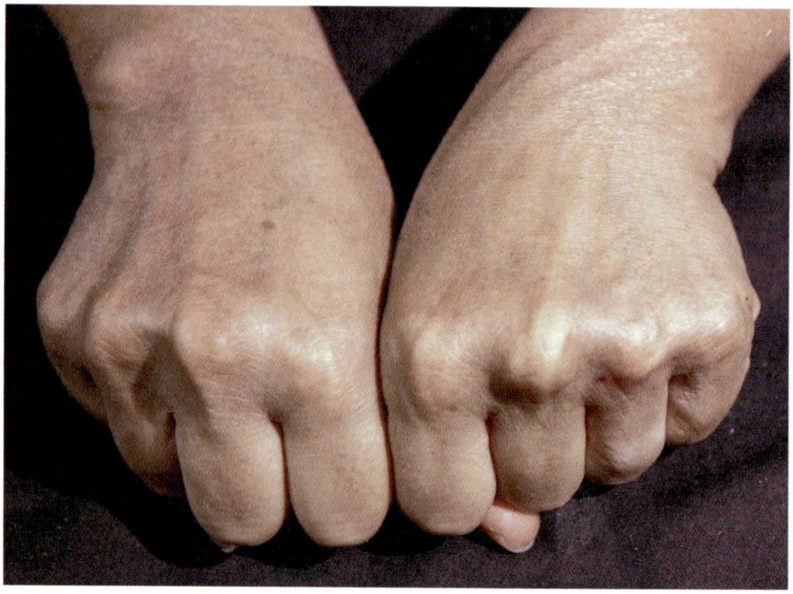

Interdigital injections with a needle of about 1 ml of rather fluid medium G′ hyaluronic acid, followed by vigorous massage. The needle is always introduced into the interdigital spaces.

CLINICAL CASES

CLINICAL CASE 3

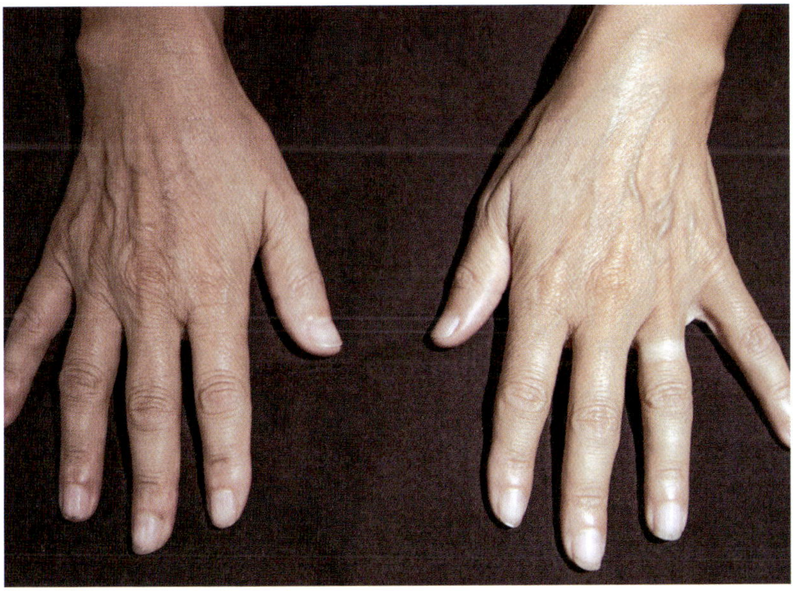

BEFORE

AFTER

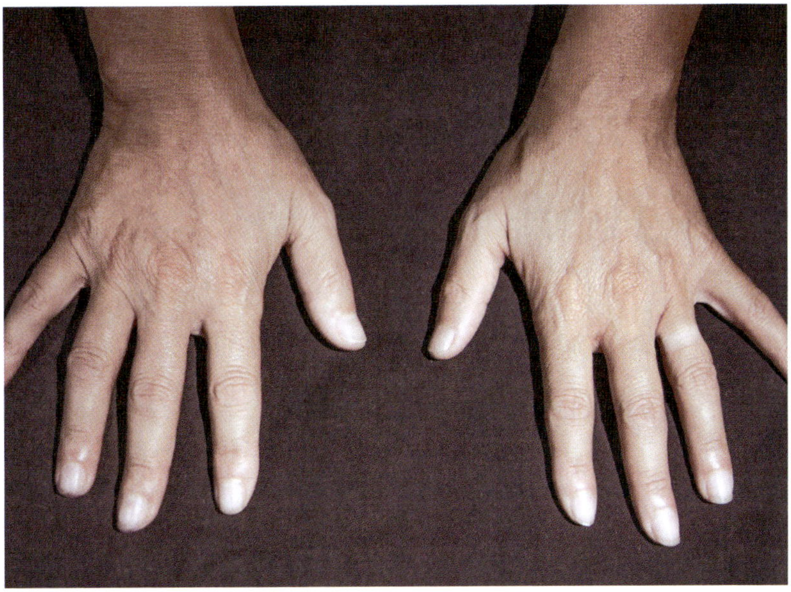

40-year-old woman, smoker. Lean hands but with relatively little damage. Corrective injection of calcium hydroxyapatite in the interdigital spaces with 27 G/40 mm micro-cannulae. Good level of satisfaction.

14

FILLER-RELATED COMPLICATIONS

Lucia Calvisi and Giuseppe Sito

Classification of complications

According to the figures of the International Society of Aesthetic Plastic Surgery (ISAPS) for 2017, the use of dermal fillers is rising sharply worldwide, especially with regard to hyaluronic acid infiltration; the use of fillers has exceeded 3 million treatments, with an increase of 2.9% compared to 2016 and 85% compared to 2012. This can be explained by the versatility and relative safety with which the procedure is carried out.

Although the incidence of complications is low and the majority of complications are minor, it goes without saying that the increase in the number of procedures also translates into an increase in the number of complications. Complications can be classified accor-

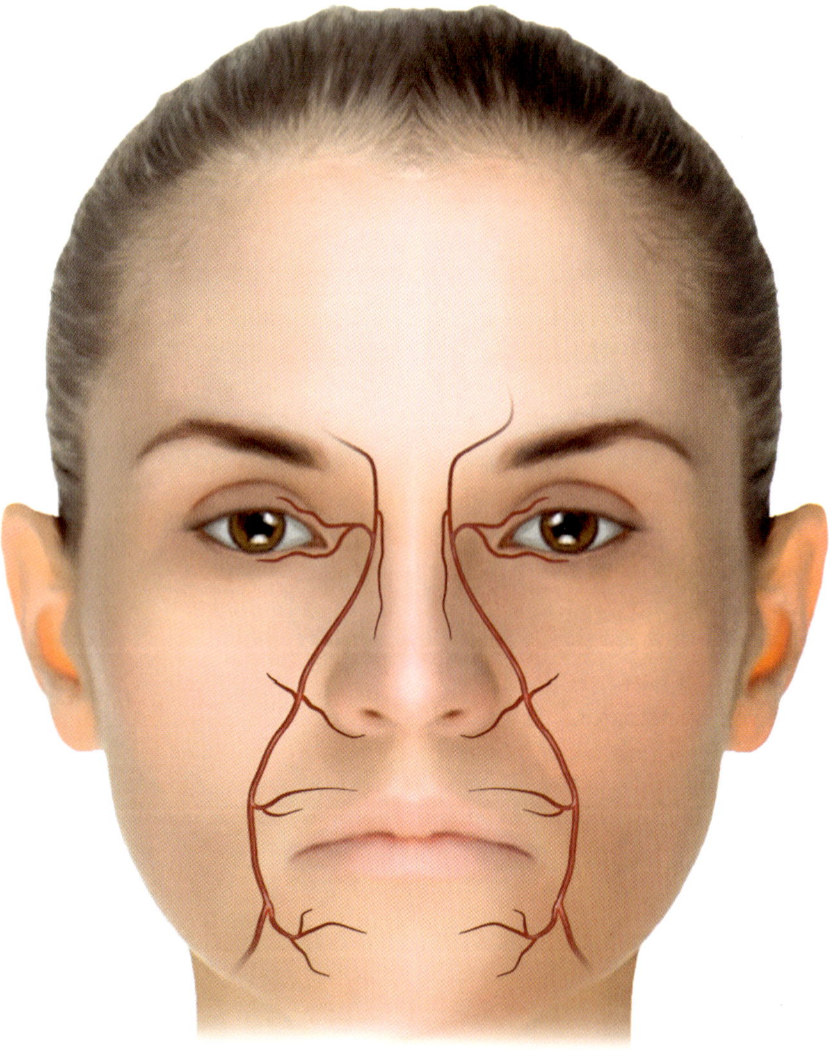

Figure 1 Vascular anatomy of the face (synopsis)

ding to their degree of severity (mild, moderate, severe), their nature (ischaemic or non-ischaemic) (fig. 1) and, even better, on the basis of the time of onset (early or late). We speak of early complications when they arise in the first 24 hours after the procedure, late when they arise between 24 hours and 4 weeks afterwards and delayed if they arise after 4 weeks. Usually complications that arise between 24 hours and 4 weeks after the procedure are treated together.

Early complications

Bruises. Bruising is the most common complication and, although patients are always unhappy about it, the marks disappear within a few days. There are areas of the face where bruising is more frequent than others, such as the perioral or periocular areas, and this is due to the rich vascularisation of the area. Bruises tend to form more easily following the use of a needle rather than a cannula and with injection into the dermis or immediate subdermal plane using a fan technique.
Bruises can be treated with ice packs, arnica and vitamin K cream.
The risk of bruising can be reduced by injecting slowly; should the bruise still appear it can be reduced by compressing the area with a gauze dressing.
Numerous studies report an increased risk of bruising in patients who take oral anticoagulants, such as Warfarin or Coumadin, or who have taken NSAIDs during the week before the procedure.
To reduce the risk of bruising and swelling, it is advisable to:
> avoid strenuous exercise for 24-48 hours after the procedure;
> avoid saunas or exposure to intense heat for 24-48 hours;
> use arnica cream or vitamin K cream for 3-4 days before the procedure;
> use the same creams for 3-4 days after the procedure.

Swelling. Transient post-procedure swelling is a normal consequence of the injection of filler and varies depending on the type and quantity of product used. Irrespective of this, certain patient-dependent factors, such as dermographism, may have an influence.
Some areas, such as the lips and periorbital region, are more susceptible to swelling than others.
Normal post-procedure swelling should not be confused with antibody-mediated angioedema, which is an extremely rare complication.
The recommended treatment of swelling is:
> arnica and bromelain 3-4 days before the procedure;
> application of ice 5-10 minutes before the procedure;
> application of ice after the procedure and, in case of severe swelling, 1 mg/kg/day of Prednisone for about three days plus a gastroprotectant.

Erythema. A certain amount of redness of the skin is absolutely normal immediately after the injection.

Infections. Any type of procedure that breaks the skin can cause skin infections. Acute infections occur with the appearance of inflammation or abscesses at the site of injection and are generally due to *Streptococcus pyogenes*.

The recommended treatment is:
> Amoxicillin plus clavulanic acid, 3 times a day for 15 days;
> Ciprofloxacin 500, 2 times a day for 2-4 weeks.

Reactivation of herpes. Dermal fillers can cause the reactivation of herpes simplex in sufferers.
Patients with a positive history of more than three episodes of herpes simplex a month should take 1g/day of Valaciclovir on the day before the procedure and for three days afterwards. In patients with active lesions, wait until the lesions have healed before going ahead with the procedure.

Dysesthesia, paraesthesia and anaesthesia. Although rare during aesthetic procedures, damage to nerve structures may occur as a result of direct trauma or tissue compression by the product. Nerve damage may be transient or permanent.
The most common site is the infraorbital nerve; less common is Bell's paralysis or mandibular nerve dysfunction, which can last for several weeks.

Nodules. These are one of the most common complications associated with fillers. They can be inflammatory, non-inflammatory or infectious.
As a general rule, recently formed, painless nodules are usually the result of malpractice or the injection of excess filler, injection too close to the surface or the use of product which is unsuitable for the area in question.
If nodules appear, we generally recommend:
> monitoring;
> if they are not inflammatory, treatment with hyaluronidase (with the limitations imposed in different countries).

Vascular compromise. This is a major complication resulting from the accidental intra-arterial injection of the filler. The absolute number of cases of vascular compromise by hyaluronic acid fillers compared to fat injection procedures is identical; however, considering that hyaluronic acid fillers are more commonly used, it can be deduced that complications from fillers using autologous fat are more common.
Early recognition of this type of complication is essential to avoid skin necrosis. The two main symptoms are a change in colour (white) and pain in the event of arterial occlusion, while in the case of venous occlusion, the pain is less marked and can be delayed. Pain may sometimes be absent if the filler formulation contains anaesthetic.
The characteristic evolution of a vascular complication is the blanching of the skin. This is usually immediate and visible during injection, lasting for a few seconds, followed by purplish mottling (*livedo reticularis*) which usually lasts for 15-20 minutes. Livedo is followed by blue-blackish discoloration which is visible for hours. This leads to the formation, after a few days, of vesicles and, if it goes untreated, of necrosis (figs. 2-4).
The treatment must be quick and aimed at restoring blood flow: vigorous massage of the area treated, hot compresses, nitroglycerin and hyaluronidase patches

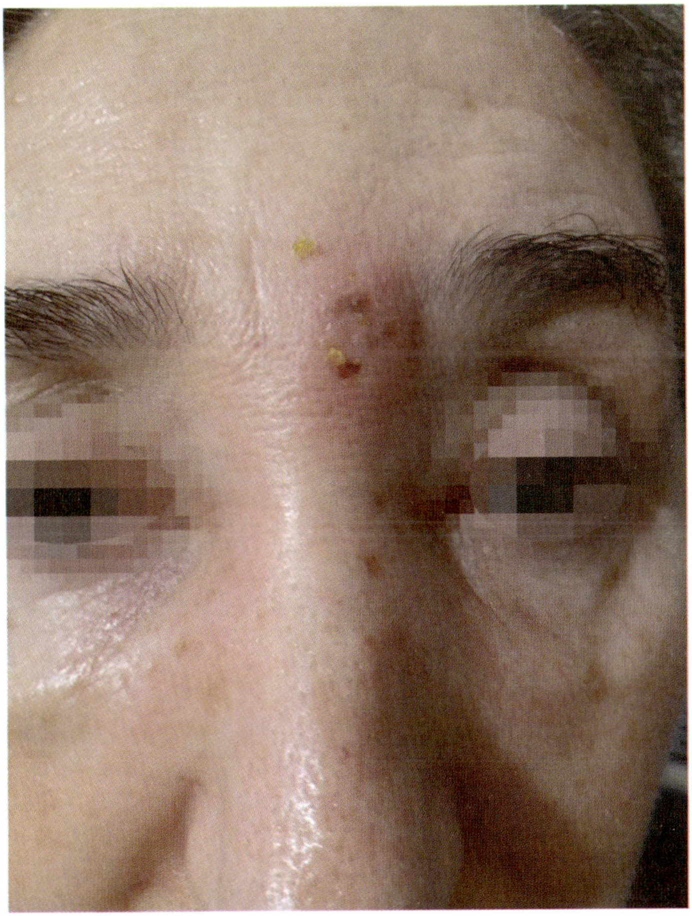

Figure 2 Ischaemic area of the glabella and start of the nasal ridge on the left

are the recommended therapies.
High dosages of hyaluronidase (200-300 U) are recommended every 2-3 hours until the clinical situation has been resolved, injecting not only where the filler has been administered but throughout the ischemic area.
To prevent the onset of vascular complications, always aspirate before injecting, use fine gauge needles or cannulae in the case of risk areas, inject small amounts of product into each injection site and use a gentle retrograde injection technique.

Occlusion of the retinal artery. This may occur following the injection of fillers into the glabella, nose or tear trough. The mechanism is a retrograde occlusion of the ophthalmic artery. Ischemia of the retinal artery is caused by embolism. The main symptom is blindness, occurring a few seconds after injection, and this is usually painless. It is necessary to intervene quickly because if the occlusion of the retinal artery continues for more than 60-90 minutes, the damage is irreversible.
The therapeutic measures to be taken are:

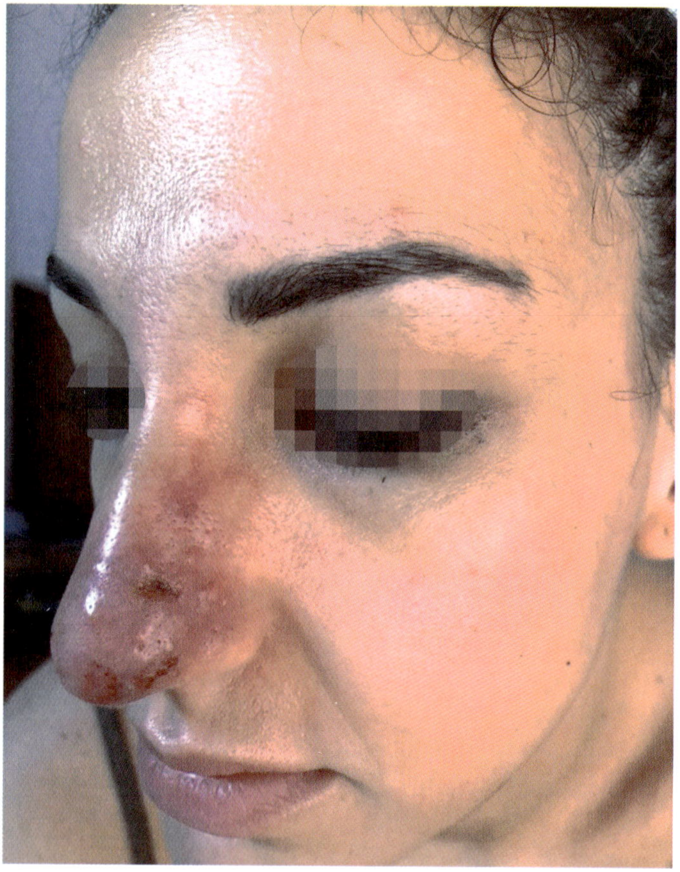

Figure 3 Ischemia of the nasal pyramid with small areas of necrosis, probably due to accidental injection into the facial artery where it divides into the alar artery of the nose

> one drop of thymololol 0.5% and/or acetazolamide 500 mg in tablet form;
> sublingual nitroglycerin or acetylsalicylic acid;
> intravenous mannitol;
> retrobulbar injection of hyaluronidase.

Late complications

Bruises. Although bruises are usually early complications, they occasionally persist and remain purple. In this case they can be treated with a dye laser.

Non-antibody-mediated swelling. Reactions usually occur one day after injection, but very occasionally they may occur after one day and last for months. These cases are not responsive to antihistamines and the best approach is to remove the triggering agent, i.e. the hyaluronic acid.

Malar swelling. This is a serious complication which has been reported after tear trough fillers (figs. 5-6).
Injection of the filler can cause swelling due to increased barrier permeability of the malar septum or by direct lymphatic compression if too much product is injected.

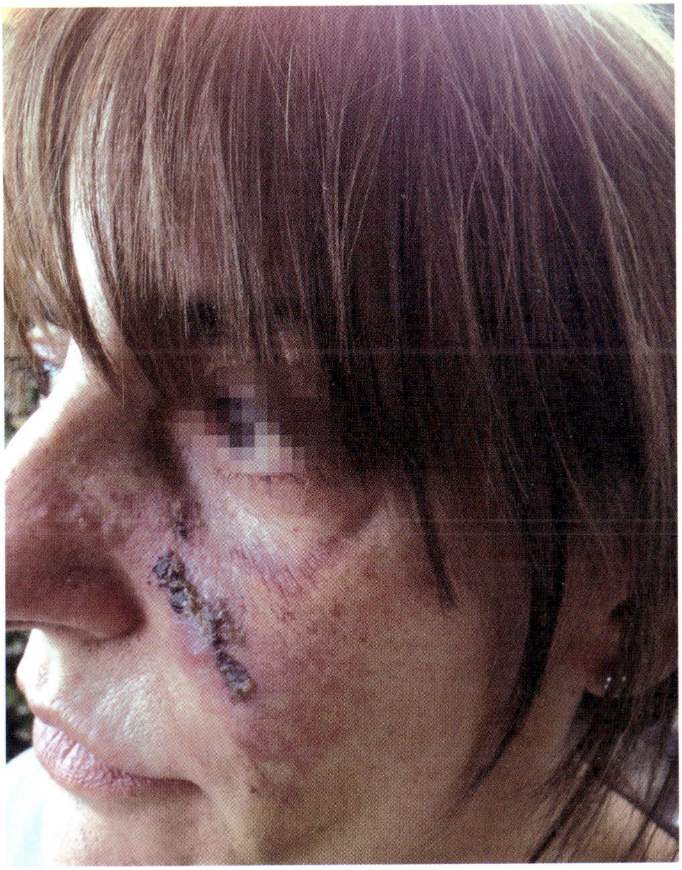

Figure 4 Ischemia and necrosis of the nasolabial fold along the facial artery, which has been accidentally injected

The most effective therapeutic approach consists in the use of hyaluronidase.

Neovascularization. The trauma caused by the needle and excessive massage can cause the formation of capillaries and arterioles. The best treatment in this case is with laser.

Tyndall effect. This occurs when a filler of inadequate density is injected too close to the surface. A bluish-grey colour appears on the skin and can persist for years if left untreated. Hyaluronidase is the most appropriate choice of therapy.

Chronic infections. These usually appear two or three weeks after the procedure. The first line of treatment is to drain the infection and take a course of antibiotics.

Nodules. Late onset nodules are negative for bacteria, but it seems that bacterial biofilm of the skin is involved. Treatment requires the use of hyaluronidase and an oral antibiotic such as Ciprofloxacin, 500 mg twice a day for 2-4 weeks, or the combination of Clarithromycin 500 mg plus Moxifloxacin 400 mg twice a day for 10 days.

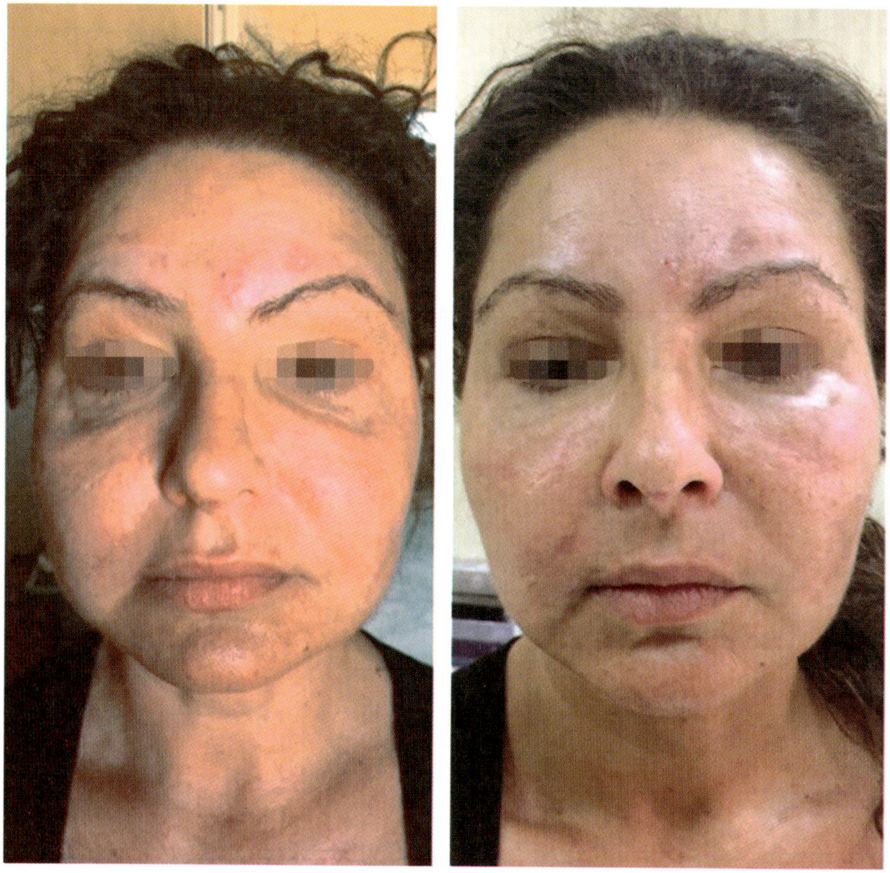

Figure 5 Considerable swelling of the lower eyelids due to the injection of unsuitable filler

Foreign body granuloma. This is due to a very rare immune reaction. The treatment of choice is hyaluronidase.

Conclusions

The use of dermal fillers has become extremely popular in recent years. Although the procedure is fairly safe, the occurrence of sometimes serious adverse events is reported in literature.
It is therefore essential for the practitioner to recognise them quickly and treat them properly.

Bibliography

1. Lee W, Koh IS, Oh W, Yang EJ. Ocular complications of soft tissue filler injections: A review of literature. J Cosmet Dermatol. 2020;19(4):772-781.
2. Shoughy SS. Visual loss following cosmetic facial filler injection. Arq Bras Oftalmol. 2019;82(6):511-513.
3. Sito G, Manzoni V, Sommariva R. Vascular Complications after Facial Filler Injection: A Literature Review and Meta-analysis. J Clin Aesthet Dermatol. 2019;12(6):E65-E72.

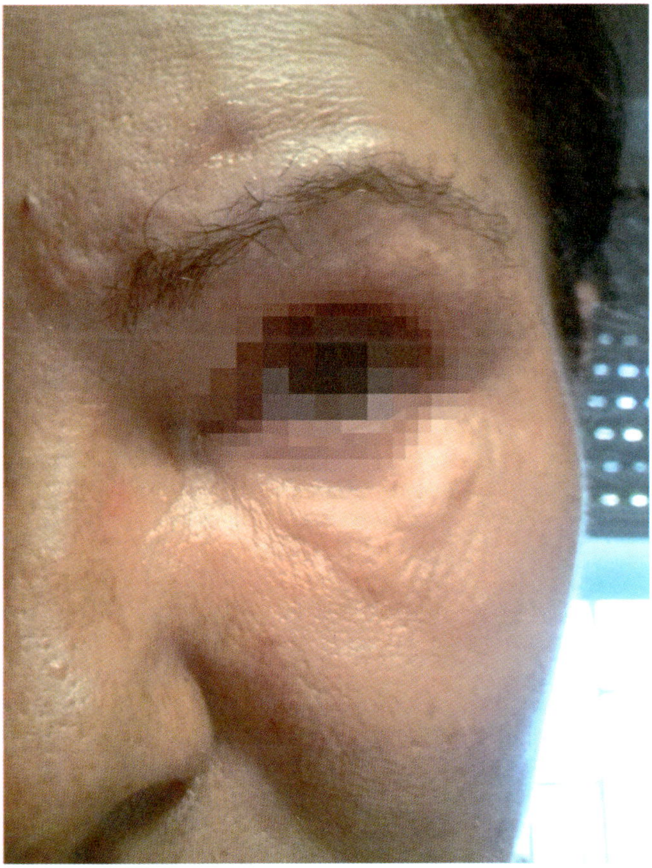

Figure 6 Visible overcorrection of the lower eyelid treated with unsuitable filler. It should be stressed that the skin on the lower eyelid is the thinnest in the whole body

4. Surek CC, Said SA, Perry JD, Zins JE. Retrobulbar Injection for Hyaluronic Acid Gel Filler-Induced Blindness: A Review of Efficacy and Technique. Aesthetic Plast Surg. 2019 Aug;43(4):1034-1040.
5. Snozzi P, van Loghem JAJ. Complication Management following Rejuvenation Procedures with Hyaluronic Acid Fillers-an Algorithm-based Approach. Plast Reconstr Surg Glob Open. 2018 Dec 17;6(12):e2061.
6. Heydenrych I, Kapoor KM, De Boulle K, Goodman G, Swift A, Kumar N, Rahman E. A 10-point plan for avoiding hyaluronic acid dermal filler-related complications during facial aesthetic procedures and algorithms for management. Clin Cosmet Investig Dermatol. 2018 Nov 23;11:603-611.
7. Jeong GJ, Kwon HJ, Park KY, Kim BJ. Pulsed-dye laser as a novel therapeutic approach for post-filler bruises. Dermatol Ther. 2018 Nov;31(6):e12721.
8. Singh P, Vijayan R, Nikkhah D. Filler Rhinoplasty: Evidence, Outcomes,

and Complications. Aesthet Surg J. 2018 Oct 15;38(11):NP165-NP167.
9. de Lacerda D. Prevention and management of iatrogenic blindness associated with aesthetical filler injections. Dermatol Ther. 2018 Nov;31(6):e12722.
10. Vidič M, Bartenjev I. An adverse reaction after hyaluronic acid filler application: a case report. Acta Dermatovenerol Alp Pannonica Adriat. 2018 Sep;27(3):165-167.
11. Vedamurthy M. Beware What You Inject: Complications of Injectables-Dermal Fillers. J Cutan Aesthet Surg. 2018 Apr-Jun;11(2):60-66.
12. Rivers JK, Mistry BD. Soft-Tissue Infection Caused by Streptococcus anginosus After Intramucosal Hyaluronidase Injection: A Rare Complication Related to Dermal Filler Injection. Dermatol Surg. 2018 Nov;44 Suppl 1:S51-S53.
13. Thanasarnaksorn W, Cotofana S, Rudolph C, Kraisak P, Chanasumon N, Suwanchinda A. Severe vision loss caused by cosmetic filler augmentation: Case series with review of cause and therapy. J Cosmet Dermatol. 2018 Oct;17(5):712-718.
14. Sung WI, Tsai S, Chen LJ. Ocular Complications Following Cosmetic Filler Injection. JAMA Ophthalmol. 2018 May 10;136(5):e180716.
15. Urdiales-Gálvez F, Delgado NE, Figueiredo V, Lajo-Plaza JV, Mira M, Moreno A, Ortíz-Martí F, Del Rio-Reyes R, Romero-Álvarez N, Del Cueto SR, Segurado MA, Rebenaque CV. Treatment of Soft Tissue Filler Complications: Expert Consensus Recommendations. Aesthetic Plast Surg. 2018 Apr;42(2):498-510.
16. Iverson SM, Patel RM. Dermal filler-associated malar edema: Treatment of a persistent adverse effect. Orbit. 2017 Dec;36(6):473-475.
17. Kim H, Cho SH, Lee JD, Kim HS. Delayed onset filler complication: Two case reports and literature review. Dermatol Ther. 2017 Sep;30(5).
18. Ibrahim O, Overman J, Arndt KA, Dover JS. Filler Nodules: Inflammatory or Infectious? A Review of Biofilms and Their Implications on Clinical Practice. Dermatol Surg. 2018 Jan;44(1):53-60.
19. Urdiales-Gálvez F, Delgado NE, Figueiredo V, Lajo-Plaza JV, Mira M, Ortíz-Martí F, Del Rio-Reyes R, Romero-Álvarez N, Del Cueto SR, Segurado MA, Rebenaque CV. Preventing the Complications Associated with the Use of Dermal Fillers in Facial Aesthetic Procedures: An Expert Group Consensus Report. Aesthetic Plast Surg. 2017 Jun;41(3):667-677.
20. Zhu GZ, Sun ZS, Liao WX, Cai B, Chen CL, Zheng HH, Zeng L, Luo SK. Efficacy of Retrobulbar Hyaluronidase Injection for Vision Loss Resulting from Hyaluronic Acid Filler Embolization. Aesthet Surg J. 2017 Dec 13;38(1):12-22.
21. Chiang YZ, Pierone G, Al-Niaimi F. Dermal fillers: pathophysiology, prevention and treatment of complications. J Eur Acad Dermatol Venereol. 2017 Mar;31(3):405-413.
22. Signorini M, Liew S, Sundaram H, De Boulle KL, Goodman GJ,

Monheit G, Wu Y, Trindade de Almeida AR, Swift A, Vieira Braz A; Global Aesthetics Consensus Group. Global Aesthetics Consensus: Avoidance and Management of Complications from Hyaluronic Acid Fillers-Evidence- and Opinion-Based Review and Consensus Recommendations. Plast Reconstr Surg. 2016 Jun;137(6):961e-71e.

23. Woodward J, Khan T, Martin J. Facial Filler Complications. Facial Plast Surg Clin North Am. 2015 Nov;23(4):447-58.
24. Carruthers JD, Fagien S, Rohrich RJ, Weinkle S, Carruthers A. Blindness caused by cosmetic filler injection: a review of cause and therapy. Plast Reconstr Surg. 2014 Dec;134(6):1197-201.